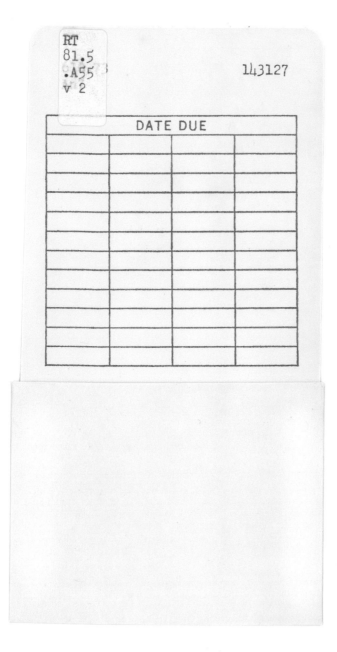

DATE DUE			

ANNUAL REVIEW of
Nursing Research

Volume 2, 1984

ANNUAL REVIEW of Nursing Research

Volume 2, 1984

Harriet H. Werley, Ph.D.
Joyce J. Fitzpatrick, Ph.D.

Editors

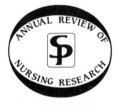

SPRINGER PUBLISHING COMPANY
New York

Order ANNUAL REVIEW OF NURSING RESEARCH, Volume 3, 1985 prior to publication and receive a 10% discount. An order coupon can be found after the index.

Springer Publishing Company, Inc.
200 Park Avenue South
New York, New York 10003

84 85 86 87 88 / 10 9 8 7 6 5 4 3 2 1

ISBN 0-8261-4351-2
ISSN 0739-6686

Annual Review of Nursing Research is indexed in *Cumulative Index to Nursing and Allied Health Literature*.

Printed in the United States of America

Contents

Preface

The *Annual Review of Nursing Research (ARNR)* series was initiated last year (1983) to provide critical, integrative reviews of research in the various content areas of nursing. The enthusiastic responses first to poster sessions on the *ARNR* series conducted by the editors at a number of professional or scientific meetings, then later to the display of the Volume 1, 1983 page proofs at several meetings, and finally the symposium on the series at the Council of Nurse Researchers' Conference attest to the recognized importance of this series. Chapter authors are requested not simply to catalogue research but to write a critical review that will be helpful to readers in terms of assessing the research and judging what further needs to be done; they also are asked to suggest research directions based on their review. In addition, authors are asked to share with readers the scope of their coverage and the criteria used in selecting the studies to be included in their review. Writing a critical, integrative review chapter is far more difficult than writing an ordinary research article, and no doubt the authors of the first few volumes have had the most difficult task. Authors of succeeding volumes can profit from the work of those before them. We expect that, increasingly, authors may move beyond the descriptive cataloguing of research and write an evaluative chapter. It is from these evaluative chapters that students and scholars will profit most, as they use these Annual Review volumes to keep abreast of research in various areas and to develop their own research.

Topical areas needing coverage initially have precluded planning for repeat chapters in the same areas so that subsequent research may be reviewed, but we will be starting this in Volume 4. Volumes 3 and 4 are in progress; negotiations are being made with authors for Volumes 5, 6, and 7; and development of a long-term plan to include the time frame for repeating selected topics is being discussed.

The need for the *ARNR* series will grow as the number of prepared researchers increases, the number who remain active in research grows, and professionals—both nurses and others—learn of the existence and the value of the series. In addition, faculty in the growing number of doctoral programs in nursing no doubt will use the volumes as teaching tools, and doctoral students will see the value of the content, as well as the critical, integrated mode of writing. Hopefully, faculty will use this latter aspect in teaching, so that all graduate students will learn to do evaluative, integrative reviews of the literature pertinent to their dissertation or thesis.

The format established for the *ARNR* series in Volume 1 will be continued. Each volume, therefore, will have research review content for practitioners, administrators or managers of nursing care delivery systems, nurse educators, those interested in the profession per se, those interested in areas needing research stimulation, and those interested in critical reviews of research in other lands, written by authors from the particular country. Part III, Research on Nursing Education, which was not included in Volume 1, is included here. The first chapter from a foreign land also appears in this volume.

As can be noted from Volume 2 Table of Contents, the research reviewed in the nursing practice area primarily pertains to the family. Suzanne L. Feetham deals with family research from a nursing perspective; Regina P. Lederman's content is pregnancy, anxiety, and maternal health; Angela Barron McBride is concerned with the experience of parenthood; Nola J. Pender covers health promotion and illness prevention; and Jean E. Johnson's content is coping with elective surgery. In the nursing care delivery area, Norma M. Lang and Jacqueline F. Clinton deal with quality of nursing care, and Marion E. Highriter's review pertains to research on public health nursing. The area of nursing education is covered by reviews of research on the teaching–learning process by Rheba de Tornyay, nursing students by Patricia M. Schwirian, and the nursing curricula by Marilyn L. Stember. Research on the profession of nursing is represented by Margaret R. Grier's review of information processing in nursing practice, while other research includes a chapter on nursing research and health policy analysis by Nancy Milio and a critical review of research in Scotland by Lisbeth Hockey and Margaret O. Clark.

We are most grateful to the investigator-authors who have examined the research in their areas and shared their views for the benefit of the readers. We also are grateful to the Advisory Board members for advice we seek periodically and for their assistance in reviewing chapters in draft form; in addition, we value the chapter reviews done by a number of anonymous reviewers who are competent in the various areas. We appreciate Roma Lee Taunton's invaluable assistance in reviewing chapter drafts; she becomes a coeditor for Volume 4. We also appreciate the secretarial assistance of Catherine R. Sweet, later Margaret M. Igl, at the University of Wisconsin-Milwaukee School of Nursing, and of Bertha Willis at Case Western Reserve University School of Nursing.

Readers' reactions to the volumes and specific chapters are welcomed. We also welcome expressions of interest in contributing a critical review chapter in the author's area of research.

Contributors

Margaret O. Clark, R.G.N.
Chief Scientist Office
Scottish Home and Health
  Department
Edinburgh, Scotland

Jacqueline F. Clinton, Ph.D.
School of Nursing
University of Wisconsin-
  Milwaukee
Milwaukee, Wisconsin

Rheba de Tornyay, Ed.D.
School of Nursing
University of Washington
Seattle, Washington

Suzanne L. Feetham, Ph.D.
Children's Hospital National
  Medical Center
Washington, D.C.

Margaret R. Grier, Ph.D.
College of Nursing
University of Illinois at Chicago
Chicago, Illinois

Marion E. Highriter, D.S.Hyg.
School of Public Health
University of North Carolina
Chapel Hill, North Carolina

Lisbeth Hockey, O.B.E., Ph.D.
Formerly Director of
Nursing Studies Research Unit
University of Edinburgh
Edinburgh, Scotland

Jean E. Johnson, Ph.D.
School of Nursing
University of Rochester
Rochester, New York

Norma M. Lang, Ph.D.
School of Nursing
University of Wisconsin-
  Milwaukee
Milwaukee, Wisconsin

Regina P. Lederman, Ph.D.
School of Nursing
University of Wisconsin-Madison
Madison, Wisconsin

Angela Barron McBride, Ph.D.
School of Nursing
Indiana University
Indianapolis, Indiana

Nancy Milio, Ph.D.
School of Nursing and
School of Public Health
University of North Carolina
Chapel Hill, North Carolina

Nola J. Pender, Ph.D.
School of Nursing
Northern Illinois University
DeKalb, Illinois

Patricia M. Schwirian, Ph.D.
College of Nursing
Ohio State University
Columbus, Ohio

Marilyn L. Stember, Ph.D.
School of Nursing
University of Colorado Health
  Sciences Center
Denver, Colorado

Forthcoming

ANNUAL REVIEW OF
NURSING RESEARCH, Volume 3

Tentative Contents

ANNUAL REVIEW of
Nursing Research

Volume 2, 1984

PART I

Research on
Nursing Practice

CHAPTER 1

Family Research:
Issues and Directions for Nursing

SUZANNE L. FEETHAM
CHILDREN'S HOSPITAL NATIONAL MEDICAL CENTER
WASHINGTON, D. C.

CONTENTS

In this chapter the development of family research is reviewed and a critical review of nursing research on families is presented. Conceptual and methodological issues are analyzed in relation to future directions for family

Susan Murray, R.N. was of invaluable help in searching the literature and compiling the references.

3

research. Recommendations are made about the knowledge base necessary for nursing, and the methods to gain this knowledge as pertains to families. The conceptualization for the categories of research presented in this chapter was derived from an extensive review of the literature related to family theory, from family research within nursing and other disciplines, and from nursing practice.

FAMILY RESEARCH

Theoretical Development

Several conceptual and theoretical frameworks have been used by researchers in a variety of disciplines to study families. Inductive theory building related to families was first attempted in the late 1950s and early 1960s (Burr, Hill, Nye, & Reiss, 1979). The early theoretical categories identified included structure-function, symbolic interaction, developmental, and family solidarity. In the early 1970s, systems and exchange theories, among others, were added. In the mid 1970s a national effort by family theorists (Burr et al., 1979) resulted in the identfication of 22 theoretical categories. These categories included generations in the family, family and fertility, wife-mother employment, men's work and men's families, social processes and power in families, communication in couples and families, and family process and child outcomes. Some nurse researchers have used these theoretical categories in their studies of families. However, these researchers did not use the 22 theoretical categories consistently enough to permit the classification of the research reported in this chapter within these categories.

Trends in Family Research

In addition to the directions for theory development in family research, methodological trends also were apparent in the research within nursing and other disciplines (Broderick, 1970; Knafl & Grace, 1978; Litman, 1974; Safilios-Rothschild, 1970; Wakefield, Allen, & Washchuck, 1979). One trend in family research has been that the families selected for study were often those identified as pathological or abnormal. Examples of studies focused on the family with pathology included those examining the responses of family members to the illness of other family members. This examination of the family with pathology may not be applicable to the normal family and may not provide information on how normal families maintain themselves (Knafl & Grace, 1978).

Another trend in family research was the attention to the internal family dynamics to the exclusion of the interdependence of the family and its individual members with the larger elements of the social structure. This research approach implies that cause and effect occur and remain with the family (Wakefield et al. 1979). A third trend, consistent with the attention to the internal family dynamics, was the use of the mother as the primary data source. The result was that the so-called family research was not research on the family but was research on the mother's perception of the family or individual family members (Feetham, 1981; Gilliss, 1983; Litman, 1974; Safilios-Rothschild, 1970).

In the Litman (1974) classic review of family research and health, Sussman (1953, 1959), a family sociologist, was recognized as instrumental in the efforts to examine the role of the family in health and illness. Studies of the relationships of the family to health and illness followed the same trends as the other research on families. By focusing on the individual as the unit of measure, and examining the family with physical and/or mental pathology, less knowledge was generated about the normal, well-functioning family.

Nursing and the Family

In the last decade, there was increasing attention to the family in both nursing practice and research as evidenced in the nursing literature. A potential deterrent to this increase was that research on families was not presented as a research direction in the review articles published in *Nursing Research* in 1977 (Barnard & Neal, 1977; Highriter, 1977; Sills, 1977). Another trend was the beginning development of conceptual frameworks for nursing and the family (Fawcett, 1975; Friedman, 1981; Knafl & Grace, 1978; Lancaster, 1980; Melson, 1980; Whall, 1981). Fawcett (1977) and Knafl and Grace (1978) reported their beginning efforts to test these frameworks. The models for nursing proposed by Rogers (1970), King (1971), and Roy (1976) did not address clearly the place of the family as a unit for nursing (Fawcett, 1975; Whall, 1981). Recently the authors of the major nursing models reviewed their own models within the context of family (Clements & Roberts, 1983). These reviews provided some clarification for studying families. Analysis of both these theoretical and methodological trends was used in the formulation of the criteria for critique of research on families included in this chapter.

CRITERIA FOR ANALYSIS OF FAMILY RESEARCH

The following criteria, identified by the author, were derived from: (a) the nursing research literature, (b) a review of family theory and research on families from nursing and other disciplines, and (c) the nursing practice literature. Some criteria are general and apply to all nursing research and others are specific to research on families. The criteria for research on families were adapted from the work of Wakefield et al. (1979). The criteria were applied to provide consistency in the critiques and to provide direction for future nursing research related to families.

Conceptualization of Family

A criterion for family research is that there is a conceptualization of the family as a basis for the research. The literature from nursing and other disciplines is replete with articles about the family. However, on close examination of this literature, the concept of family is often not defined within the framework of the research, nor is the family a basic unit of analysis in the research.

Family Functioning and Structure

Another criterion for family research is the probability that knowledge about functioning and/or structure of the family will result from the research. Most studies in the nursing literature, while including family within the title, did not include the family in the conceptualization of the study. Also, the family system was not the basic unit of analysis. Even when the family system was included in the conceptualization of the studies, in most instances, the research was not conducted within the family unit.

Definition of Family

The presence of an operational definition of family within the context of the study is another criterion for family research. The specific definition is not as important as the presence of a definition. The investigator may define family in its more generic sense as the nuclear, biological, and/or legal group; or family could be defined by the study subjects in terms of their functional relationships to others.

Nursing Research

A criterion for all nursing research is the identification of the relevance of the study to nursing. The investigators of most of the studies reviewed for this chapter did not identify the relevance to nursing in either the support of the significance of the study or in the presentation of the research implications.

Partial and Full Theoretical Models

The presence of a theoretical or conceptual model was another criterion used to critique the studies for this chapter. Although the model issue applies to all nursing research, family research was used as an example. The majority of studies on the family had a primary limitation in that either a partial or no theoretical or conceptual model was used in the report of the research. When researchers used a partial model, limited variables were examined without identifying their relationship to the whole. Within the context of family research, Wakefield et al. (1979) identified the partial model as conservative and negating the true influence of the interdependence of individuals within the family and the family as a system.

The researchers' use of a partial model implies that a linear cause and effect occurs and remains within the family, and assumes that family phenomena are a function of the small group or family (Wakefield et al., 1979). Examples of studies using a partial model are those in which investigators examine only internal family dynamics, and/or conceptualize and examine single variables as if they had primary significance in the variance accounted for in the phenomena under study. Also, in studies derived from a partial model, the study variables are treated as if they were unrelated to environmental influences.

In contrast, researchers using a full theoretical or conceptual model attend to the following criteria: (a) the interdependence of the individual within the family, the family system, and the environment; (b) the environment defined as the natural environment and the human-built (i.e. society, culture, health care system) environment (Morrison, 1974); and (c) the family or family system as a mediator between the individual and society. Multivariate interaction can be inferred as the family is neither the total etiology of problems within society or individual, and an individual family member is not the single causation of family pathology.

In the studies reviewed for this chapter, the investigators described a full theoretical model in a small portion of studies. For example, Roberts and Feetham (1982) used the family ecological framework, recognizing the interdependence between the child, family, and environment. Fawcett (1977) derived her study of body image during pregnancy from an open systems model also recognizing the interaction of multiple variables. Researchers, in review articles from other disciplines, supported the importance of the full theoretical model in family research (Litman, 1974; Murphy, 1980).

Many methodological issues are inherent in the testing of full conceptual or theoretical models in nursing research. Suggestions are given in this chapter about building on the knowledge of families gained from studies using partial or no theoretical models to formulate and test full models for nursing research on families.

Scientific Merit

In addition to the above criteria, the criterion of scientific merit also was used to examine the studies. The criteria for scientific merit included: conceptual clarity; consistency of discussion of the relationships among variables and how they were operationalized and measured; and appropriateness of the methodology, including reliability and validity of the instruments, sampling, and data analysis.

For most studies included in this chapter, the researchers did not meet the criteria discussed above. However, the studies were reviewed if they were thought to be examples of potential areas for nursing research on families and/or the investigator used methods appropriate to the study of the family as a basic unit of measure.

REVIEW OF FAMILY RESEARCH IN NURSING

Conceptual Categories of Research

The conceptual categories for this chapter were developed by the author from the analysis of nursing research on families, recognizing the work of other disciplines. The conceptual or theoretical categories in this chapter are not inclusive and could be defined in many ways. The major categories identified for this chapter are: (a) the family or family characteristics as the unit of research, (b) the family as the environment of the individual, (c) the external environment and the family, (d) family-related research, and (e) nursing intervention with families. Of these categories, the largest number of investigators reported studies pertaining to the first category, family characteristics.

Family Characteristics

The investigators examined several characteristics including the roles of family members, the factors influencing family roles, family solidarity, communication patterns, and family structure. Roles of family members were the family characteristic most often reported. In these studies, role change was usually a dependent variable, with illness of a family member as the independent variable.

Anderson (1981) used participant observation to study family role change in four families of children with chronic illness and 12 families of well children. Using the construct of normalization, Anderson found that parents semantically defined their children as normal, but the parents' verbal accounts were inconsistent with the observed family practices. A strength of the study was the use of qualitative methods for data collection; quantitative methods might have masked these discrepancies. Anderson did not include a conceptualization of family, but concluded that nurses need to direct interventions to the family system rather than to individuals.

The method of data collection was a strength in Benoliel's (1970) study of nine families and their children with diabetes. In this study of roles, total family interviews were used to examine the meaning of diabetes as a social crisis in the family. Subject selection was designed to assure a range in the variables of age of onset, sex, and socioeconomic status of the family.

The process and rationale for data collection were described fully. Benoliel concluded that the study results supported the use of the total family interview to examine families.

Stember (1977) reported on family role change using a sample of 80 couples. Data were obtained by interviewing hospitalized adults and their spouses, obtaining questionnaire responses from attending physicians, and reviewing charts. The investigator measured the dependent variable—familial stress—through a response index, stressor index, and a general question asking the respondents to rate the level of stress. No information was given on the instruments; reliability and validity coefficients of the multiple indicator coefficients were reported. The investigator appropriately reported the support of 4 of the 13 hypotheses with caution. The amount of hospital experience, severity of the illness, length of time the family had lived at the same residence, and duration of the illness were related to family stress. A strength was that the investigator implied a full model for family research by the multiple variables identified and the use of path analysis as a corollary to causal modeling. A limitation was that nursing was not mentioned in the report.

The theoretical framework of adult family roles was used in a research program by Knafl and Grace (1978) to examine family beginnings, childbearing, childrearing, and child-launching families. The purpose of the research program was to provide baseline information about family life, across the life cycle, essential to practitioners. The investigators' motivation for the research was the need for studying families on the family's terms, the need for baseline data on the development of normal families, and the need for holistic studies of family life processes. The need for a full theoretical model was implicit. Most data were collected by interviews, using instruments developed for this research program. Reliability and validity tests of the instruments were not reported. Descriptive discussion was used to report the results of the 17 studies. Later research reported by some of the authors of the original book did not build explicitly on the initial work (Knafl, 1982; Knafl & Dixon, 1983).

White (1977) identified the roles of the family in relation to the development of the child as the theoretical basis for a study of maternal satisfaction. The family was not used as an independent or dependent variable, and the mother and child were data sources. The dependent variable was maternal satisfaction derived from interviews of 104 mothers who were part of an 11-year longitudinal study of neonatal perceptions. The reliability and validity data of the two interview forms, developed by the researcher, were not presented. Content analysis was used to classify the interview data. White reported that maternal satisfaction related significantly to the absence of mental disorder in first-born children at age 10 to 11 years. No explicit reference to nursing was made in the report.

White and Dawson (1981) were most consistent in their identification and measure of family characteristics. They examined the effect of the at-risk infant on 99 families. The construct—family solidarity—was measured in three groups of parents when the infants were three and six months of age. Four categories of the construct were: togetherness, communication, team performance, and both the instrumental and expressive dimensions of ritual. Groups were parents of low-risk, moderate-risk, and high-risk infants. The investigators implied a full theoretical model, recognizing the interdependence of the multiple variables. No significant differences were found on major variables among the three groups. Strengths of the study included the use of reliable and valid instruments and appropriate analysis. Limitations were the extensive use of univariate analysis and the broad conceptual leaps made to nursing in the conclusions, when this relationship was not identified earlier.

Aiken (1982) defined family structure as a concept in a study pertaining to patient need for and participation in cancer support groups. The purpose of this study of 24 men treated for cancer was to explore one aspect of the ill individual's rationale for use of psychological support groups. The limitations of this exploratory pilot study were listed clearly, including the use of a 20-item interview schedule developed by the investigator. The instrument's reliability and validity were not reported. Appropriate analysis was used for the small sample. The hypotheses were not supported as age, family structure, and time since diagnosis were not related significantly to group attendance. This small study was an appropriate systematic effort by a clinic nurse to assess which patients benefitted from a support group.

Davis (1980) used family structure as the underlying concept for home interviews in a study of decision making for home care in 30 families with disabled adults. The investigator referenced several related family theories with limited interpretation of these references in relation to the study. Data were analyzed using content analysis. Since the methodology was not presented, the ability to interpret the results and identify the relevance to nursing was limited.

Hurley (1981) examined the family characteristic of communication patterns, using a convenience sample of 68 couples. She used the construct of family power to investigate the relationship between marital communication patterns and an assessment index of the power structure of the dyad. Although the power literature Hurley cited was appropriate, the concept of power has received limited attention in recent family research. The methods were described clearly, including reliability and validity of the instrument used, as well as the process to protect human subjects. Data analysis was appropriate for the type of data and sample size. The relevance to nursing was mentioned in both the support of the problem and in relation to the recommendations. Hurley stressed that characteristics of the family environment have not been examined and research by nurses on communication patterns among family members could contribute to nursing assessment of families.

The characteristic of family coping was one variable examined by Ventura (1982) in a study of 200 mothers and fathers of 100 two to three month old infants. Low but significant correlations between family coping patterns, parent functioning, and infant temperament were reported. A strength of this study was the use of instruments with evidence of reliability and validity that related to the concepts identified in the review of the literature. A unifying conceptual framework might have guided the investigator to multivariate analysis rather than the multiple single t-tests and correlations used to test the research questions.

There was no pattern found in the research on family characteristics except the consistent presence of several limitations. The first limitation was that the studies were unrelated to each other, with no investigator building on other nursing research. There also was limited use of instruments tested in other nursing or related research. Another major limitation of these studies was that the relevance to nursing was seldom explicit.

Family as Environment of the Individual

Several investigators examined the family within the context of the relationship of the environment to the individual. This is an important concept in the study of the family and is consistent with the criteria for a full model for research on the family.

In a well-designed study, Tinelli (1981) examined the family as one component of the individual's environment. Sixty-three children, with parental consent, completed instruments on family concept and self-esteem. Both instruments had evidence of reliability and validity, and measured constructs presented within the theoretical framework for the study. Data analysis was appropriate to the design and sample. The two hypotheses were supported in that children with higher self-esteem reported higher family satisfaction, and perceived their families as more considerate, loyal, close, and communicative. One strength of the study was the use of instruments that measured perceptions. The study was consistent with a full model for research on the family in that it was derived from systems theory and included recognition of the interdependence of the child, family, and environment. This was an excellent example of an investigator realistically examining a few variables within a broad theoretical framework. Implications for nursing practice were presented.

MacCarthy and Morison (1972) also studied the family as part of the environment of the individual. Family functioning determined by a child center social worker was one independent variable in an epidemiological study of the incidence of preschool morbidity. The sample included 23 families and 34 children. Family was defined operationally in this study. Although there was an apparent lack of relationship of the family functioning variable to the group results, there was a higher incidence of episodic illness of children in families where the social worker believed family therapy was indicated. The interpretation and application of the results were limited due to methodological and conceptual problems.

Garlinghouse and Sharp (1968) examined the relationships among bleeding episodes in the child with hemophilia, the child's self-concept, and family stress. A convenience sample of 18 children with hemophilia and their 14 mothers was used. Family stress was conceptualized as social stress and measured by a life experiences questionnaire. The reliability and validity of the questionnaire was referenced. The investigators reported an inverse relationship between self-concept and bleeding episodes when family stress was held constant. When family stress was high, the relationship between self-concept and bleeding episodes tended to break down. This study is an example of a partial model. The analysis was appropriate to the design and research question.

Two studies were reported in which the investigators examined families of patients in coronary care units as part of the individual's environment. Brown (1976) measured the effect of family visits on the blood pressure and heart rate of 50 newly admitted patients. From limited data in a poorly designed study, Brown suggested that family visits had a detrimental effect on the patients. In another study, the family members of 12 patients in an 18-bed coronary care unit (CCU) were assigned to a control or experimental group to examine the effect of family preparation on the state anxiety level of the patient (Doerr & Jones, 1979). Although a standardized anxiety scale was used, the sample, design, and methods were not sufficient to support the conclusion that family preparation significantly reduced the amount of anxiety transferred from the family member to the CCU patient.

The need for the examination of the concept of the family as the environment of the individual was indicated from these studies. Although the investigators did not provide a clear conceptual framework of the family and often lacked reliable and valid measures of the family as a unit, the studies were examples of the potential for this important conceptualization of the family.

External Environment and the Family

Another area of family research was the examination of the health care system as a part of the external environment of the family. In such research, investigators would meet the criteria of a full model by recognizing the interdependence of the family with the environment, including the relationships with the larger social structure of the health care system. These investigators contributed to the knowledge of the relationships between the health system and the family.

LaFargue (1972) replicated aspects of earlier work on the relationship of perceived prejudice of health care providers and the seeking of health care by black families. The small sample of 10 families precluded analysis to examine the relationship of the variables. Strengths of the study included building on previous research, the use of tested instruments, and the investigator's clear delineation of the study limitations.

Potter (1979) examined the relationship between 75 family member's perceptions of stress from three different intensive care unit (ICU) environments, with the independent variables of the family members' age, sex, education, and past ICU experience. The investigator developed a 24-item questionnaire using a five-point Liker-type scale, with content validity determined during pilot testing. Strengths were that Potter built on previous nursing studies, delineated the relevance for nursing practice, and listed the limitations, including possible intervening variables. Inappropriate analysis was selected for the data and research question. Future researchers could clarify the conceptualization and improve on the methodology to increase knowledge about the family system.

Another concept of the health care system is family-centered care. Over the last decade, investigators examined the health care workers' role conception in relation to family-centered care (Porter, 1979), the concept of family-centered care in community health (Yauger, 1972), and the delivery of family-centered care in pediatric and maternity centers (Sonstegard & Egan, 1976). Few investigators defined the family unit, used family theory or concepts in the conceptualization of the study, or examined the family as the unit of measure. In the future, investigators examining family-centered care could contribute knowledge about the family and family functioning by applying the above criteria for family research.

Nursing Interventions with Families

The testing of nursing interventions with families is essential for nursing. Through such studies nurses can delineate nursing's unique contribution to health care and to families. Welch (1981) reported two studies in which she examined the expectations of family members for nursing interventions of adults with cancer ($N = 25$ and $N = 41$). The investigator built on previous nursing research, using literature related to role transition and the reorganization of family interactions during family illness. Other strengths were that Welch presented the relevance to nursing practice, and the limitations of the study were stated. From these limited data and analysis, Welch concluded that the diagnosis of cancer can cause serious disorganization within a family unit. In her study of men with cancer, as reviewed above, Aiken (1982) examined the need for and participation in cancer support groups. This study was an attempt to identify nursing interventions that were most effective with this group of patients.

In a family-related study, researchers examined the need for family education in the care of terminally ill cancer patients (Grobe, Ilstrup, & Ahmann, 1981). Structured interviews were used with 27 patients with advanced cancer, 28 of their family members, and 29 additional family members of deceased patients. The appropriate statistic was used to test associations between variables. The investigators reported that identified education needs were related to physical care, disparities existed between the expectations of the patient and family members, and education of the family for patient management was likely to support the goal of home care.

High-risk families were the reported care recipients in a longitudinal study to test three types of nursing interventions (Barnard, Snyder, & Spietz, in press). Strengths of this multivariate study were that instruments with evidence of reliability and validity were used, and the researchers built on a program of clinical research. The investigators reported the adaptation of the helping process with supportive nursing acts for 60 high-risk mothers and infants. In the future, to provide further testing of this nursing intervention model, path analysis of data could be done to identify those variables and nursing actions most predictive of positive family outcomes. Although each of the intervention studies lacked a clear conceptualization and measure of the family, they were important attempts to examine nursing interventions.

Family-Related Research

The potential to contribute knowledge about the functioning of families, family structure, and family roles is a criterion for family research. In several studies, investigators examined variables that were components of the family but either did not include a conceptualization of family in the study, or had no measures of family. Therefore, the potential for the investigators' contributing knowledge regarding the family was limited. The studies in which the investigators failed to discuss family concepts but examined components of families were not included in this review (Meleis & Swendsen, 1978; Palermo, 1980; Uphold & Susman, 1981).

The criteria for family-related research were met more clearly by the investigators of several studies (Adams, 1968; Fawcett, 1977; Hoskins, 1979; Mack, 1952; MacElveen, 1972). The same variables such as marital relationships and responses of spouses were examined, but the investigators gave recognition to the construct of family and tended to reference family theorists. However, a common pattern by the investigators was that family theory was referenced as part of the theoretical base of the study, but this concept was not developed through the definition of variables studied. These studies were included in the critique since the investigators had more potential for contributing knowledge of family functioning. The studies were considered examples of underdeveloped family research.

In the first issue of *Nursing Research,* Mack (1952) reported on the personal adjustment of the chronically ill elderly in-home care. The relationship of four factors to the adjustment of the aged were examined using a convenient, stratified sample of 84 ill adults and 100 controls. One of the four factors examined was family attitudes. Although appropriate statistical analysis was described under study methods, the data were reported only through the investigator's interpretive discussion. A relationship between family attitudes and adjustment was reported.

Family composition was used as a measure of interaction by Adams (1968) in an experimental study of 300 patients in a public health nursing program. Adams reported that nurses supported aging, chronically ill adults in their efforts to remain in their home, and help patterns between the aged and family interaction were demonstrated. MacElveen (1972) used family concepts in the conceptualization of her study of 21 home dialysis patients, their partners, and a staff member. However, the variables she examined— cooperation, adherence to the medical regime, wellness, activity, and morale—were not specific family variables.

Several investigators reported the responses of individual family members to other ill family members. The investigators presented the issues related to responses of families with ill members, but the construct of family was not conceptualized clearly. The investigators either did not use the family as a research variable or used a variable other than family as the dependent variable (Bond, 1982; Knafl, 1982; Knafl & Dixon, 1983; Leavitt, 1975; Silva, 1978, 1979).

Hoskins (1979) met the criteria of family-related research in her study of 16 marital dyads. The variables of level of activation, body temperature, and interpersonal conflict were examined. Older references, related to interpersonal conflict within the family system, formed the basis of the conceptual support of the study. A strength of the research was that the relevance to nursing was presented, and the need for a full theoretical model was supported. The expected relationships among the variables were not found. The investigator developed her own instrument although other tested instruments existed. Reliability and validity for the new instruments were not reported.

One study was an excellent example of research derived from a full model. Using a unified open systems framework, Fawcett (1977) examined patterns of change in the body image of 50 married couples before and after pregnancy. The purpose of the research was to develop and test a theoretical model and hypotheses from an abstract conceptual framework of nursing. The linkage of the research questions to the family framework was presented, but the relationship to each phase of the study was not apparent. In future research, a clearer consistent measure of the family model would contribute to the knowledge of families. The research was well designed and appropriately reported, except for this factor.

Family Research Methods

There was evidence in the nursing literature of researchers' efforts to develop and systematically test measures of the family. A possible reason for the limited number of available instruments was that only in the past decade have nurses addressed the family as a conceptual entity. Specialists in nursing spoke of the importance of families, but limited efforts were made to develop conceptual frameworks with the family central to nursing practice. The most well-known nurse theorists focused on the individual (Clements & Roberts, 1983; Whall, 1981). A second reason for the lack of measures may be that nurse researchers have not reported consistent use of instruments developed and tested by other disciplines (McCubbin & Patterson, 1981; Moos, 1974; Olson, Bill, & Portner, 1978; Stein & Riesman, 1980, Straus, 1964).

Another reason was the complexity of developing such measures of the family. Gilliss (1983) supported this issue stating that research on the family was complicated by difficulties of measuring the aggregate and its component parts. There was lack of agreement as to what should be measured as well as to how both the parts and the sum should be measured (Aldous, 1978; Feetham, 1981; Gilliss, 1983). Some answers to the methodological issues may come from the development of full conceptual or theoretical nursing models that identify the family as both the central unit and the context for the behaviors of the individual members.

There were several reports in the nursing literature of tools for family assessment (Gregory, 1975; Harrison, 1976; Meister, 1977; Sciarillo, 1980; Tapia, 1972). These reports were derived from the clinical practice of nurses and the nurses' systematic documentation of the needs and responses of families to nursing intervention. Because these assessment tools came from practice with an attempt to identify a conceptual base for the tools, it is reasonable to speculate that with further testing some of these tools might be validated for nursing. Unfortunately, only one of these tools was reported to have had further testing (Hymovich, 1979, 1981, 1983).

Hymovich (1981) developed her instrument to examine the effect of a child's chronic illness on family developmental tasks and parent coping strategies and to measure the outcome of intervention. Hymovich referenced relevant literature related to responses of families or parents of children with chronic illness; however, the conceptual framework for her research and for the instrument was not clear. From three studies ($N = 40$), Hymovich identified areas for content analysis that were applied to interview data from 23 parents. The 300-item instrument was then piloted on a very small sample of 29 parents representing 25 families. There was reported evidence of content validity and internal reliability; the instrument was considered to be in developmental stages.

Roberts and Feetham (1982) developed an instrument to assess family functioning across three areas of relationships between: (a) the family and broader social units, (b) the family and subsystems, and (c) the family and each individual. The instrument was tested in studies of families with children with health problems and in studies of families with healthy infants (Feetham & Humenick, 1982). The instrument was developed within a program of research using a full conceptual model. Appropriate tests of reliability and validity were conducted. In addition to the original conceptualization as a measure of family functioning, the researchers also used the instrument to measure social support (Feetham & Humenick, 1982).

Several instruments were reported in a series of studies conducted within a research program related to adult roles (Knafl & Grace, 1978); the instruments were interview schedules. The investigators did not identify tests for reliability and validity. Further tests of these instruments were not found in the nursing literature.

Stacey (1978) used ethnography to study intergenerational relationships in seven families. Behavior and relationships with older family members were described to provide information of how families function. Stern (1981) also used field methods in a study of 40 Filipino childbearing families. Field methods were recommended to provide a richer data base, including systematic documentation of how normal families functioned.

A major methodological issue in family research is that a full theoretical model implies that the sum of the variables studied is more than the sum of the parts. At this time, even the multivariate analysis techniques are additive. In time, other options for analyses may become available.

SUMMARY AND FUTURE RESEARCH DIRECTIONS

In the last decade, nurses have given increasing attention to the relationships of families and nursing as evidenced in the literature. In this chapter, criteria for family research were proposed. The publications were critiqued and conceptualized within the categories of family characteristics, the family as the environment of the individual, the external environment and the family, nursing interventions with families, and family-related research. Conceptual and methodological issues also were addressed.

Nurse researchers have a contribution to make in relation to knowledge of the family. Nurses investigating the family need to continue to build on knowledge and research of other disciplines while developing full theoretical nursing models and examining the family as the unit of analysis. Researchers using a full model may examine a limited number of variables in a single study. The researcher's interpretation of the full model guides the researcher in the selection of variables for study; this results in the researcher examining a few variables to test pieces of the full model. Investigators also need to identify components or behaviors of the individual and family system that are most predictive of positive outcomes of the family and individual family members. Researchers need to examine how families help each other, how they cope, and how they grow. With identification of these predictor variables, nurses can focus on prevention.

A single definition of family by nurses is not essential. It is essential that each investigator define family within the context of the research. Nurse researchers may substantiate a category of relationships that meet the roles and functions of family but do not meet the biological or legal definition of family. These relationships may constitute a person's "chosen" family, which nurse researchers may identify as an important resource in nursing interventions (Howard, 1976).

Measures of family health or well-being have not been a central concept in nursing research (O'Brien, 1979). Efforts by nurse researchers directed toward the definition and predictors of family well-being are relevant to nursing practice (Meister, 1984). Family health or well-being is more than the sum of each family member's health status (Litman, 1974). Researchers who examine concepts common to healthy families, or to families growing and developing in spite of illness within the family, will help identify predictors of family health. Such a direction in family research would focus on family strengths.

In charting a direction for research on families, nurse researchers also must build on previous research in nursing and other disciplines. A single conceptualization or model for nursing research on families is not required. However, it is imperative that each model have internal consistency, with a clear definition and measure of the family unit. These models should meet the criteria for family research and meet the criteria for a full model, recognizing the interdependence with the human-built and natural environment. Nurses' research on families carries the same patterns of strengths and limitations as family research in other disciplines. Nurse researchers can provide leadership and make major contributions to the knowledge of families. Nurses direct their practice toward the health of individual family members. With nurses also extending their focus to the family system, they are in an excellent position to identify and test research questions and examine variables most predictive of the health and well-being of the family.

REFERENCES

Adams, M. Older patients and their care: Interaction with families and public health nurses. In *American Nurses' Association, Fourth Nursing Research Conference*. New York: American Nurses' Association, 1968.

Aiken, S. Family structure and utilization of cancer support groups. *Oncology Nursing Forum*, 1982, 9(1), 22–26.

Aldous, J. *Family careers, developmental change in families*. New York: Wiley, 1978.

Anderson, J. M. The social construction of illness experience: Families with a chronically-ill child. *Journal of Advanced Nursing*, 1981, 6, 427–434.

Barnard, K. E., & Neal, M. V. Maternal-child nursing research: Review of the past and strategies for the future. *Nursing Research*, 1977, 26, 193–200.

Barnard, K., Snyder, C., & Spietz, A. Supportive acts for high-risk infants and families. In K. Barnard & P. Brandt (Eds.) *Social support and infants at risk*. New York: Alan R. Liss, in press.

Benoliel, J. A. The developing diabetic identity: A study of family influence. In M. V. Batey (Ed.), *Communicating nursing research* (Vol. 3). Boulder, Colo: Western Interstate Commission for Higher Education, 1970.

Bond, S. Communicating with families of cancer patients 1. The relatives and doctors. *Nursing Times*, 1982, 78, 962–965.

Broderick, C. B. Beyond the five conceptual frameworks: A decade of development in family theory. *Journal of Marriage and the Family*, 1970, 33, 139–159.

Brown, A. J. Effect of family visits on the blood pressure and heart rate of patients in the coronary-care unit. *Heart and Lung,* 1976, *5,* 291–296.

Burr, W. R., Hill, R., Nye, F. I., & Reiss, J. L. (Eds.). *Contemporary theories about the family* (Vol. 1). *Research based theories.* New York: Free Press, 1979.

Clements, I. W., & Roberts, F. B. (Eds.). *Family health—A theoretical approach to nursing care.* New York: Wiley, 1983.

Davis, A. J. Disability, home care and the care-taking role in family life. *Journal of Advanced Nursing,* 1980, *5,* 475–484.

Doerr, B. C., & Jones, J. J. Effect of family preparation on the state anxiety level of the CCU patient. *Nursing Research,* 1979, *28,* 315–316.

Fawcett, J. The family as a living open system: An emerging conceptual framework for nursing. *International Nursing Review,* 1975, *22,* 113–116.

Fawcett, J. The relationship between identification and patterns of change in spouses' body images during and after pregnancy. *International Journal of Nursing Studies,* 1977, *4,* 199–213.

Feetham, S. Critique of study—The impact of the infant at risk on family solidarity. In R. Lederman & B. Raff (Eds.), *Perinatal parental development: Nursing research and implications for newborn health.* New York: Alan R. Liss, 1981.

Feetham, S., & Humenick, S. The Feetham Family Functioning Survey. In S. Humenick (Ed.), *Analysis of current assessment strategies in the health care of young children and childbearing families.* New York: Appleton-Century-Crofts, 1982.

Friedman, M. M. *Family nursing theory and assessment.* New York: Appleton-Century-Crofts, 1981.

Garlinghouse, J., & Sharp, L. The hemophilic child's self-concept and family stress in relation to bleeding episodes. *Nursing Research,* 1968, *17,* 32–37.

Gilliss, C. The family as a unit of analysis: Strategies for the nurse researcher. *Advances in Nursing Science,* 1983, *5*(3), 50–59.

Gregory, D. Family assessment and intervention plan. *Pediatric Nursing,* 1975, *1*(4), 23–29.

Grobe, M. E., Ilstrup, D., & Ahmann, D. Skills needed by family members to maintain the care of an advanced cancer patient. *Cancer Nursing,* 1981, *4,* 371–375.

Harrison, L. L. Nursing intervention with the failure-to-thrive family. *MCN, The American Journal of Maternal Child Nursing,* 1976, *1,* 111–116.

Highriter, M. E. The status of community health nursing research. *Nursing Research,* 1977, *26,* 183–192.

Hoskins, C. N. Level of activation, body temperature, and interpersonal conflict in family relationships. *Nursing Research,* 1979, *28,* 154–160.

Howard, J. *Families.* New York: Simon & Schuster, 1976.

Hurley, P. M. Communication patterns and conflict in marital dyads. *Nursing Research,* 1981, *30,* 38–42.

Hymovich, D. P. Assessment of the chronically ill child and family. In D. P. Hymovich & M. U. Barnard (Eds.), *Family health care* (Vol. 1). (2nd ed.). New York: McGraw-Hill, 1979.

Hymovich, D. P. Assessing the impact of chronic childhood illness on the family and parent coping. *Image*, 1981, *13*, 71–74.

Hymovich, D. P. The chronicity impact and coping instrument: Parent questionnaire for use by clinicians and researchers. *Nursing Research*, 1983, *32*, 275–281.

King, I. M. *Toward a theory for nursing.* New York: Wiley, 1971.

Knafl, K. A. Parents' views of the responses of siblings to a pediatric hospitalization. *Research in Nursing and Health*, 1982, *5*, 13–20.

Knafl, K. A., & Dixon, D. M. The role of siblings during pediatric hospitalization. *Issues in Comprehensive Pediatric Nursing*, 1983, *6*, 13–22.

Knafl, K. A., & Grace, H. K. *Families across the life cycle studies for nursing.* Boston: Little, Brown, 1978.

LaFargue, J. P. Role of prejudice in rejection of health care. *Nursing Research*, 1972, *21*, 53–58.

Lancaster, J. *Community mental health nursing: An ecological perspective.* St. Louis: Mosby, 1980.

Leavitt, M. The discharge crisis: The experience of families of psychiatric patients. *Nursing Research*, 1975, *24*, 33–40.

Litman, T. J. The family as a basic unit in health and medical care: A social-behavioral overview. *Social Sciences and Medicine*, 1974, *8*, 495–519.

MacCarthy, J., & Morison, J. An explanatory test of a method of studying illness among preschool children. *Nursing Research*, 1972, *21*, 319–326.

MacElveen, P. M. Cooperative triad in home dialysis care and patient outcomes. In M. V. Batey (Ed.), *Communicating nursing research* (Vol. 5). Boulder, Colo.: Western Interstate Commission for Higher Education, 1972.

Mack, M. J. The personal adjustment of chronically ill old people under home care. *Nursing Research*, 1952, *1*, 9–30.

McCubbin, H., & Patterson, J. (Eds.). *Systematic assessment of family stress, resources and coping.* St. Paul, Minn.: Univ. of Minnesota, Family Social Sciences, 1981.

Meister, S. B. Charting a family's developmental status for intervention and for the record. *MCN, The American Journal of Maternal Child Nursing*, 1977, *2*, 43–48.

Meister, S. B. Family well being. In J. Campbell & J. Humphreys (Eds.), *Nursing care of victims of family violence.* Reston, Va.: Reston, 1984.

Meleis, A. I., & Swendsen, L. A. Role supplementation: An empirical test of a nursing intervention. *Nursing Research*, 1978, *27*, 11–18.

Melson, G. F. *Family and environment—An ecosystem perspective.* Minneapolis: Burgess, 1980.

Moos, R. *Family environment scale.* Palo Alto: Consulting Psychologists Press, 1974.

Morrison, B. The importance of a balanced system. *Man-environment systems*, 1974, *4*, 171–178.

Murphy, M. A. The family with a handicapped child: A review of the literature. *Journal of Development and Behavioral Pediatrics*, 1980, *3*, 73–82.

O'Brien, R. A. A conceptualization of family health. In *American Nurses' Associa-*

tion clinical and scientific sessions. New York: American Nurses' Association, 1979.

Olson, D., Bill, R., & Portner, J. *FACES.* St. Paul, Minn.: University of Minnesota, Family Social Sciences, 1978.

Palermo, E. Remarriage: Parental perceptions of steprelations with children and adolescents. *Journal of Psychiatric Nursing and Mental Health Services,* 1980, *18,* 9–13.

Porter, L. S. Health care workers' role conceptions and orientation to family-centered child care. *Nursing Research,* 1979, *28,* 330–337.

Potter, P. Stress and the intensive care unit: The family's perception. *Missouri Nurse,* 1979, *48*(4), 5–8.

Roberts, C., & Feetham, S. L. An instrument for assessing family functioning across three areas of relationship. *Nursing Research,* 1982, *31,* 231–235.

Rogers, M. E. *An introduction to the theoretical basis of nursing.* Philadelphia: F. A. Davis, 1970.

Roy, C. *Introduction to nursing: An adaptation model.* Englewood Cliffs, N.J.: Prentice-Hall, 1976.

Safilios-Rothschild, C. The study of family power structure: A review 1960–1969. *Journal of Marriage and the Family,* 1970, *32,* 539–552.

Sciarillo, W. G., Jr. Using Hymovich's framework in the family-oriented approach to nursing care. *MCN, The American Journal of Maternal Child Nursing* 1980, *5,* 242–248.

Sills, G. M. Research in the field of psychiatric nursing 1952–1977. *Nursing Research,* 1977, *26,* 207–210.

Silva, M. C. How the patient's spouse views the operation. *Surgical Rounds,* 1978, *1,* 42–43.

Silva, M. C. Effect of orientation information on spouse's anxieties and attitudes toward hospitalization and surgery. *Research in Nursing and Health,* 1979, *2,* 127–136.

Sonstegard, L., & Egan, E. Family-centered nursing makes a difference. *MCN, The American Journal of Maternal Child Nursing,* 1976, *1,* 249–254.

Stacey, S. Parents and children growing old. *Australian Nursing Journal,* 1978, *7,* 36–39.

Stein, E. K., & Riesman, C. K. The development of an impact on family scale: Preliminary findings. *Medical Care,* 1980, *18,* 465–472.

Stember, M. Familial response to hospitalization of an adult member. In M. V. Batey (Ed.), *Communicating nursing research* (Vol. 3). Boulder, Colo.: Western Interstate Commission for Higher Education, 1977.

Stern, P. N. Solving problems of cross-cultural health teaching: The Filipino childbearing family. *Image,* 1981, *13,* 47–50.

Straus, M. Measuring families. In H. Christensen (Ed.), *Handbook of marriage and the family.* Chicago: Rand McNally, 1964.

Sussman, M. B. The help pattern in the middle class family. *Sociological Review,* 1953, *18,* 22–28.

Sussman, M. B. The isolated nuclear family: Fact or fiction. *Social Problems,* 1959, *6,* 333–340.

Tapia, J. The nursing process in family health. *Nursing Outlook,* 1972, *20,* 267–270.

Tinelli, S. The relationship of family concept to individual self-esteem. *Issues in Mental Health Nursing,* 1981, *3,* 251–270.

Uphold, C. R., & Susman, E. J. Self-reported climacteric symptoms as a function of the relationship between marital adjustment and childbearing stage. *Nursing Research,* 1981, *30,* 84–88.

Ventura, J. Parent coping behaviors, parent functioning, and infants temperament characteristics. *Nursing Research,* 1982, *31,* 269–273.

Wakefield, R. A., Allen, C., & Washchuck, G. (Eds.). *Family research: A source book, analysis and guide to federal funding* (Vol. 1). Westport, Conn.: Greenwood Press, 1979.

Welch, D. Planning nursing interventions for family members of adult cancer patients. *Cancer Nursing,* 1981, *4,* 365–370.

Whall, A. L. Nursing theory and the assessment of families. *Journal of Psychiatric Nursing and Mental Health Services.* 1981, *19,* 30–36.

White, L. J. Maternal satisfaction and the mental health of firstborn children. In M. V. Batey (Ed.), *Communicating nursing research* (Vol. 10). Boulder, Colo.: Western Interstate Commission for Higher Education, 1977.

White, M., & Dawson, C. The impact of the at-risk infant on family solidarity. In R. Lederman & B. Raff (Eds.), *Birth defects: Original article series* (Vol. 17). New York: March of Dimes Birth Defects Foundation, 1981.

Yauger, R. A. Does family-centered care make a difference? *Nursing Outlook,* 1972, *20,* 320–323.

CHAPTER 2

Anxiety and Conflict in Pregnancy: Relationship to Maternal Health Status

REGINA P. LEDERMAN

SCHOOL OF NURSING

UNIVERSITY OF WISCONSIN—MADISON

CONTENTS

Supported in part by the Division of Nursing, Bureau of Health Professions, Health Resources and Services Administration, United States Public Health Service under Grant Nos. NU 00521 and NU 00931.

Early investigators exploring the psychosomatic or psychobiologic basis of reproductive outcomes focused on the study of anxiety in pregnancy. While complications of pregnancy and childbirth have been associated with anxiety, neither the duration and pattern of variation in the three trimesters, nor the behavioral correlates of anxiety, were considered. Increasingly, pregnancy is recognized as a critical developmental stage, one that challenges the adaptive and integrative capacity of the expectant woman and her family. A developmental conceptualization of pregnancy implies a continuum of reproductive health and adaptation, in which prenatal adaptation may influence the childbirth process, subsequent maternal adjustment, and maternal-infant relationships in the postbirth period.

In this chapter, the scope and prevalence of anxiety and fears in pregnancy are reviewed, as well as their significance for adaptation. Developmental tasks and conflicts inherent in pregnancy also are reviewed, in addition to personality dimensions within the mother, her relationship with significant others, and the development of a parenthood role during pregnancy. Patterns of developmental task achievement are reviewed for their relevance first to prenatal adaptation and then to physiological and psychosocial reproductive health outcomes. Longitudinal multifactorial studies necessarily are cited more than once. When comparison among the studies is limited by disparities in design, they are cited and discussed individually. Nurses have contributed to the literature on prenatal developmental tasks and they are in key clinical positions to recognize and study relationships between psychophysiological reproductive problems and maternal-fetal health status.

ANXIETY AND FEAR IN PREGNANCY

Anxiety may be defined as an emotional state characterized by feelings of tension, nervousness, worry, apprehension, and heightened autonomic nervous system activity. Speilberger, Gorsuch, and Lushene (1970) differentiated between state anxiety as a transitory emotional condition, and trait anxiety as a stable individual difference in anxiety proneness. Spielberger and Jacobs (1978) also differentiated between stress and threat. Whereas stress denotes objective stimulus properties of a situation, threat refers to an individual's perception of a situation as more or less dangerous or personally threatening to him or her. Many research reports do not reflect these differences.

Functional Anxiety

It has been purported that the adaptive processes of pregnancy and child-birth necessarily involve anxiety (Uddenberg, Fagerström, & Hakanson-Zaunders, 1976). Entwisle and Doering (1981) conducted two interviews with 120 women in last trimester pregnancy and 60 of their husbands to "chronicle and describe" experiences as a couple changes into a "family"; they surmised that the "work of worrying," described by Janis (1958), is a healthy and desirable reaction to pregnancy. A correlation of .41 was obtained between Taylor Manifest Anxiety Scale (MAS) scores and total worry scores related to pregnancy and childbirth. On the other hand, Lederman, Lederman, Work, and McCann (1979), who interviewed 32 primigravidas in the last trimester of pregnancy, found only low positive relationships between trait anxiety and personality dimensions in pregnancy related to role development and relations with significant others. Trait anxiety appears to be related more to a tendency to perceive threat and worry than to the process of developmental role achievement and reorganization of close family relationships.

Researchers suggested that some anxiety is good in pregnancy, that it indicates a woman is confronting and working through inevitable conflict. Leifer's (1980) follow-up of 19 married subjects spanned the three trimesters, and showed that anxiety about the fetus and deformity is indicative of a concern about well-being and the formation of a protective emotional bond with the fetus. Winget and Kapp (1972) measured anxiety and threat in dream content and found that women with higher anxiety had shorter labors. The researchers concluded that dreams containing content on the anticipation of events in labor and coping responses enabled the mother to become better prepared for childbirth.

Denial

In general, denial—as opposed to low or moderate levels of anxiety and conflict—resulted in inadequate preparation, although it may have reduced anxiety. In a longitudinal multidisciplinary study of 57 primigravid subjects, Shereshefsky and Yarrow (1973) reported that denial early in pregnancy was associated with serious adaptational problems later in pregnancy and the postpartum. Denial, noted in 68% of the subjects, was observed when problem-free reports were given in interviews, but psychological tests revealed depression, anxiety, and insecurity. The researchers acknowledged that the high rate of denial in their study may be attributed to the conduct of interviews jointly with husbands and wives, as well as the subject's inability to confront the conflicts of pregnancy. Shainess (1968) observed that denial reported in first trimester pregnancy was later manifested in the form of somatic complaints and complications in the second and third trimesters, (i.e., denial of existence shifted to psychosomatic behavioral manifestations).

Regression

Pregnancy is frequently purported to involve regressive phenomena wherein earlier developmental conflicts are revived, particularly those pertaining to the mother, thereby permitting more mature confrontation and a higher level of integration than was achieved at an earlier stage. This regression is often termed fruitful. Shereshefsky and Yarrow (1973), however, did not find any unusual regressive patterns, and Leifer (1980) reported little resurgence of past intrapsychic conflict as found by Bibring (1966) and Benedek (1970). Although most researchers recognized pregnancy as a period of reexamination of the mother-daughter relationship and of fears associated with bodily vulnerability and integrity, it was not always accompanied by regressive behavior.

Content and Trimester Changes

Researchers also focused on patterns of anxiety and changes in content over time. Hanford (1968) proposed a model wherein anxiety was high in the first trimester after a woman discovered she was pregnant and faced radical changes in her life, followed by a decrease in the second trimester, and a surge in the last one to two months of third trimester pregnancy. A "nonnormal" model was conceptualized in which the high anxiety of the first trimester continues unabated through the second trimester and is associated with complications such as abortion, preeclampsia, premature delivery, and prolonged labor. The normal pattern proposed by Hanford was supported by the research results of Shereshefsky and Yarrow (1973) and Lubin, Gardener, and Roth (1975), who found a decrease in anxiety from first to second trimester and intensified anxiety by the eighth and ninth month. Other researchers (Chertok, 1969; Grimm, 1961) also noted increased anxiety in the last one to two months of pregnancy.

    The content of first trimester pregnancy often involves a cost analysis of what is given and what is taken away by pregnancy (Rubin, 1975) and resolution of the conflict, "I or the child" (Deutsch, 1945). The task of the first trimester is acceptance of the pregnancy, the fetus, and oneself as a mother-to-be. The first trimester, thus, is accompanied by a focus on the self and, as Shereshefsky and Yarrow (1973) noted, an emphasis on the importance of the immediate reality of pregnancy itself. Quickening in the second trimester marks a shift in focus to the child, its well-being and care, acceptance by family members, fantasied interactions, and a growing love and attachment (Ballou, 1978; Rubin, 1975; Shereshefsky & Yarrow, 1973). Shereshefsky and Yarrow noted that the transition from the third to seventh month was marked by less anxiety about the infant, clearer visualization of oneself as a mother, increased feelings of well-being, increased husband-wife adjustment and validation as a couple, and generally decreased anxiety. The third trimester is a period of increased awareness of maternal-fetal vulnerability and danger as delivery approaches, as well as preparation for separation of the fetus and readiness to receive the child. Two prospective studies using third trimester interviews showed that most of the mothers' concerns focused on fetal well-being and the approaching labor and delivery (Areskog, Uddenberg, & Kjessler, 1981; Standley, Soule, & Copans, 1979)

Some researchers reported that primigravidas had more fears, anxieties, and concerns than multigravidas (Areskog et al., 1981; Burstein, Kinch, & Stern 1974; Heymans & Winter, 1975; Light & Fenster, 1974), but others disagreed (Jarrahi-Zadeh, Kane, Van de Castle, Lachenbruch, & Ewing, 1969; Lederman & Lederman, Note 1). Light and Fenster (1974) found that primigravidas were more concerned about maternal responsibility, pain in childbirth, and birth defects, whereas multigravidas expressed more concern about care of the family. Heymans and Winter (1975) noted that fears pertaining to the infant and labor occurred more commonly among primigravidas, whereas Areskog et al. (1981) observed that the most severe fears were reported by multigravidas with a previous traumatic delivery. Burstein et al. (1974) found that expectant mothers who knew others who had a previous miscarriage had higher general and pregnancy-related anxiety scale scores.

In addition to parity and history, timing of assessment may also be important. Areskog et al. (1981) reported that 23% of their prospective sample had moderate or severe fears, but in two other retrospective studies, investigators (Heymans & Winter, 1975; Light & Fenster, 1974) reported fear and anxiety in approximately 80% of the sample. While retrospective reports may be confounded by inaccuracies of memory and the postbirth health of the mother and neonate, Heymans and Winter (1975) suggested that they more accurately reflect fears pertaining to injury and death, which mothers may be too frightened to confront or reveal prenatally.

Many researchers agreed that older, better educated subjects have less anxiety and fear than their younger counterparts (Burstein et al., 1974; Standley et al., 1979). Concerns about finances may also be substantial in some expectant families. Light and Fenster (1974) reported that 47% of their sample cited such a concern. Specific information on another important factor, marital status, was lacking in most studies cited above. In this regard, Heymans and Winter (1975) reported that 50% of their subjects told their fears to their husbands and 31% of the sample received reassurance by him. Since marital status and the quality of the marital relationship may influence anxiety states, these factors should be considered in the design of future research.

Anxiety and Depression

The relationship between prenatal anxiety and depression also was examined. In a well-designed and thorough statistical analysis, Lubin et al. (1975) followed 93 middle-class, married primigravidas and multigravidas through each of three trimesters of pregnancy to obtain repeated measures on anxiety, depression, and somatic symptoms. No differences were found in depressive mood or anxiety in any trimester or subject group. A significant difference was noted for the amount of somatic symptoms in multiparas with a previous abortion. For this group, somatic symptoms were increased significantly above the mean for other groups, but decreased to a comparable mean in the third trimester. Significant relationships also were noted between anxiety and somatic symptoms, although they were not significant between somatic symptoms and depressive moods.

A number of investigators reported a relationship between prenatal and postnatal anxiety and depression. Zajicek and Wolkind (1978) obtained first trimester interview measures of emotional difficulty, defined as impairment in daily functioning and relationships, from 138 cohabitating subjects. Subsequent adjustment was evaluated at 7 months of pregnancy and again postpartally at 4 and 14 months. The results showed that 81% of the subjects who reported emotional problems in the past had difficulties during pregnancy, compared to 10% with no previous emotional problems. Of the subjects experiencing continuous pregnancy and prepregnancy difficulties, 50% had emotional difficulties at 4 months postpartum and 64% at 14 months; these subjects were pregnant at a young age and without planning, had more health problems, and felt more restricted by their pregnancies. In a somewhat similar study, Meares, Grimwade, and Wood (1976) obtained prenatal measures of anxiety and neuroticism from 129 married women of varying parity and length of pregnancy, as well as postpartum measures of depression. Subjects who were depressed or treated for a previous postpartum depression had significantly higher prenatal anxiety and neuroticism scores. Thus, high levels of anxiety in pregnancy tended to predict puerperal depression.

Other researchers (Jarrahi-Zadeh et al., 1969), who obtained pre- and postnatal questionnaire scale measures of neuroticism, anxiety, and depression, reported higher scores from 86 subjects in pregnancy than in the early postpartum period; multiparas obtained higher scores on depression than primiparas. Rees and Lutkins (1971), utilizing the Beck Depression Inventory at various points in the pregnancy and postpartum, found that the overall incidence of depression remained relatively uniform throughout the antenatal period and during the 12 months following delivery. Group means for depression, however, tended to decrease postpartally, but the differences were not statistically significant. Westbrook (1978a) used women's recollections of a completed pregnancy and childbirth and also found, retrospectively, significantly higher diffuse and cognitive anxiety (reaction to an inability to anticipate experiences) in pregnancy compared to the labor and postpartum periods. The foregoing investigators suggested there is a continuum of anxiety before and during pregnancy that is associated with neuroticism and depression, which predicts postpartum depression. On a continuum, there generally appeared to be more emotional disequilibrium prenatally than postnatally. For some subjects, anxiety may have been a state-specific phenomenon that was limited to the nine months of pregnancy.

Measurement Factors

It appears that anxiety and the measurement of anxiety in pregnancy is influenced by a number of factors and these include: age, education, parity, gravidity, socioeconomic status, previous obstetrical experience, health and health history, marital status and relationship, trimester of pregnancy, prospective or retrospective data collection, the measurement instrument utilized, the gravida's personal strength and history of coping with critical experiences, and social desirability in relation to prevalant cultural norms. Future investigators should give careful consideration to these factors in planning research designs, and also should differentiate between assessments of state and trait anxiety. Studies of anxiety will form a better basis for intervention if demographic, sociologic, developmental, and physiologic variables are incorporated into research designs.

PERSONALITY DIMENSIONS AND DEVELOPMENTAL CONFLICTS IN PREGNANCY

The developmental process in pregnancy is largely defined by the changes in oneself, as well as in the relationship to one's husband, parents, and the coming child. Leifer (1980), in a longitudinal study of primigravidas, indicated that most subjects believed pregnancy was essential in order to prepare psychologically for motherhood and to prepare their marriage for parenthood. In 1945, Deutsch—on the basis of vast clinical experience— stated that the course of pregnancy was dependent on the woman's emotional maturity and a favorable social, economic, and marital environment.

Some developmental tasks are related to preparation of oneself and one's body for the trial of labor and delivery. As previously noted, several studies indicated substantial anxiety pertaining to labor during the prenatal period. An increasing preoccupation with the body and bodily functions was noted by Deutsch (1945), as were heightened sensory-bodily experiences by Rubin (1975). Other factors that may have an impact on adaptation to pregnancy include high levels of stress and specific life circumstances, such as adequacy of finances and employment, illness or death of family members, relocation, and the availability of supportive persons and resources. The developmental processes and life stresses cited have been the subject of systematic investigations which are reviewed in the next section.

Maternal Characteristics and Attitudes of Acceptance or Rejection of Pregnancy

Planning and acceptance of pregnancy are variables frequently included in pregnancy-adaptation research, although the assessment measures vary considerably from one study to another. Caplan (1959) reported that 85% of his study group revealed some initial rejection of pregnancy, but by the end of the first trimester 85 to 90% accepted it. Shereshefsky and Yarrow (1973) reported that 73% of their primigravid sample planned the pregnancy. Two-thirds of the sample followed by Entwisle and Doering (1981) reported pregnancy was planned completely, and 34% that it was planned somewhat. Planning, however, was not related to the wife's attitude toward being pregnant in the Entwisle and Doering study, nor to pregnancy adaptation in the Shereshefsky and Yarrow study. Thus, it appears that planning and acceptance need to be differentiated, and that there is a significant increase in acceptance from early knowledge of pregnancy to the end of the first trimester. Unplanned pregnancy in the Shereshefsky and Yarrow study correlated with youthfulness of the couple, shorter marriage, the husband's dissatisfaction with his job, his lack of response to pregnancy, and a less positive maternal mood at the the three-month prenatal period.

Pohlman (1968), who conducted a number of studies on birth planning, advised caution in interpreting evidence of rejection or acceptance of pregnancy. Planning of pregnancy for sociocultural reasons may not be associated with acceptance of the baby and parenthood. Primigravidas who find themselves pregnant before they are ready may be more amenable to acceptance if social and financial circumstances are deemed adequate. Multiparas, on the other hand, who feel they have more children than they want may not be able to overcome feelings of rejection. Acceptance for such women might better be termed resignation, which is achieved by rationalization, if at all. Pohlman (1968) suggested there is some stability in parental attitude regarding acceptance over the course of pregnancy.

Doty (1967) provided a further explanation for primigravid and multigravid differences. Doty studied the relationship of maternal characteristics to acceptance of pregnancy by administering mailed questionnaires on attitude, anxiety, and personality to 200 subjects. The results showed that multigravidas of lower social position indicated significantly more emotional disturbances and rejection of pregnancy and fewer physical symptoms than primigravidas and middle-class multigravidas. Multigravidas, as a whole, expressed significantly more rejection of the maternal role and less fear of pregnancy and childbirth than primigravidas.

Lederman et al. (1979), who assessed acceptance of pregnancy, found that it correlated with other personality dimensions and with state anxiety and progress in labor. Primigravidas who had difficulty in accepting pregnancy also had greater anxiety in the relationship with their mother and in the identification of a motherhood role, as well as greater fears about labor; they also were less prepared for labor and experienced higher anxiety and a longer duration of labor.

Other studies showed a relationship between anxiety pertaining to pregnancy and pregnancy symptoms. Green (1973), who followed 71 prenatal subjects in second trimester pregnancy, found that good prenatal adjustment was associated with fewer psychosomatic anxiety symptoms, general good health, and less anxiety. Shereshefsky and Yarrow (1973) found a correlation between medical symptoms and the overall reaction to pregnancy. Personality problems, or psychological conflict, were high in every instance where women had 11 or more medical symptoms. A higher level (number) of physical pregnancy-related symptoms was associated with lower emotional health (Grossman, Eichler, & Winickoff, 1980) and with a lesser desire for pregnancy (Klein, Potter, & Dyk, 1950).

Inquiry also was directed to the possible predictiveness of prenatal emotional state and somatic complaint patterns to delivery status and infant health. Zemlick and Watson (1953) reported that initial acceptance or rejection of pregnancy correlated with attitude toward the baby. Goshen-Gottstein (1966) found that women with an early rejection of pregnancy had more fears concerning their babies. In the Shereshefsky and Yarrow study (1973), pregnancy adaptation was associated with ego strength and nurturance of the gravidas, which in turn predicted postpartum measures of acceptance and confidence in the maternal role.

Doty (1967) also studied prenatal attitude and subsequent offspring well-being at six months. Attitudes in pregnancy were predictive of maternal dependency and infant behavior problems; negative attitudes were correlated positively with infant problems such as feeding, crying, and physical health, and these problems were significantly more prevalent in primiparas than multiparas. Primiparas were considered more dependent and anxious regarding their infant and themselves both during and after pregnancy. Doty theorized that emotional stress in pregnancy (negative attitude) might combine additively with postnatal maternal disturbances (rejecting childrearing attitudes) and might compound offspring behavioral disturbance. Doty suggested that more serious attention should be paid to the assessment and counseling of pregnant women.

One other measure influencing adaptation, but not as frequently cited, was health of the mother and her health history. Shereshefsky and Yarrow (1973) noted that a history of serious illness and accidents was associated with accentuated dependency needs and anxiety about doctors, medical procedures, and hospitalization. Thus, a number of maternal characteristics and attitudes influenced acceptance and adaptation to pregnancy, and there was some indication of long-range consequences after birth.

The Gravida's Relationship with Her Mother

The psychoanalytic position postulated that the gravida's relationship with her mother was at the center of the psychological problems of pregnancy. Bibring (1961, 1966) followed 15 primigravidas in each trimester of pregnancy, in labor and delivery, and postpartally up to one year, with interviews and projective psychological tests. Bibring's analysis indicated that the gravida formed a new identification with her mother during pregnancy, a new respect, and a new relationship in which the gravid daughter was an adult equal. The daughter also showed greater tolerance and acceptance of her own mother.

Ballou (1978), who conducted interviews and projective test assessments with 12 primigravidas through pregnancy and up to three months postpartum, placed strong emphasis on the significance of reconciliation with the mother. Reconciliation was described as a gradual progressive process wherein women, by the third trimester, saw their childhood as good, their mothers as giving, and the mother-child relationship as gratifying. Ballou's work confirmed and built upon Benedek's (1970), which emphasized gaining a sense of one's mother and of being mothered as a prerequisite to attaining a wholesome sense of one's child and the role of mother. As important as reconciliation was, when the relationship with the mother was marked with hostility, Ballou found that a nurturant husband could reassure a doubting wife and thus assuage and attenuate the negative influence of a poor mother-daughter relationship.

Other researchers examined the relationship with the mother or aspects of it and its influence on labor and delivery and postpartum adaptation. Levy and McGee (1975) reported that 60 primigravidas who received no information from their mothers concerning the mother's childbirth experience were unprepared and had a poorer evaluation of labor and delivery than women receiving information. Extreme evaluations from the mother, whether positive or negative, resulted in a poorer opinion of childbirth by the gravida than women who received only moderately negative or positive evaluations from their mothers. Extreme evaluations, by either creating too high a level of confidence or anxiety, tended to preclude the necessary preparation by the gravida for childbirth. By examining communication patterns, these investigators were able to glean and interpret complex information pertaining to the relationship with the mother and the labor experience. In this regard, Lederman et al. (1979) and Lederman (in press) found that an available reassuring mother was a constructive model, one which the gravida tended to emulate, thereby enhancing her own sense of maternal confidence. The relationship with the mother correlated with the primigravida's identification of her own motherhood role, childbirth preparation, and the resolution of fears concerning labor and delivery, as well as measures of progress in labor. Shereshefsky and Yarrow (1973) found that the relationship with the mother was related to husband-wife adaptation and self-confidence in the maternal role, but not to any of the three major maternal and infant outcome variables. Furthermore, Shereshefsky and Yarrow found the relationship to the mother was constant over the course of childhood, pregnancy, and the postpartum, and they suggested, in contrast to other reports, that the mother-daughter relationship does not change much.

Nilsson, Uddenberg, and Almgren (1971) and Nilsson and Almgren (1970) conducted an extensive study of paranatal emotional adjustment in 165 women. Similar to the results reported by Shereshefsky and Yarrow (1973), Lederman et al. (1979), Lederman (in press), and Nilsson et al. (1971) reported that women with a high degree of perceived similarity with the mother generally showed fewer signs of adjustment difficulty. They more often planned their pregnancy, were more prepared for motherhood, had fewer postpartum symptoms, and generally had a less complicated perinatal period.

In a subsequent study, Uddenberg and Fagerström (1976) compared the deliveries of primiparous daughters of reproductively well-adjusted and maladjusted mothers. Daughters of maladapted mothers had a higher incidence of obstetric pathology including significantly more toxemia, premature rupture of membranes, and both very short and very long labors. The researchers indicated that longer labors were associated with denial and repression of conflict, while the very fast labors were associated with a high number of conflicts that were dealt with during pregnancy. Thus, the authors provided evidence that indicates it is the method of coping with conflict, perhaps more than the conflict itself, that is significant. Further investigation in this area (Uddenberg, 1974) showed that power and closeness in the relationship with the mother also determined the strength of her influence, whether positive or negative, on the daughter's adaptation; these factors should not be overlooked in future research on the relationship of the gravida with her mother.

Considering the importance of the relationship with the mother, Cohen (1979) indicated, in his review of the literature, professional concern with loss of the mother before puberty. In this connection, Rubin (1975) stated that the lack of a female support system in itself constituted a risk factor. The research literature generally showed that the relationship with the mother was significant, but that this significance was dependent on communication patterns, power and closeness in the relationship, and the part that other significant persons play—particularly the husband—as a nurturant figure.

Relationship with Husband

The marital relationship has not been included regularly as a variable in studies on pregnancy adaptation and reproductive outcome, and past studies produced inconsistent results. Shereshefsky and Yarrow (1973) found only low or no correlations between the marital relationship and measures of pregnancy adaptation. On the other hand, Wenner and colleagues (Wenner, Cohen, Weigert, Kvarnes, Ohaneson, & Fearing, 1969) found the marital relationship to be the most significant factor influencing the course of pregnancy. Wenner et al. (1969) and Bibring (1961, 1966) concluded that an interdependent and egalitarian relationship is most conducive to adaptation, versus exaggerated dependent or independent relationships. In contrast, Gladieux (1978) found that couples with traditional, but mutually acceptable, marital relationships had fewer problems than couples with a contemporary relationship and more independent pursuits. Entwisle and Doering (1981) noted that a first pregnancy creates marital strain if the work role is the primary role for one or both partners.

Wenner et al. (1969) studied pregnancy problems and the dynamics of adaptive responses, and found that common prenatal fears and anxiety symptoms were more intense and preoccupying in the subjects with poor marriages. Wenner et al. concluded that, although characteristics of the gravida and her environment are important, success in the marital relationship is the most significant predictor of pregnancy adaptation. Like Ballou (1978), Wenner et al. felt that while practical considerations often were cited by subjects as influencing the course of pregnancy, problems with the marriage and other anxieties were more pertinent. Grossman et al. (1980) agreed that marital satisfaction and an egalitarian lifestyle, particularly for primigravidas, were associated with fewer pregnancy symptoms and better adaptation. In the Grossman et al. study, prenatal marital adjustment was marked by increased closeness, a sense of growth emotionally, and efforts by the couple to make room for a new family member. Grossman et al. also concluded that the marital relationship as well as past adaptive coping patterns were the most important variables influencing adaptation.

Westbrook (1978b) specifically investigated the relationship between the husband and the gravida's reactions to childbearing and early motherhood. Conducting the study retrospectively to obtain a large sample, the investigators used pictorial scenes representing the childbearing year and multidimensional scaling to classify positive and negative responses. Higher than normal scores were obtained on several anxiety scales, indicating that childbearing is a time of profound affective arousal. Women with positive marital relationships had the least disturbed reaction, less rejection of pregnancy, less problems in labor, and they were perceived to be the most calm group. Women with ambivalent relationships surprisingly had the least traumatic labor. Although they had expressed rejection of pregnancy, they were considered to be the warmest mothers; 83% had a positive relationship with the baby. It was felt that these women concentrated on the child throughout pregnancy and labor versus their body and the pregnancy experience. A self-oriented group, described as ignoring other people, failed to refer to the husband in their responses and showed no maternal warmth; they were particularly anxious about bodily injury. A fourth group characterized as negative experienced rejection of the child and/or pregnancy, in contrast to the ambivalent group, and continued to express rejection and high anxiety after delivery. Westbrook (1978b) stressed the need for evaluation of the marital relationship during pregnancy and timely intervention. Deutscher (1970) also underscored the need for attention to the marital relationship to help spouses recognize each other's fears and doubts and be supportive of each other.

Lederman et al. (1979) and Lederman (in press) assessed empathy, mutuality, and support for one another in the marital relationship. Few gravidas expressed problems forthrightly, even when they were present. Accuracy of responses was enhanced by inquiry into changes in the relationship, including sexual adaptation, since the advent of pregnancy. A poor marital relationship was associated with admission to the obstetric unit in the very early latent phase of labor, the administration of sedatives and tranquilizers for pronounced anxiety in early labor, and a prolonged duration of labor.

Overall, in most reports investigators suggested that the marital relationship appeared to influence adaptation to pregnancy. The literature, however, was more uniform and consistent in recognizing the significance of the relationship for postpartum adaptation (Lederman, Lederman, Work, & McCann, 1981; Russell, 1974; Shereshefsky & Yarrow, 1973).

Development of a Parental Role and Fetal Attachment

The development of a parental orientation and the formulation of a motherhood role during pregnancy was considered in longitudinal, prospective, psychological and sociological investigations, but these studies were few in number. This task was often defined in terms of giving (Lederman, in press; Rubin, 1975; Wenner et al., 1969). Giving referred to an analysis of costs and rewards in the first trimester, an exploration of concrete acts of giving and receiving in the second trimester, and specific preparations for the child and childbirth in the third trimester (Rubin, 1975).

Four relevant categories of maternal giving were developed by Wenner et al. (1969). At the first ideal level, Wenner et al. equated giving with the capacity for motherliness or tenderness (that is, the ability to derive pleasure from giving and to give in a manner that certifies and dignifies the needs of others). A second, less ideal category referred to the mother's ability to derive pleasure from giving only by merging with the recipient, and she responded only to those needs that resembled her own. In a third style of giving the mother derived pleasure by subjugating herself to the recipient and she responded dutifully to all needs, unable to sort out those to meet or treat otherwise. A fourth category related to women who generally were unable to derive pleasure from giving; they often were deprived and giving was equated with losing. Women with a more mature conceptualization of giving demonstrated more hope, confidence, and general coping ability versus less mature responses that were associated with anxiety, physical symptoms, depression, anger, and extreme fears for the well-being of oneself and the fetus.

Leifer (1980) also proposed a developmental pattern across trimesters that bore similarity to the one proposed by Rubin (1975). In the first trimester, the mother increasingly visualized herself as a mother; in the second trimester, she read and visited other mothers to learn about the motherhood role. By the third trimester, the mother had developed a sense of relatedness to the baby and was ready to have her baby. Mothers who used the pregnancy to initiate a relationship with the fetus had a more positive mood during pregnancy, higher self-esteem, higher attachment to the baby, and less motherhood stress. Those well-informed about childbirth related to the baby with relative ease. Ballou (1978) also noted that the development of a sense of her child was associated with increased feelings of competence and effectiveness. These processes, in turn, validated the gravida's sense of herself as a mother and enhanced her empathic understanding of the child.

Lederman et al. (1979) found that the gravida's identification of a motherhood role, which included measures of her potential to be nurturant and empathic in relation to a child, was related significantly to her acceptance of the pregnancy, as well as the relationship with her mother. Extreme anxiety or conflict concerning motherhood was related to fears about labor and to slower progress in all phases of labor.

The Shereshefsky and Yarrow (1973) measure of the women's ability to visualize herself as a mother, which was similar to the Lederman et al. (1979) measure of Identification of a Motherhood Role, correlated with prenatal measures of ego strength and nurturance. However, only the motherhood visualization variable correlated with maternal postpartum adaptation and with measures of responsiveness to the infant, infant alertness, husband-wife adaptation, and family adaptation in general. It is noteworthy that Shereshefsky and Yarrow (1973) and Wenner et al. (1969)

both indicated that an interest in children was related to prenatal and postnatal adaptation. Both of these studies demonstrated that the dimension of nurturing was an important, but not sufficient, variable to predict postnatal adaptation and the relationship with the child. Thus, while there were similarities in the way one related to significant others in general, as Ballou (1978) demonstrated, an evaluation of pregnancy adaptation and its predictiveness to the postpartum period must consider specifically the mother's progressive efforts to identify a motherhood role, as well as other pertinent variables. The literature showed it is also important to evaluate the mother's interest in children, her knowledge about children, her anticipation regarding the relationship with her child, and the realistic nature of all these conceptions.

Other investigators addressed expectant mothers' progressive attachment to the fetus during pregnancy. Cranley (1981) administered a fetal attachment questionnaire to gravidas at 35 to 40 weeks gestation. No significant relationships were reported either for the demographic variables or the measure of trait anxiety with fetal attachment. It may be, as Spielberger and Jacobs (1978) suggested, that specific prenatal state anxiety (versus general trait anxiety) is a more relevant measure of the anxiety occurring in pregnancy. Self-assessed stress caused by the mother's ill health or difficulties during pregnancy (which may reflect state anxiety), correlated negatively ($r = -.41$) with the Cranley measure of fetal attachment. In a second stage of the study, Cranley sought husband responses regarding the strength of the marriage and found positive associations between the marital relationship and the paternal-fetal attachment scale scores. A measure of social support also correlated ($r = .51$) with maternal-fetal attachment. It thus appeared that maternal stress, the quality of the marital relationship, and the availability of social support had a bearing on the extent of maternal-fetal attachment. Cranley presented important information which suggested that fetal awareness can be enhanced by a number of teaching methods, and this, in turn, may enhance fetal attachment as well.

Evidence for the value of specifically assessing fetal attachment is also presented by Robson and Moss (1970), who found that "early attachers"— those mothers who experienced immediate warmth and attachment to the newborn—experienced unusually high fetal attachment during pregnancy. These fetal attachment studies further underscored the need to assess specifically the gravida's awareness and conceptualization of the fetus, as well as her role in relation to the fetus.

There seems to be substantial agreement among researchers that identification of a motherhood role and measures of fetal attachment are particularly salient, not only for pregnancy adaptation, but for normal progress in labor and adaptation to the postpartum—to motherhood and the mother-child relationship.

Life Stresses and Behavior Influencing
Pregnancy Adaptation and Outcome

Although not specifically addressed above, a number of researchers identified specific life stresses such as financial strain, unemployment, relocation, illness, and loss of significant family members as having an influence on pregnancy adaptation and outcome (Cohen, 1979; Grossman et al., 1980; Helper, Cohen, Beitenman, & Eaton, 1968; Nadelson, 1973; Shere-shefsky & Yarrow, 1973; Yamamoto & Kinney, 1976). Grossman et al. (1980) reported that financial stress takes its toll on the marriage. Shere-shefsky and Yarrow (1973) additionally reported a negative relationship between life stress and nurturance.

The numerous factors associated with a maladaptive response to pregnancy included prior adverse experiences in childbirth, problematic or inadequate support—particularly from the husband and mother—inadequate preparation for childbearing and parenthood, maternal health problems, a previous history of psychiatric treatment or hospitalization or of difficulty in coping with developmental challenges, a poor marital relationship, loss of the mother at a young age and without replacement by a substitute or surrogate mother, failure to show reality-based perceptions of the fetus, failure to develop an emotional attachment to the fetus or absence of any thoughts or fantasies about the fetus, inability to anticipate life changes as a mother or a relationship with the neonate, considerable ambivalence or rejection of pregnancy in the third trimester, and limited formulation of a motherhood role.

COMPLICATIONS IN PREGNANCY

The complications discussed below are limited to those occurring primarily in the latter half of pregnancy, or near term, which are a threat to both the mother and fetus. In addition to studies in which investigators focused on complications in general, prematurity and pre-eclamptic toxemia are reviewed specifically, and they are discussed separately even though they may not be mutually exclusive events.

Prematurity

In studies of prematurity, researchers generally used the criterion of weight less than 2,500 grams, although it is recognized that other criteria define maturity, such as gestational age, neurological responses, and neuromotor development. Most investigators used a retrospective design and the weakness of such a design was often acknowledged. Nevertheless, there was some consistency among the findings regarding personality characteristics and stressful life events associated with prematurity. At 3 to 4 days postpartum, Newton and colleagues (Newton, Webster, Blau, Maskrey, & Phillips, 1979) administered a modified life-events scale to three gestation groups: less than 33 weeks, 33 to 36 weeks, and 37 weeks or more. The number of major life events in the week immediately preceding the onset of labor was significantly higher in the two preterm groups. The groups were all matched for age, gravidity, and parity, and the results were independent of social class.

In another retrospective study (Blau, Slaff, Easton, Welkowitz, Springarn, & Cohen, 1963), 30 women who delivered prematurely were matched with 30 controls who were examined in a psychiatric interview and with a number of psychological, intelligence, and attitude tests. The major finding was that premature delivering mothers had more negative attitudes toward pregnancy that exceeded the ambivalence commonly found in most women. They were also more emotionally immature. They became pregnant unwillingly, rejected the pregnancy, and attempted induced abortion. Gunter (1963) reported findings similar to those of Blau et al. Gunter examined stressful life events in addition to obtaining objective and projective psychological measures and public health nurse home visit evaluations. The premature group of 20 black married women was more immature and also more dependent and helpless than the 20 matched controls delivering at term. They experienced significantly more life and pregnancy stressors, had more gynecological problems, and more psychosomatic and neuropsychiatric symptoms. They were also more often neglected or deserted by their own mothers.

Creasy, Gummer, and Liggins (1980) developed a system for predicting preterm birth, using a risk factor matrix based on obstetric history, present health status, and social stress variables. Subjects at risk were followed with weekly visits, but most of the improvement in prevention was attributed to early and effective long-term tocolytic therapy for women who went into preterm labor. The overall incidence of prematurity was reduced, and this was attributed to the supportive care given by nurses.

The few studies focused on the psychophysiological roots of prematurity indicated that life stress during pregnancy was a common factor. The research results indicated that under such circumstances the pregnancy was either rejected, or the woman was too dependent and immature to cope with the stress of pregnancy and other life events.

Preeclampsia and Other Complications

Several early researchers examined anxiety in pregnancy and the overall occurrence of complications in pregnancy. Grimm and Venet (1966) conducted an extensive study of 105 normal pregnant women throughout the maternity cycle to determine the relationship of early emotional adjustment and attitudes toward later adjustment in parturition and the puerperium. The investigators did not control for age, parity, education, or occupation. Few significant results were found, but some were noteworthy. The researchers reported that primigravidas were not more anxious than multigravidas. Neuroticism was not related to other prenatal circumstances or concerns, but there was a relationship between neuroticism, depression, and adjustment in the postpartum period, which was similar to other reports (Meares, Grimwade, & Wood, 1976; Rees & Lutkins, 1971). Concerns and fears expressed early in pregnancy were indicative of reactions in labor and the authors were able to conclude, similar to Gorsuch and Key (1974), that early pregnancy attitudes were predictive of later attitudes.

Gorsuch and Key (1974) studied life stress and anxiety before and during pregnancy. Prepregnancy measures of life stress and trait anxiety were obtained retrospectively during the pregnancy, while serial measures of state anxiety and life stress were obtained throughout pregnancy from 118 low-income gravidas. There was no mention of control for age, parity, or marital status; marital status at the time of clinic admission was related significantly to later findings of abnormality in pregnancy. Anxiety early in pregnancy, but not later, differentiated groups with and without subsequent pregnancy and labor complications. In contrast to anxiety, the life stress measure at the second and third trimester, but not the first, was associated with pregnancy complications. The researchers pointed out that neither trait nor state anxiety were related to the life stress measure, that the stress measure predicted complications regardless of the level of anxiety, and that events during pregnancy were more critical and predictive than before pregnancy. It was somewhat surprising that the level of anxiety between the abnormal and normal groups was similar during the second and third trimesters and that it was rather constant during the latter six months of gestation.

In addition to measuring stressful events, the team of Nuckolls, Cassel, and Kaplan (1972) also measured life change and support. For the 170 subjects followed at 32 weeks gestation, neither high life change scores before or during pregnancy, nor psychosocial assets, were related to complications in pregnancy or labor. However, of the women with high life change scores, those with high psychosocial assets had only one-third the complications of women with low psychosocial assets. The results demonstrated the significance of adequate support when needed during periods of high stress.

In another study of stressful life situations and antenatal complications (Hetzel, Bruer, & Poidevin, 1961), a prolonged labor group experienced more stress related specifically to pregnancy, and more unfavorable and indifferent reactions to pregnancy than a normal labor group. The prolonged group, as well as a group of toxemic patients, reported more economic and occupational stressful life situations, but it should be noted that complications also were reported as a source contributing to stress scores. In toxemic patients, the husband was more often considered to be an inadequate provider, which, according to the authors, indicated rejection of the pregnancy. A number of other studies provided similar findings regarding responses to pregnancy and problems in the relationship with the husband.

In a retrospective study conducted by Coppen (1958), the toxemic group had a more disturbed attitude toward pregnancy accompanied by psychiatric symptoms and high neuroticism scores on the Maudsley Personality Inventory (MPI). In contrast, Yost and Kimball (1970) did not find higher MPI scores for the group of abnormal subjects. Coppen reported more emotional disturbances associated with the family in the toxemic group, but not significantly more neurotic symptoms in childhood. Glick, Royce, and Salerno (1964), however, reported an abnormal childhood in patients with preeclampsia, with evidence of emotional disorders and the need for psychiatric treatment. Brown (1964), in a similar but somewhat more extensive personality follow-up of toxemic patients, found significant correlations between the severity of toxemia and the husband's involvement, but not between severity and any other personality measures. Brown concluded that the toxemic group experienced greater social disturbance but no personality differences, as had been reported by Ringrose (1961a, 1961b) and Coppen (1958).

Studies by two research teams are particularly noteworthy for their prospective design (Glick et al., 1964; Pilowsky & Sharp, 1971). Pilowsky and Sharp administered a number of personality, pregnancy, and parental attitude scales to 80 married primiparas, 18 of whom subsequently developed toxemia. The results of Pilowsky and Sharp showed that toxemia patients had a lesser desire for pregnancy—as was shown by Hetzel et al. (1961)—less verbal intelligence, and more depression. As in a number of other studies, several problems were found upon testing of the husband as well, including a lack of ego strength and a lesser ability to tolerate frustration. Pilowsky and Sharp (1971) concluded that further study of intrafamily dynamics was warranted with toxemic patients. Findings by Glick et al. (1964) of separation from the husband, due to divorce, widowhood, or separation during a previous pregnancy, supported the recommendation of Pilowsky and Sharp.

Uddenberg and Fagerström (1976) examined relationships of the gravida with her mother rather than with the husband. Reproductively maladaptive mothers, as defined by these researchers, had daughters with a higher incidence of obstetric pathology. Eight cases of toxemia were observed, all in daughters of reproductively conflicted mothers.

Future investigators studying prenatal complications need to demonstrate more carefully that the sampling methods and measures logically follow and are appropriate to the research question. Retrospective data collection and convenience sampling, which were the predominant methods used, confounded accuracy (as well as confidence) in the results. Data collection periods should also be consistent and uniform across subjects, rather than based chiefly on a criterion of convenience.

There also needs to be a more concerted effort in formulating theoretical frameworks or foundations to guide research. Often there was insufficient evidence of forethought and theoretical consideration of possible patterns of relationships among the dependent and all of the independent variables selected for study. Designs tended to be either too general and global (e.g., an excessive battery of psychologic tests) or too singular and narrow (e.g., frequency of signs and symptoms associated with pregnancy such as nausea, gastric acidity). Research findings that supported the unique and developmental nature of pregnancy and the multiple factors influencing development pointed to a need for multivariate designs and serial data collection throughout the reproductive or maternity cycle.

Perhaps one of the most promising areas for further investigation is the marital relationship and its impact on mental and reproductive health. Several investigators identified problems in the relationship with the husband as a factor in prenatal complications. It was shown that women most often turn to their husbands for support during pregnancy and that, postpartally, mothers seek the husband more than any other person as a resource on infant care concerns (Pridham, Note 2). The husband is likely to be, or expected to be, the greater part of the mother's support system. Existing research results are limited, but further investigation into the dynamics and changes in the marital relationship during expectant parenthood, as well as intervention methods to enhance supportive relationships are suggested.

COMPLICATIONS OF LABOR AND DELIVERY

In this section the focus is on the relationship between attitudinal and developmental factors in pregnancy and maternal adaptation and complications in labor and delivery. Emphasis is placed on health outcomes and on prenatal predictors of health status.

Anxiety and Complications

A number of early investigators (Davids & DeVault, 1962; Kapp, Horstein, & Graham, 1963; McDonald & Christakos, 1963; McDonald, Gynther, & Christakos, 1963; McDonald & Parham, 1964) supported a relationship between prenatal anxiety and complications in childbirth, while a few researchers failed to find such significant relationships (Grimm & Venet, 1966). In addition, in a review Stott (1963) argued convincingly for the effect of prenatal stress in wartime and the postwar years on neonatal central nervous system malformations and the lesser likelihood that these could have been due to malnutrition.

McDonald and Christakos (1963) administered the Institute for Personality and Ability Testing (IPAT) anxiety scale to married clinic subjects of mixed gravidity and reported a significant positive correlation between anxiety and duration of labor. McDonald and Christakos (1963) reported that this same abnormal group also obtained higher mean scores on the Taylor MAS and on a majority of MPI scales. Less use of repressive type defense mechanisms were observed in the abnormal group at the seven-month prenatal data collection period. McDonald and Parham (1964) reported similar results with an unmarried group of 160 primigravidas; in this study the abnormal group tended to deny their feelings, while the normal group discussed them more openly. Davids and DeVault (1962) also administered a broad battery of psychological tests to 50 subjects in the seventh month of pregnancy. A blind review of hospital records served to classify subjects in normal and complicated labor groups. This abnormal group obtained higher mean scores on the Taylor MAS. There were no differences for age, intelligence, socioeconomic status, or parity, but marital status was not controlled and the effect of this important variable was not known. In addition, some of the complications found in the abnormal group did not appear immediately relevant, for example, short cord and prominent ensiform process. Likewise, some of the complications included in the study by McDonald and Parham (1964), for example, benign breast mass, were also somewhat questionable. Furthermore, the researchers did not indicate whether subjects were screened for prenatal medical complications that could account for high anxiety and labor complications.

Several years later, Crandon (1979) conducted a similar study. Crandon administered the IPAT anxiety self-analysis form to 146 gravidas in the third trimester of pregnancy and, on the basis of anxiety scores above or below 7, groups of low and high anxiety were defined. The anxiety scores correlated with the incidence of preeclampsia, prolonged labor, precipitate labor, forceps delivery, primary postpartum hemorrhage, manual removal of the placenta, and clinical fetal distress. Some complications again—for example, manual removal of the placenta—seemed distantly related to emotional state. As in the research by McDonald and coworkers and by Davids and DeVault (1962), the complications categories in Crandon's study raised some questions in this reviewer's mind about whether the researchers were "stuffing the ballot box."

Developmental Conflicts and Complications

In an early study to consider the influence of developmental conflicts on outcome of pregnancy, Kapp et al. (1963) compared normal and prolonged labor subjects on retrospective interview measures including the relationship of the mother and father, the gravida's adjustment to pregnancy, her concept of labor, and attitude to marriage and motherhood. The subjects were primiparas, matched for race and marital status, and the interviewers were blind to subject grouping. The results showed that the prolonged labor group obtained significantly higher scores on all the psychosocial factors. However, some aspects of the blind review by the authors were not clear. The postdelivery collection of data may also have influenced the results.

Other investigators studied labor complications using a prospective design. Engstrom, af Geijerstam, Holmberg, and Uhrus (1964) investigated whether psychosocial factors before and during pregnancy could influence the outcome of pregnancy. The interview schedule paralleled some of the psychosocial factors investigated by Kapp et al. (1963), such as social, marital, and financial attitudes; fear of pregnancy, labor, and delivery; response to the fetus; and motherhood conflicts. An emotionally negative attitude during delivery occurred twice as often in patients assessed as negative in one of two prenatal interviews, and these negatively responding patients experienced a higher percentage of uterine inertia and fetal asphyxia at delivery.

Later researchers also attempted to design studies focused on the roots of conflict and anxiety, and the relationship to length of labor. Uddenberg et al. (1976) indicated that women reporting many neurotic symptoms during pregnancy experienced a generally short labor, while those reporting few symptoms experienced longer labors. The researchers suggested that conflicts regarding reproduction, motherhood, and an ability to communicate and admit anxiety may result in a longer duration of labor. Winget and Kapp (1972) similarly found that subjects relaying fewer dreams with manifest anxiety content had a longer duration of labor. These results were similar to those found by McDonald and Christakos (1963), which related denial—rather than the overt expression of hostility and anxiety—to prolonged labor.

The expression of anxiety and hostility, however, appeared to be different from negative attitudes toward pregnancy, as indicated by Kapp et al. (1963), Engstrom et al. (1964), and Pilowsky (1972). Pilowsky administered psychological tests and a semistructured interview to 82 married primiparas in the second trimester. A sample of 45 husbands also were tested. The results showed that women who were likely to have complications, judged for severity by an obstetrician, were those who manifested an early negative attitude to pregnancy, showed unusual concern for the condition of the child, had less confidence in the doctors caring for them, saw their employment as disrupted, and had more contacts with women who had complicated pregnancies. They also described their mothers' health as poor and they themselves complained of a greater number of somatic symptoms and anxiety. These results were iterated in several previously cited studies. Pilowsky suggested that the high symptom and anxiety scores were indicative of early decompensation and pregnancy experiences with more of the attributes of crisis.

Norr, Block, Charles, and Meyering (1980) conducted one of the very few studies comparing the birth experience of multigravidas with primigravidas. Of 249 subjects, the primigravidas in the sample experienced significantly more complications, used more analgesia and anesthesia in labor, had less spontaneous deliveries, and experienced more blood loss and lacerations at delivery. Multiparas, however, experienced more discomfort during pregnancy, received less support from their husbands during labor, and also sought less contact with their babies during the hospital stay. These differences should be considered in studies using subject samples of mixed parity.

Lederman, Lederman, Work, and McCann (1978, 1979)—in addition to an in-depth investigation of prenatal personality variables relevant to adaptation in pregnancy and parturition—also sought to determine the biochemical correlates for both anxiety and uterine contractile activity in labor. The results in labor showed that state anxiety at the onset of active labor or Phase 2 correlated with endogenous plasma epinephrine. Higher epinephrine levels were related significantly to lower contractile activity at the onset of active labor and to longer labor in Phase 2 (3–10 cm. cervical dilatation). Psychological variables measured in pregnancy were correlated significantly with variables measured at the onset of active labor. For example, conflict concerning the Acceptance of Pregnancy and the Identi- fication of a Motherhood Role showed the most significant relationships with anxiety, epinephrine, and uterine activity at the onset of active-phase labor and with the length of labor in Phase 2 and Phase 3 (second stage labor). Beck, Siegel, Davidson, Kormeier, Breitenstein, and Hall (1980) also found that state anxiety on admission to the labor unit, but not prenatal trait anxiety, was predictive of labor duration. The trait anxiety measure in pregnancy correlated with the state anxiety measure in active labor and with uterine activity.

In addition to Lederman et al. (1978, 1979), two other research teams—one focusing on attitude toward the baby (Laukaran & van den Berg, 1980) and the other on attitudes toward pregnancy (Zemlick & Watson, 1953)—found that prenatal maternal attitude was a significant predictor of perinatal outcomes. Zemlick and Watson (1953) followed a small sample of 15 married primigravid subjects and showed that prenatal anxiety—particularly in late third trimester pregnancy—and attitudes of rejection of pregnancy and motherhood were related to adjustment during delivery and the postpartum period. Laukaran and van den Berg (1980), on the other hand, conducted a large-scale prospective study of 8,000 gravi- das, and analyzed responses to the question, "How do you feel about having a baby now?" Negative maternal attitudes were more often associated with perinatal (fetal) death, severe congenital anomalies, a higher perinatal mortality rate, and more postpartum infection and hemorrhage. The negative group also presented more psychosocial complaints related to anxiety and more accidental injuries during pregnancy, as well as a greater need for analgesics during labor. These results held when potentially confounding factors such as parity, age of mother, and socioeconomic status were controlled. Although investigators often did not distinguish between attitudes toward the pregnancy, the baby, and parenthood, the research cited—as well as research on motivation for pregnancy (Flapan, 1969; Pohlman & Pohlman, 1969)—indicated that it was important to do so.

Another group of researchers (Standley, Soule, & Copans, 1979) focused on identifying specific dimensions of prenatal anxiety rather than attitudes, and their influence on pregnancy outcome. Anxieties about pregnancy, birth, and parenting were related significantly to the administration of anesthesia during childbirth and to motor maturity of the neonate. It is possible that these two findings—anesthesia and neonatal motor maturity—also were interrelated.

It is of interest to note that background factors of age, education, and preparation for childbirth in Standley et al. (1979) were correlated negatively with anxieties about pregnancy and childbirth, but that Zax, Sameroff, and Babigian (1977) did not find that subjects' general anxiety was affected by a program of preparation for childbirth. Sosa, Kennell, Klaus, Robertson, and Urrutia (1980) examined only the effects of a "doula" (supportive lay person) in labor and found that subjects with a "doula" had a shorter duration of labor than a control group and fewer perinatal problems (such as Cesarean section and fetal meconium staining) than the control group. In a somewhat similar vein, Davenport-Slack and Boylan (1974) found that wanting the husband in the labor room was associated with a shorter labor. And Cogan, Henneborn, and Klopfer (1976) found that the support of significant others, particularly the husband, and confidence in the form of childbirth preparation were related to the amount of reported pain experienced in childbirth.

Erickson (1971, 1976a, 1976b) conducted studies to examine the relationship between psychological variables and specific childbirth complications and identified a sequence of complications occurring in labor. The psychological variables most often discriminating between subjects in the experimental (complications) and control groups were fears for self and baby, and dependency. These variables were associated with prolonged first and second stage labor and uterine inertia, assisted head rotation, low forceps delivery, and Apgar scores from 5 to 7. The author suggested that these events formed a sequence of complications that were initiated by psychological stresses in pregnancy.

Life Stress, Coping, Social Support, and Complications

Other factors that were found to influence pregnancy outcome included life stress in relation to the frequency of complications, and adoption of the sick role in relation to prolonged labor (Rosengren, 1961). While Gorsuch and Key (1974) found that life stress during (but not before) pregnancy correlated with the frequency of complications, Jones (1978) found a negative correlation between life stress and labor complications. It is possible, as Jones suggested, that individual differences in stress perception, coping, and support might have accounted for the findings. An alternative explanation for the results obtained by Jones is that the sample was drawn entirely from an inpatient residential facility of healthy, but indigent, women. These subjects might have experienced less stress in this environment than the one they came from, and thus less complications in labor as well. Moore (1977), who also assessed life stress in a sample of 147 primigravidas of low socioeconomic status, found that high life change and a negative expectation about motherhood correlated with the total number of pregnancy, delivery, and neonatal abnormalities. In addition, life stress was associated with prenatal complications in other studies previously cited.

Summary and Discussion

In summary, the research seems to support Rubin's (1975) contention that all the fears and conflicts of pregnancy come together in the critical experience of labor and delivery. Numerous investigators found some association between anxiety, developmental conflicts, negative attitudes toward motherhood, specific fears about labor and delivery, and subsequent complications in childbirth, including prolonged labor, forceps delivery, maternal injury (laceration), fetal distress, low Apgar score, and others. While some investigators did not indicate controls for potentially confounding variables, such as prenatal complications, marital status, gravidity, parity, age, education, and socioeconomic status, several other researchers did address these factors in the study design.

Only a few authors acknowledged the difficulty of collecting data in labor (Chertok, 1969; Morris, 1978). The difficulty was quite apparent in the reliance of a majority of investigators on the medical record for their collection of data. While some data could be relied upon for collection in this way, other data—such as length of labor—were more subject to inaccuracy. The length of first stage labor included a long and less clinically significant latent stage of labor, as well as a more significant active phase from 3 to 10 cm. cervical dilatation. The onset of labor was frequently difficult to determine accurately, and may have been in error by several hours or more. The length of second stage labor was also subject to considerable confounding due to its comparative brevity, the availability of medical personnel at the appropriate time interval, and other factors, such as intervention with forceps-assisted delivery. Consideration of medications administered to enhance labor—such as oxytocin—and other medications that may influence length—such as analgesics and anesthesia—also must be taken into account. A partial solution is to evaluate length in three recognized obstetrical phases of labor. The best solution is for medical-surgical investigators to collect and evaluate their own data, although the difficulties incurred by this solution are recognized. This solution may make prospective studies more difficult to implement, and this may limit sample size, but the alternative is less accurate and less reliable data.

Other factors that need consideration in future investigations are the development of categories of complications versus a heterogeneous random listing and consistency in the definition of terms across studies—particularly stress and anxiety, length of labor parameters, and labor complications. There is also a need for uniform testing periods, and for general acknowledgment and control of confounding factors. New instruments will be developed inevitably as research continues, but it is important that these instruments be developed in accordance with recognized and well-established measurement principles, and these must be reported for examination by other investigators. There is a need for more prospective versus retrospective studies, and for empirical designs, with future research building on past studies so that comparative evaluation is made more feasible.

CONCLUSIONS AND RESEARCH DIRECTIONS

More systematic and scientific approaches to the conduct of research are needed. The complexity of interactions inherent in psychophysiological research will require multidisciplinary and multivariate research designs. It will become increasingly necessary to scrutinize carefully the research literature to identify critical independent variables and relevant theoretical frameworks to guide research designs and methods. A stepwise or hierarchical program of research, and the careful selection of instruments rather than reliance on an arbitrary battery of psychosocial and developmental tests, are necessary for manageability, interpretability, and generalizability of the results produced. In developmental and psychophysiological research it will be particularly important to study patterns of relationships and the consistency of changes over time. Serial measurements of anxiety and development in the successive trimesters of pregnancy will permit such an examination of change, as well as the determination of the long-term correlates of maternal-fetal health status. Such an approach will allow normal and abnormal patterns of behavior to be distinguished. Thus, it will be equally important to select carefully the measurement instruments and the times of data collection. Another important consideration will be measurement of the intensity and duration of emotional states, such as anxiety and depression, as well as the psychosocial assets and liabilities related to health outcomes. The influence of other possible contributing variables to stress states and health outcomes, such as age, health, parity, nutrition, socioeconomic status, and childbirth events also must be considered and controlled.

It is possible that different factors are associated with adaptation in the different phases of pregnancy, labor and delivery, and the postpartum. For example, the marital relationship, financial status, and the availability of various support systems may have a different impact on pregnancy versus the postpartum period. Thus, researchers must consider the differential influence of various psychosocial factors on adaptation, while at the same time identifying relationships among relevant factors and change over time. A related area of investigation involves identifying short-term versus long-term effects of stress, and determining which effects are amenable to correction with optimal parenting and home environmental conditions and which require other solutions. It also would be helpful to continue to conduct individual family member studies such as motherhood adaptation studies, as well as interactive family studies of husband, wife, and sibling adaptation over the course of pregnancy and the postpartum period. It should not be assumed that any one assessment approach or model is necessarily better than any other until the evidence for such an interpretation is available. Future intervention studies should be based on the results of developmental and psychophysiological studies, and should contemplate changes in the organization of health care delivery and changes in health and social policy in institutions serving parents and children.

REFERENCE NOTES

1. Lederman, R. P., & Lederman, E. *The development of a prenatal self-evaluation questionnaire for the measurement of seven psychological dimensions.* Paper presented at the meeting of the American Nurses' Association Council of Nurse Researchers, San Antonio, Texas, December, 1979.
2. Pridham, K. F. *Information needs and problem-solving behavior of parents of new babies.* Paper presented at the March of Dimes Nursing Roundtable on Social Support and Familes of Vulnerable Infants. Lake Wilderness, Wash.: University of Washington Conference Center, October, 1982.

REFERENCES

Areskog, B., Uddenberg, N., & Kjessler, B. Fear of childbirth in late pregnancy. *Gynecologic and Obstetric Investigation,* 1981, *12,* 262–266.
Ballou, J. W. *The psychology of pregnancy.* Lexington, Mass.: Lexington Books, 1978.
Beck, N. C., Siegel, L. J., Davidson, N. P., Kormeier, S., Breitenstein, A., & Hall, D. G. The prediction of pregnancy outcome: Maternal preparation, anxiety and attitudinal sets. *Journal of Psychosomatic Research,* 1980, *24,* 343–351.
Benedek, T. The psychobiology of pregnancy. In E. J. Anthony & T. Benedek (Eds.), *Parenthood: Its psychology and psychopathology.* Boston: Little, Brown, 1970.
Bibring, G. A study of the psychological processes in pregnancy and the earliest mother-child relationship, Parts I and II. *The Psychoanalytic Study of the Child,* 1961, *16,* 9–24.
Bibring, G. Recognition of psychological stress often neglected in OB care. *Hospital Topics,* 1966, *44,* 100–103.
Blau, A., Slaff, B., Easton, K., Welkowitz, J., Springarn, J., & Cohen, J. The psychogenic etiology of premature birth. *Psychosomatic Medicine,* 1963, *25,* 201–211.
Brown, L. B. Anxiety in pregnancy. *British Journal of Medical Psychology,* 1964, *37,* 37–58.
Burstein, I., Kinch, R. A., & Stern, L. Anxiety, pregnancy, labor and the neonate. *American Journal of Obstetrics and Gynecology,* 1974, *118,* 195–199.
Caplan, G. *Concepts of mental health and consultation: Their application in public health social work* (DHEW Publication No. 373). Washington, D.C.: U.S. Government Printing Office, 1959.
Chertok, L. *Motherhood and personality: Psychosomatic aspects of childbirth.* Philadelphia: Lippincott, 1969.
Chertok, L., Mondzain, M. L., & Bonnaud, M. Vomiting and the wish to have a child. *Psychosomatic Medicine,* 1963, *25,* 13–18.

Cogan, R., Henneborn, W., & Klopfer, F. Predictors of pain during prepared childbirth. *Journal of Psychosomatic Research*, 1976, *20*, 523–533.

Cohen, R. L. Maladaptation to pregnancy. *Seminars in Perinatology*, 1979, *3*(1), 15–24.

Coppen, A. J. Psychosomatic aspects of pre-eclamptic toxaemia. *Journal of Psychosomatic Research*, 1958, *2*, 241–265.

Crandon, A. J. Maternal anxiety and neonatal wellbeing. *Journal of Psychosomatic Research*, 1979, *23*, 113–115.

Cranley, M. S. Roots of attachment: The relationship of parents with their unborn. *Birth Defects: Original Article Series*, 1981, *17*(6), 59–83.

Creasy, R. K., Gummer, B. A., & Liggins, G. C. System for predicting spontaneous preterm birth. *Obstetrics and Gynecology*, 1980, *55*, 692–695.

Davenport-Slack, B., & Boylan, C. H. Psychological correlates of childbirth pain. *Psychosomatic Medicine*, 1974, *36*, 215–223.

Davids, A., & DeVault, S. Maternal anxiety during pregnancy and childbirth abnormalties. *Psychosomatic Medicine*, 1962, *24*, 464–470.

Deutsch, H. *Psychology of women* (Vol. 2). New York: Grune & Stratton, 1945.

Deutscher, M. Brief family therapy in the course of first pregnancy: A clinical note. *Contemporary Psychoanalysis*, 1970, *7*, 21–35.

Doty, B. A. Relationships among attitudes in pregnancy and other maternal characteristics. *Journal of Genetic Psychology*, 1967, *111*, 203–217.

Engstrom, L. af Geijerstam, G., Holmberg, N. G., & Uhrus, K. A prospective study of the relationship between psycho-social factors and course of pregnancy and delivery. *Journal of Psychosomatic Research*, 1964, *8*, 151–155.

Entwisle, D. R., & Doering, S. G. *The first birth*. Baltimore: Johns Hopkins University Press, 1981.

Erickson, M. T. Risk factors associated with complications of pregnancy, labor, and delivery. *American Journal of Obstetrics and Gynecology*, 1971, *111*, 658–662.

Erickson, M. T. The influence of health factors on psychological variables predicting complications of pregnancy, labor and delivery. *Journal of Psychosomatic Research*, 1976, *20*, 21–24. (a)

Erickson, M. T. The relationship between psychological variables and specific complications of pregnancy, labor and delivery. *Journal of Psychosomatic Research*, 1976, *20*, 207–210. (b)

Flapan, M. A paradigm for the analysis of childbearing motivations of married women prior to birth of the first child. *American Journal of Orthopsychiatry*, 1969, *39*, 402–417.

Gladieux, J. D. Pregnancy—The transition to parenthood. In W. B. Miller & L. F. Newman (Eds.), *The first child and family formation*. Chapel Hill, N.C.: University of North Carolina Population Center, 1978.

Glick, I. D., Royce, J. R., & Salerno, L. J. Psychophysiologic factors in the etiology of pre-eclampsia. *Psychosomatic Medicine*, 1964, *26*, 632. (Abstract)

Gorsuch, R. L., & Key, M. K. Abnormalities of pregnancy as a function of anxiety and life stress. *Psychosomatic Medicine*, 1974, *36*, 352–362.

Goshen-Gottstein, E. R. *Marriage and first pregnancy*. London: Tavistock, 1966.

Green, R. T. Perceived styles of mother-daughter relationship and the prenatal adjustment of the primigravida (Doctoral dissertation, George Washington University, 1973). *Dissertation Abstracts International*, 1973, *34*, 2305B. (University Microfilms No. 73-25, 094).

Grimm, E. R. Psychological tension in pregnancy. *Psychosomatic Medicine*, 1961, *23*, 520-527.

Grimm, E. R., & Venet, W. R. The relationship of emotional adjustment and attitudes to the course and outcome of pregnancy. *Psychosomatic Medicine*, 1966, *28*, 34-49.

Grossman, F. K., Eichler, L. S. & Winickoff, S. A. *Pregnancy, birth and parenthood*. San Francisco: Jossey-Bass, 1980.

Gunter, L. M. Psychopathology and stress in the life experiences of mothers of premature infants. *American Journal of Obstetrics and Gynecology*, 1963, *86*, 333-340.

Hanford, J. M. Pregnancy as a state of conflict. *Psychological Reports*, 1968, *22*, 1313-1342.

Helper, M. M., Cohen, R. L., Beitenman, E. T., & Eaton, L. F. Life-events and acceptance of pregnancy. *Journal of Psychosomatic Research*, 1968, *12*, 183-188.

Hetzel, B. S., Bruer, B., & Poidevin, L. O. S. A survey of the relation between certain common antenatal complications in primiparae and stressful life situations during pregnancy. *Journal of Psychosomatic Research*, 1961, *5*, 175-182.

Heymans, H., & Winter, S. T. Fears during pregnancy. An interview study of 200 postpartum women. *Israel Journal of Medical Sciences*, 1975, *11*, 1102-1105.

Janis, I. L. *Psychological stress*. New York: Wiley, 1958.

Jarrahi-Zadeh, A., Kane, F. J., Jr., Van de Castle, R. L., Lachenbruch, P. A., & Ewing, J. A. Emotional and cognitive changes in pregnancy and early puerperium. *British Journal of Psychiatry*, 1969, *115*, 797-805.

Jones, A. C. Life change and psychological distress as predictors of pregnancy outcome. *Psychosomatic Medicine*, 1978, *40*, 402-412.

Kapp, F. T., Horstein, S., & Graham, V. T. Some psychological factors in prolonged labor due to inefficient uterine action. *Comprehensive Psychiatry*, 1963, *4*, 9-18.

Klein, H. R., Potter, H. W., & Dyk, R. B. *Anxiety in pregnancy and childbirth*. New York: Hoeper, 1950.

Laukaran, V. H., & van den Berg, B. J. The relationship of maternal attitude to pregnancy outcomes and obstetric complications: A cohort study of unwanted pregnancy. *American Journal of Obstetrics and Gynecology*, 1980, *136*, 374-379.

Lederman, R. P. *Psychosocial adaptation in pregnancy: Assessment of seven dimensions of maternal development*. Englewood Cliffs, N.J.: Prentice-Hall, in press.

Lederman, R. P., Lederman, E., Work, B. A., Jr., & McCann, D. S. The relationship of maternal anxiety, plasma catecholamines, and plasma cortisol to progress in labor. *American Journal of Obstetrics and Gynecology*, 1978, *132*, 495-500.

Lederman, R. P. Lederman, E., Work, B. A., Jr., & McCann, D. S. Relationship of psychological factors in pregnancy to progress in labor. *Nursing Research*, 1979, *28*, 94–97.

Lederman, E., Lederman, R. P., Work, B. A., Jr., & McCann, D. S. Maternal psychological and physiological correlates of fetal-newborn health status. *American Journal of Obstetrics and Gynecology*, 1981, *139*, 956–958.

Leifer, M. *Psychological effects of motherhood: A study of first pregnancy.* New York: Praeger, 1980.

Levy, J. M., & McGee, R. K. Childbirth as a crisis: A test of Janis' theory of communication and stress resolution. *Journal of Personality and Social Psychology*, 1975, *31*, 171–179.

Light, H. K., & Fenster, C. Maternal concerns during pregnancy. *American Journal of Obstetrics and Gynecology*, 1974, *118*, 46–50.

Lubin, B., Gardener, S. H., & Roth, A. Mood and somatic symptoms during pregnancy. *Psychosomatic Medicine*, 1975, *37*, 136–146.

McDonald, R. L., & Christakos, A. C. Relationship of emotional adjustment during pregnancy to obstetrical complications. *American Journal of Obstetrics and Gynecology*, 1963, *86*, 341–348.

McDonald, R. L., Gynther, M. D., & Christakos, A. C. Relations between maternal anxiety and obstetric complications. *Psychosomatic Medicine*, 1963, *25*, 357–363.

McDonald, R. L., & Parham, K. J. Relation of emotional changes during pregnancy to obstetric complications in unmarried primigravidas. *American Journal of Obstetrics and Gynecology*, 1964, *90*, 195–201.

Meares, R., Grimwade, J., & Wood, C. A possible relationship between anxiety in pregnancy and puerperal depression. *Journal of Psychosomatic Research*, 1976, *20*, 605–610.

Moore, D. Identification of women at obstetrical risk from measures of prenatal psychological stress (Doctoral dissertation, George Peabody College for Teachers, 1977). *Dissertation Abstracts International*, 1977, *38*, 2377A–2378A. (University Microfilms No. 77–25, 119).

Morris, N. Stress in labour. In L. Carenza, P. Pancheri, & L. Zichella (Eds.), *Clinical psychoendocrinology in reproduction.* London: Academic Press, 1978.

Nadelson, C. "Normal" and "special" aspects of pregnancy. *Obstetrics and Gynecology*, 1973, *41*, 611–620.

Newton, R. W., Webster, P. A. C., Blau, P. S., Maskrey, N., & Phillips, A. B. Psychosocial stress in pregnancy and its relation to the onset of premature labour. *British Medical Journal*, 1979, *2*, 411–413.

Nilsson, A. & Almgren, P. E. Para-natal emotional adjustment. A prospective investigation of 165 women. II. The influence of background factors, psychiatric history, parental relations, and personality characteristics. *Acta Psychiatrica Scandinavica*, 1970, *220*(2, Supplement), 65–141.

Nilsson, A., Uddenberg, N., & Almgren, P. E. Parental relations and identification in women with special regard to para-natal emotional adjustment. *Acta Psychiatrica Scandinavica*, 1971, *47*(1), 57–81.

Norr, K. L., Block, C. R., Charles, A. G., & Meyering, S. The second time around: Parity and birth experience. *Journal of Obstetric, Gynecologic, and Neonatal Nursing,* 1980, *9,* 30–36.

Nuckolls, K. B., Cassel, J., & Kaplan, B. H. Psychosocial assets, life crisis and the prognosis of pregnancy. *American Journal of Epidemiology,* 1972, *95,* 431–441.

Pilowsky, I. Psychological aspects of complications of childbirth: A prospective study of primiparae and their husbands. In N. Morris (Ed.), *Psychosomatic medicine in obstetrics and gynaecology.* Basel: Karger, 1972.

Pilowsky, I., & Sharp, J. Psychological aspects of pre-eclamptic toxemia: A prospective study. *Journal of Psychosomatic Research,* 1971, *15,* 193–197.

Pohlman, E. W. Changes from rejection to acceptance of pregnancy. *Social Science and Medicine,* 1968, *2,* 337–340.

Pohlman, E. W., & Pohlman, J. M. *The psychology of birth planning.* Cambridge, Mass.: Schenkman, 1969.

Rees, W. D., & Lutkins, S. G. Parental depression before and after childbirth: An assessment with the Beck Depression Inventory. *Journal of the Royal College of General Practitioners,* 1971, *21,* 26–31.

Ringrose, C. A. D. Further observations on the psychosomatic character of toxemia of pregnancy. *Canadian Medical Association Journal,* 1961, *84,* 1064–1065. (a)

Ringrose, C. A. D. Psychosomatic influence in the genesis of toxemia of pregnancy. *Canadian Medical Association Journal,* 1961, *84,* 647–651. (b)

Robson, K. S., & Moss, H. A. Patterns and determinants of maternal attachment. *Journal of Pediatrics,* 1970, *77,* 976–985.

Rosengren, W. R. Social sources of pregnancy as illness or normality. *Social Forces,* 1961, *39,* 260–267.

Rubin, R. Maternal tasks in pregnancy. *Maternal-Child Nursing Journal,* 1975, *4,* 143–153.

Russell, C. S. Transition to parenthood: Problems and gratifications. *Journal of Marriage and the Family,* 1974, *36,* 294–301.

Shainess, N. Abortion: Social, psychiatric and psychoanalytic perspectives. *New York State Journal of Medicine,* 1968, *68,* 3070–3073.

Shereshefsky, P. M., & Yarrow, L. J. (Eds.). *Psychological aspects of a first pregnancy and early postnatal adaptation.* New York: Raven Press, 1973.

Sosa, R., Kennell, J., Klaus, M., Robertson, S., & Urrutia, J. The effect of a supportive companion on perinatal problems, length of labor, and mother-infant interaction. *New England Journal of Medicine,* 1980, *303,* 597–600.

Spielberger, C. D., Gorsuch, R. L., & Lushene, R. E. *Manual for the State-Trait Anxiety Inventory.* Palo Alto, Calif.: Consulting Psychologists Press, 1970.

Spielberger, C. D., & Jacobs, G. A. Stress and anxiety during pregnancy and labor. In L. Carenza, P. Pancheri, & L. Zichella (Eds.), *Clinical psychoneuroendocrinology in reproduction.* London: Academic Press, 1978.

Standley, K., Soule, A. B., & Copans, S. A. Dimensions of prenatal anxiety and their influence on pregnancy outcome. *American Journal of Obstetrics and Gynecology,* 1979, *135,* 22–26.

Stott, D. H. How a disturbed pregnancy can harm the child. *New Scientist,* 1963, *320,* 15–17.

Uddenberg, N. Reproductive adaptation in mother and daughter. A study of personality development and adaptation to motherhood. *Acta Psychiatrica Scandinavica*, 1974, *50* (Supplement No. 254), 1–115.

Uddenberg, N., & Fagerström, C. F. The deliveries of daughters of reproductively maladjusted mothers. *Journal of Psychosomatic Research*, 1976, *20*, 223–229.

Uddenberg, N., Fagerström, C. F., & Hakanson-Zaunders, M. Reproductive conflicts, mental symptoms during pregnancy and time in labour. *Journal of Psychosomatic Research*, 1976, *20*, 575–581.

Wenner, N. K., Cohen, M. B., Weigert, E. V., Kvarnes, R. G., Ohaneson, E. M., & Fearing, J. M. Emotional problems in pregnancy. *Psychiatry*, 1969, *32*, 389–410.

Westbrook, M. T. Analyzing affective responses to past events: Women's reactions to a childbearing year. *Journal of Clinical Psychology*, 1978, *34*, 967–971. (a)

Westbrook, M. T. The reactions to child-bearing and early maternal experience of women with differing marital relationships. *British Journal of Medical Psychology*, 1978, *51*, 191–199. (b)

Winget, C., & Kapp, F. T. The relationship of the manifest content of dreams to duration of childbirth in primiparae. *Psychosomatic Medicine*, 1972, *34*, 313–320.

Yamamoto, K. J., & Kinney, D. K. Pregnant women's ratings of different factors influencing psychological stress during pregnancy. *Psychological Reports*, 1976, *39*, 203–214.

Yost, M. A., Jr., & Kimball, C. P. Personality factors in pre-eclampsia of pregnancy. *Obstetrics and Gynecology*, 1970, *36*, 753–757.

Zajicek, E., & Wolkind, S. Emotional difficulties in married women during and after the first pregnancy. *British Journal of Medical Psychology*, 1978, *51*, 379–385.

Zax, M., Sameroff, A. J., & Babigian, H. M. Birth outcomes in the offspring of mentally disordered women. *American Journal of Orthopsychiatry*, 1977, *47*, 218–230.

Zemlick, M. J., & Watson, R. I. Maternal attitudes of acceptance and rejection during and after pregnancy. *American Journal of Orthopsychiatry*, 1953, *23*, 570–584.

CHAPTER 3

The Experience of
Being a Parent

ANGELA BARRON MCBRIDE
INDIANA UNIVERSITY SCHOOL OF NURSING

CONTENTS

Recently both the name and the focus of many departments of maternity nursing were changed so the emphasis is on parenthood over the years and not just on labor and delivery. Instead of viewing motherhood in its most biologic sense, the focus increasingly has been on the developmental challenge of parenthood for both sexes (McBride, 1973). The most recent nursing research roundtable funded by the March of Dimes Birth Defects Foundation (Lederman, Raff, & Carroll, 1981) included presentations and discussion of patterns of parental development in both naturalistic and clinical settings. The growth and development strains of affiliative relationships are regarded as phenomena of prime concern to nursing (American Nurses' Association, Note 1). Given the fact that the nursing profes-

Elizabeth Jeannine Gale was of invaluable help in searching the literature and screening the listings of research-based articles. Work on this review was facilitated by the author's National Kellogg Fellowship to study Stages in Being a Parent. Requests for both a full description of the methods used to survey the literature in this area and a summary of the 53 key studies that constitute the core of this review should be sent to Angela Barron McBride, Department of Psychiatric/Mental Health Nursing, Indiana University School of Nursing, 610 Barnhill Drive, Indianapolis, Ind. 46223.

sion has an investment in parental development, how can research on the experience of being a parent be characterized? This review includes first a brief statement of the approach used to develop this chapter, then comments on the overall nature of the nursing literature in this area. Fifty-three studies are then summarized and analyzed for their contributions to the field. Finally, recommendations are made regarding future research.

METHOD OF REVIEW

Once all of the nursing indexes through July and August 1982 were scrutinized for articles on the experience of being a parent, pertinent references were read in order to ascertain whether they were data-based. For an article to qualify as a research report, the sample had to be described and there had to be evidence of some method of data collection.

Only those studies that included a description of some aspect of the parents' experience *after* the immediate postpartum period were considered. No studies of breastfeeding per se or some other specific task were included, since the focus was on the experience of parents, and not on parents' accomplishment of a specific procedure. Only studies of parents' behavior that involved asking parents about their experience were included in the review, so children's assessments of their parents' behavior (e. g., Yanni, 1982) were not regarded as equivalent to accounts of the parents' own experience.

NURSING AND THE EXPERIENCE OF BEING A PARENT

Many think pieces, reviews of the literature, discussions of the needs of parents with special children, and descriptions of programs for parents are part of the nursing literature on the experience of being a parent, but these fall short of qualifying as research reports. A number of think pieces, for example, included consideration of parenthood as a developmental crisis (Donner, 1972) or as an experience with distinct phases (Hrobsky, 1977; Streff, 1981). Mothering (Perdue, Horowitz, & Herz, 1977), fathering (Kiernan & Scoloveno, 1977), and the lot of parents of tomorrow (Cronenwett, 1980; Gilmore, 1966; McBride, 1975) were discussed in terms of sex roles, choices, and nursing's response to changing family structures.

There were several distinct subcategories within the literature on the experience of being a parent. One was directed at how nursing can meet the needs of parents with a retarded, sick, or dying child (Freiberg, 1972; Goldfogel, 1970; Lowenberg, 1970; Mann, 1974; Rajokovich, 1969; Zamerowski, 1982). Butani (1974) reviewed the literature on reactions of mothers to the birth of an anomalous child; Gordeuk (1976) summarized motherhood when the child was less than perfect. Horan (1982) described an attributional approach to parents' reactions to the birth of an infant with a defect.

Another subcategory within this literature was the description of existing programs for parents. Bishop (1976) recounted how she assessed parenting capabilities using three kinds of information: mothers' (primary caretakers') physical and emotional energy, support systems available to mothers, and mothers' current level of parenting. Lockhart (1982) described the development of a series of parenting classes for couples who adopt children. McAbee (1977) developed a tool for teaching rural parents basic concepts and appropriate parenting based on Erikson's developmental stages. Role acquisition and role mastery were features of two other programs (Shaw, 1974; Swendsen, Meleis, & Jones, 1978).

Most of the literature was focused on maternal behavior, but concern about father emerged (Hines, 1971). Cronenwett (1982) reviewed father participation in child care. Cronenwett and Kunst-Wilson (1981) developed a transition-to-fatherhood paradigm; they also explored the relationship of the father in the context of attachment theory.

While nurse investigators have been concerned generally with facilitating the experience of being a parent, much of what their publications reflected was either an impressionistic sharing of clinical perceptions or a discussion of how theories from other fields can be applied to nursing. The emphasis was on mothering rather than on fathering or parenting, and on the adjustment of the first-time parent in the child's first year of life.

RESEARCH TRENDS

Research on the experience of being a parent is on the rise. Only two studies were published during the 1960s, 18 during the 1970s, and 33 in the first three years of the 1980s. This acceleration in interest was partially due to the fact that journals such as the *Journal of Obstetric, Gynecologic, and Neonatal (JOGN) Nursing* and *MCN, The American Journal of Maternal Child Nursing* adopted publishing policies that reflect a growing research orientation; 22 of the papers considered for this review appeared in such specialty periodicals. Twenty-two others were published in journals devoted exclusively to research or theory issues. Of the remaining nine articles, five appeared in periodicals that focused on other areas (e.g., *Journal of Psychiatric Nursing, Journal of Gerontological Nursing*), and four were published outside the United States.

Methodological Considerations

The 53 research reports analyzed for this review reflected the tendencies of authors in this area to emphasize mothering rather than fathering or parenting, and to focus on the adjustment of the parent in the child's first year of life. Twenty-nine of the studies were focused only on the experience of the mother; 18 included both mothers and fathers in their samples; 6 were concerned only with fathers. Forty-one percent of the investigators who scrutinized the experience of the mother limited their research to the experience of primiparas. Fifty-nine percent of those studies—in which the age of the parents' children was clear—featured children who were in the first year of life.

There was a strong tendency for investigators to collect data using instruments they themselves had devised. In about 57% of the studies the investigators relied exclusively on interview protocols and questionnaires that were the researchers' inventions; in 23% of the studies the investigators used a combination of both their own instruments and those devised by others; and in 21%, investigators relied exclusively on instruments developed by others. Broussard's Neonatal Perception Inventories (Broussard & Hartner, 1970), which required the mother to rate the average baby and her own baby on six criteria, were used in six studies (Hall, 1980; Jones, 1981; Lotas & Willging, 1979; Mercer, 1980; Mercer, 1981a; White & Dawson, 1981). The Brazelton Neonatal Behavioral Scale (Brazelton, 1973) was featured in three studies (C. J. Anderson, 1981; Jones, 1981; Snyder, Eyres, & Barnard, 1979); it contained 20 neurological reflex items and 27 behavioral items, and was developed to measure the interactive behavior of infants from birth to one month of age.

Some instruments developed by nurse researchers were constructed carefully. As a result of her interest in maternal attitudes about sex education, Bloch (1979) published attitude scales on the content and timing of sex education for children (CT-Attitudes) and on sex education in school (S-Attitudes). Boyd (1981) developed a Likert-type attitude scale to examine the attitudes of fathers toward participation in infant caretaking activities. Hymovich (1981) constructed an instrument to assess the impact of a child's chronic illness on family developmental tasks and parenting coping strategies and to measure the outcome of intervention. Lederman, Weingarten, and Lederman (1981) developed a postpartum self-evaluation questionnaire with eight scales to measure maternal adaptation. These investigators demonstrated concern about validity and reliability issues in their reports, but 27 (51%) of the authors of the 53 studies under scrutiny were not at all attentive to such matters. These were serious omissions, since any concern about the validity or reliability of the instruments used, no matter how general, was regarded by this writer as evidence of having dealt with validity-reliability issues. The absence of concern about validity-reliability issues in more than half of all studies was a major problem, not only because so many of the researchers relied exclusively on their own investigator-designed interview protocols and questionnaires, but also because existing instruments cannot be assumed to be valid and reliable automatically. For example, Palisin (1981) reminded us that Broussard's Neonatal Perception Inventories—the most frequently used instruments in the studies included in this review—may not be as related to each other as previously thought because of the questionable assumption that a mother's ratings on Neonatal Perception Inventory I were based on fantasy.

Another problem uncovered by this survey was the general tendency of authors not to frame a study in theoretical terms. Archbold (1980) developed her research in terms of the Strauss framework of chronic illness, Curry (1982) used the theory of symbolic interaction, Delvaux (1978) based her research on Newcomb's theory of cognitive consistency, and C. J. Anderson (1981) and Holaday (1981) used the concepts of reciprocity and attachment respectively, but these were the exceptions. In 70% of the studies, investigators made absolutely no attempt to describe the theoretical underpinnings for their research. Literature on the topic under scrutiny regularly was placed in the introduction section of an article, but relatively few researchers described explicitly how the research questions flowed from a particular model of behavior. For example, an investigator described herself or himself as studying parental attitudes, but attitude seemed to be regarded as a general word for parents' perceptions, since the resultant study was not linked to the assumptions of a particular attitude theory. Because an investigator used Likert-type scaling, the impression was sometimes conveyed that Likert's theory of attitude (Edwards, 1957, pp. 149–171) might be shaping the study, but none of the preliminary work to solicit beliefs across a continuum of opinion was in evidence. Among those who based their research on theory were several who used ground theory in organizing their study of a particular phenomenon (Gottlieb, 1978; Stacey, 1978; Stern, 1982).

Since a survey of the literature on the topic in question is one estimate of the framework from which the researcher is operating, the studies were analyzed for the names of those investigators most cited in references. These researchers did not always make use of the existing nursing literature. Thirty-six percent of the studies scrutinized showed no obvious reference to the nursing literature (i.e., no journals or books that referred to nursing were in evidence). This indicated some predisposition to cite the findings in the social and biologic sciences, and to ignore what might already be written on the topic in question in the nursing literature, or as it pertained to nursing. However, the work of nurse Rubin (1967a, 1967b) on attainment of the maternal role was cited in 27% of the studies not including her own research. The work of Klaus and Kennell (1976) was the next most cited in these studies followed by that of Bowlby (1969), Broussard (Broussard & Hartner, 1970), and Brazelton (1973).

The overwhelming majority of the studies were descriptive in nature. In many of these, investigators were concerned with how the woman grows into and in the role of mother (e. g., Bampton, Jones, & Mancini, 1981; Brown, 1975; Gottlieb, 1978; Rubin, 1967a, 1967b). There were only three studies with an experimental design. Hall (1980) studied the effect of structured teaching concerning infant behavior received two to four days after discharge on mothers' perceptions of their newborns at one month. Thirty mothers of newborns were assigned by C. J. Anderson (1981) to one of three treatment groups in order to assess the effects of an early intervention designed to familiarize mothers with the capabilities and individual characteristics of their infants on maternal responsiveness at 10 to 12 days. Curry (1982) studied the effect of skin-to-skin contact between mother and infant during the first hour following delivery on later maternal attachment behavior and self-concept.

Two other researchers studied naturally occurring differences. Lotas and Willging (1979) investigated differences in perceptions of their babies between mothers in a rooming-in setting and those in a traditional setting. Jones (1981) explored the question of whether fathers, who held their infants in the first hour of life, demonstrated more nonverbal behavior toward their infants during an observation at one month than those who did not have this early contact.

While the majority of the studies were concerned with the experience of parents with healthy children, 28% described the behavior and perceptions of parents with an ill, retarded, or dead child (J. M. Anderson, 1981; Appell, 1963; Beck, 1973; D'Antonio, 1976; Gudermuth, 1975; Holaday, 1981; Hymovich, 1981; Knafl, 1982; Knafl, Deatrick, & Kodadek, 1982; McKeever, 1981; Mercer, 1974a, 1974b; Nikolaisen & Williams, 1980; Passo, 1978; Williams & Nikolaisen, 1982). Archbold (1980) and Stacey (1978) were unique in analyzing parent-child relations when the parent was debilitated and the child was the caregiver. Bloch (1979) and Passo (1978) focused on one particular aspect of the parenting role—sex education. Feldman (1978), Knafl et al. (1982), and Woods (1980) studied the effect of work on parents' behavior.

Key Themes

What do we know as a result of this review? It is foolhardy to make any sweeping statements both because of the size of some of the samples—50% of the samples were 40 parents or less—and because different aspects of experience were investigated in the separate studies. Nevertheless, there were some themes that could be gleaned from considering all the studies as a whole.

Parents' expectations. Until recently nurses looked only for negative characteristics in newborns (Erickson, 1978), because they and the lay public alike saw all infants as totally dominated by reflexes, unaware of their surroundings, and unable to see, hear, or experience emotions. Now they are assessing actively the newborns' capabilities because the focus shifted to the various mechanisms infants developed to adapt optimally to their needs, and there is evidence that this positive appraisal, when it involves mothers, can have a positive effect on mother-child relations. C. J. Anderson (1981) found that maternal responsiveness was enhanced significantly at 10 to 12 days when mothers observed the administration of the Brazelton Neonatal Behavioral Assessment Scale (Brazelton, 1973) and were told their infants' responses. Hall (1980) informed mothers about normal infant behavior one to two days postdischarge, and found that this teaching improved their perceptions of their infants at one month postpartum. Although the instruments used in these two studies were different, the results were similar; understanding the capabilities of their infants had a positive effect on mothers' perceptions of their infants.

In a related study, Snyder et al. (1979) noted that what a mother expected of her baby was what she got. Humenick and Bugen (1981) also found that women's prenatal expectations for later infant interaction accounted significantly for the variance in their postpartum parent-infant interaction, but this tendency was less strong for fathers. Ventura (1982) discovered that parents who perceived their infant as having a more smiling, laughing temperament and as crying less, used coping behaviors designed to maintain family integrity. Rojas (1980) found that white mothers had higher expectations in personal-social and fine motor-adaptive development than did Puerto Rican mothers, and this may have had consequences for language development. Jarrett (1982) found that some mothers had a tendency to expect too much of their children too soon, then physically punished them for noncompliance long before they were biologically ready for such tasks (e.g., 86% expected bladder control by 18 months when the norm for mastery is 18 to 24 months). Mothers with the least accurate expectations of their children were those with the least amount of education, income, and psychosocial assets (Jarrett, 1982; Snyder et al., 1979). The mothers that Brailey (1978) studied were most concerned about their children being contrary or stubborn. One wonders if this finding, too, was not indirectly connected with their having some inaccurate expectations.

Parents' concerns. Another major theme in the research reviewed was that parents had concerns and needs too. Where once nurses served primarily as ombudsmen to children, they now recognized in the research questions they asked that parents were worried about their role performance. Hott (1980) found that women who experienced the crisis of an operative or anesthetized delivery had definite changes in their concept of ideal woman three to four weeks postpartum. Leonard (1981) described the stress involved in being a mother of twins; the mothers indicated they did not take time to look after themselves. Lovell and Fiorino (1979) reported that all the mothers in their study expressed concern or confusion about their parenting skills. They saw themselves as the least important member of the family, and indicated that their physical health was less than optimal, but 18 of 20 mothers reported having no established fitness regimen for themselves. Hanson (1981) found that single custodial fathers made an effort to provide more nurturing and caring for their children than they experienced from their fathers as children.

Bull (1981) found moderate to much concern in areas related to self (e.g., fatigue, being a good mother) and to the baby (e.g., feeding, signs of illness). Walker (1981) identified the needs pertaining to information, feelings, judgment, or development of adoptive parents. Mercer (1981a) noted that some anxiety and complaints about the unexpected demands of the maternal role (extensiveness of time and energy required) were a feature of all mothers' responses. Norbeck and Sheiner (1982) found that, for single mothers, the absence of a close friend and the lack of available people to call on for practical help were related to problems in parenting. Robson (1982) reported that artificially rupturing a woman's membranes was associated highly with a lack of maternal affection, and that there was an association between initial detachment and more negative scores on an attitude-toward-baby scale throughout the whole of the first postpartum year. Sumner and Fritsch (1977) found that parents of first or male infants had a much higher rate of questions. Sweeny and Davis (1979) noted that one of the major issues that seemed to bedevil all the parents they studied was: "Am I acting normally?" This central question may have been behind the concerns of most of the parents in all of the research surveyed.

Parenting sick children. Yet another theme that emerged in the research reviewed was that parents with sick children strove to see themselves and their families as coping well. J. M. Anderson (1981) described how parents with a chronically ill child regularly emphasized the normality of the child. Appell (1963) found the generally reported finding that parents of retarded children were disturbed, anxious, and unhappy individuals was not corroborated in his study. The thread that ran through his findings was the parents' persistent hope that their children would achieve normalcy. In Beck's study (1973), 84% of 38 participating parents wanted to be involved in the care of their hospitalized children. However, when both parents were employed outside the home, mothers were much more likely to miss work for the child's hospitalization than were fathers (Knafl et al., 1982). In 78% of the 59 families studied by Knafl (1982), parents reported virtually no negative behavioral or emotional changes in their other children during a sibling's hospitalization.

But there also were parents who admitted they had many problems because they were saddled with a chronically ill child. The mothers studied by D'Antonio (1976) did not view their children who were sick with cardiac problems in a positive way. They were constantly watchful and exhausted, fearing that the child would die suddenly; the needs of other family members seemed to be secondary to the wants or needs of the afflicted child. McKeever (1981) also found that the most troublesome concern could be the unpredictable nature of the chronically ill child's disease. Gudermuth (1975) and Mercer (1974a) both noticed that mothers who had children with defects experienced some difficulty in establishing mutuality with their infants. Holaday (1981) pointed out that infants with chronic illnesses cried more frequently than well infants. No matter how quickly or how often the mother responded, she could not reduce the number of cries, only the duration of the cry. This was very frustrating for the mothers.

Attainment of the maternal role. It was not particularly surprising that the nurse who accounted for the most studies reviewed in this chapter (Mercer, 1974a, 1974b, 1980, 1981a, 1981b) would also be the one who developed the most complete theoretical framework for studying one aspect of parental experience, namely, the factors that influence the attainment of the maternal role in the first year of motherhood. Mercer (1981a, 1981b) used concepts from role theory, a favorite theory of those concerned with mothering and fathering practices (Robischon & Scott, 1969), and current knowledge of the infant's development, in order to construct a complex framework. The variables with which she was concerned were: age, perceptions of the birth experience, early maternal-infant separation, social stress, support systems, self-concept and personality traits, maternal illness, childrearing attitudes, infant temperament, infant illness, culture, social class, and socioeconomic/educational level. Her objective was to determine over time the relative significance of the major variables in predicting primipara's maternal role attainment. Maternal role attainment has been a fundamental concern of nursing since the pioneering work of Mercer's mentor, Rubin (1967a, 1967b), almost two decades ago. It is now becoming the research-based, theoretically sound construct that nurse researchers have been searching for in their analysis of the experience of new mothers.

Strengths and Weaknesses

This review chapter includes content that falls between other chapters in this volume on childbearing by Lederman and on families by Feetham. The experience of being a parent is a nursing concern that stretches over an expanse of time much longer than the childbearing period per se, but is not as all-inclusive as the area of family. It is part of a lifespan developmental orientation that regards parenthood as a key role in adult development (Alpert & Richardson, 1980). Both because parenthood itself often was described as a developmental crisis (Hobbs & Cole, 1976; LaRossa & LaRossa, 1981; LeMasters, 1957; Rossi, 1968) and because of the vast literature on attachment and bonding, attention was on the functioning of the parent (usually mother) during the first child's first year of life. The nursing research in this area definitely contributed to the interdisciplinary literature both by extending this line of inquiry into health settings and by drawing attention to the situation of the parent with a sick or dying child. Moreover, nurse researchers are beginning to have something to say about the effect of mothering on a woman's own health (Uphold & Susman, 1981; Woods, 1980), and what was bound, because of demographic trends, to be a growing interest in the relationship between elderly parents and middle-aged children (Archbold, 1980; Stacey, 1978). But the nurse researchers were remiss in not showing much concern with some entire areas, for example, parenting the school-age child and adolescent, or motherhood and fatherhood as complementary, conflicting, or same roles.

The traditional approach to the study of parenting in nursing and other disciplines was focused on the effects of parenting on the child. In the last decade, however, there has been mounting interest in the effects of parenting on the parents (Lerner & Spanier, 1978; McBride, 1973, 1975, 1976). Gutmann (1975) even argued that parenthood is the key to the comparative study of the life cycle. Erikson (1950, 1959) was probably the most mentioned theorist when adult development was discussed. His seventh stage of development, generativity versus stagnation, was centered around the individual developing a sense of continuity with future generations (Troll, 1975), and as such was associated with the experience of parenthood. Though his writings regularly were cited when an author was discussing parenthood as a role in adult development, his work did not shape research the way the writings of Klaus and Kennell (1976), Bowlby (1969), Broussard (Broussard & Hartner, 1970), and Brazelton (1973) influenced study of the effects of parenting on the child. Since nonnurses are writing more and more about the various stages of parenting (Aldous, 1978; Galinsky, 1981; Rapoport, Rapoport, & Strelitz, 1977), nurse researchers should follow suit and become more concerned with the parenting experience over time.

RECOMMENDATIONS FOR FUTURE RESEARCH

Recommendations for future research flow in large measure from the critique of existing research. Investigators claiming to study parenting should not limit the sample to mothers. Study of mothers should not be limited to descriptions of the experience of primiparas. Parent-child relations beyond the child's first year of life is a vast area sorely in need of investigation. Both the effects of the parent on the child and the effects of the child on the parent should be studied in order to understand fully the experience of being a parent.

Nurse researchers need to build both on the findings of existing nursing research, demonstrated both by citing relevant nursing literature in their references and by replicating existing studies, as well as on their own work by doing follow-up research in the same area. If nursing theory is to be developed, it requires a sustained concern with defining and operationalizing key concepts and testing relationships around a particular phenomenon of concern. It is difficult to recognize common themes when analyzing an assortment of studies all conducted by different individuals using a variety of concepts and newly created, unrefined instruments. However, research over time with a specific focus conducted by one investigator can lead to the evolution of the sort of complete, complex, theoretical framework that is the ultimate objective of nursing science, and of which Mercer's work (1974a, 1974b, 1980, 1981a, 1981b) seems to be the best example to date.

Barnard (1981) closed the nursing research roundtable (on Perinatal Parental Behavior: Nursing Research and Implications for Newborn Health funded by the March of Dimes Birth Defects Foundation) with the suggestion that two concepts, anxiety and supportive relationships, emerged as important variables in those studies related to the problems of childrearing. Her perception was relevant to the research reviewed in this chapter, and underscored the need to devote future efforts to refining these concepts and operationalizing them in valid and reliable instruments. Another concept that was bandied about in the research reviewed for this chapter was attitude. Generally, it was defined in an imprecise way without any attention to the belief elicitation procedures across a spectrum of opinions that are the hallmarks of the various attitude theories (Edwards, 1957; Fishbein & Ajzen, 1975). This concept should be used in a more precise way if subsequent research on parents' attitudes is to be replicable.

Some researchers (J. M. Anderson, 1981; Gottlieb, 1978; Stern, 1982) featured in this review either described their studies as efforts to understand the experience of a set of parents using grounded theory or an ethnographic approach, or relied on the case-study method of nursing process recordings (Mercer, 1974a). These approaches were in keeping with Oiler's (1982) notion that the phenomenological approach, with its appreciation of lived experience, conforms to nursing's fundamental values. Qualitative methods are as important as quantitative methods. However, there are criteria for assessing the trustworthiness of naturalistic inquiries (Guba, 1981) just as there are criteria for assessing the trustworthiness of inquiries based on the rationalistic paradigm (e.g., persistent observation, peer debriefing, triangulation, collection of referential adequacy materials, establishing an audit trail, and practicing reflexivity).

Given that nurse researchers interested in the experience of being a parent are attracted to the use of qualitative methods, they need to familiarize themselves with how to use and describe their methods with a precision comparable to that which is the norm for quantitative methods, so that their important conclusions can be taken seriously.

Both to be applauded in the present and to be recommended for the future is the practice of following some research articles on parent-child relationships (Jarrett, 1982; Walker, 1981) with a commentary on those research findings by a practitioner (Turner-Woodson, 1982; Van Steenkiste, 1981). The vital relationship between research and practice becomes more obvious by such a juxtaposition. Efforts to describe research, then have one person critique the enterprise, with later opportunity for general discussion and rebuttal (Lederman, Raff, & Carroll, 1981) conveyed the notion that researchers can question and disagree, thereby lifting work in an entire area to a higher plane.

Nurses need to take more advantage of naturally occurring events (e.g., the Sumner and Fritsch 1977 recording of parents' telephone questions as an estimate of their concerns) in formulating their research questions and designing their studies. If nurse researchers had more of a longitudinal perspective, they might keep track of whether the same relaxation techniques developed by women to handle their labor and delivery can be of use to them as they have to deal with the inevitable sleep deprivation and tensions that accompany new motherhood. Generally, considerations of the experience of being a parent did not include behavioral estimates of a biologic nature (e.g., weight fluctuations, sleep patterns, headaches, backaches) as much as they included estimates of psychosocial functioning (e.g., fears, concerns). But the inclusion of such new variables would result in studies that could highlight just how much nurses can contribute to an understanding of parenthood by virtue of their concern with the total person.

The 53 research reports analyzed focused on mothering rather than fathering or parenting, and on the adjustment of primiparas in the child's first year of life. Three themes were noted in the research reviewed: (a) maternal expectations influence subsequent mother-child interactions; (b) parents have concerns and needs too; and (c) parents with chronically ill children strive for some semblance of normality, but may experience some difficulty in establishing a positive relationship with the child. It is recommended that future research focus on parent-child relations beyond the child's first year of life, and that nurse researchers pay greater attention to describing the methods of their naturalistic inquiries.

REFERENCE NOTE

1. American Nurses' Association. *Nursing: A social policy statement.* Kansas City, Mo.: Author, 1980.

REFERENCES

Aldous, J. *Family careers: Developmental change in families.* New York: Wiley, 1978.

Alpert, J. L., & Richardson, M. S. Parenting. In L. W. Poon (Ed.), *Aging in the 1980s: Psychological issues.* Washington, D. C.: American Psychological Association, 1980.

Anderson, C. J. Enhancing reciprocity between mother and neonate. *Nursing Research,* 1981, *30,* 89–93.

Anderson J. M. The social construction of illness experience: Families with a chronically-ill child. *Journal of Advanced Nursing,* 1981, *6,* 427–434.

Appell, M. J. Some attitudes of parents of mentally retarded children. *Journal of Psychiatric Nursing,* 1963, *1,* 487–494.

Archbold, P. G. Impact of parent caring on middle-aged offspring. *Journal of Gerontological Nursing,* 1980, *6,* 78–85

Bampton, B., Jones, J., & Mancini, J. Initial mothering patterns of low-income black primiparas. *Journal of Obstetric, Gynecologic, and Neonatal (JOGN) Nursing,* 1981, *10,* 174–178.

Barnard, K. Closing. In R. P. Lederman, B. S. Raff, & P. Carroll (Eds.), *Perinatal parental behavior: Nursing research and implications for newborn health.* New York: Alan R. Liss, 1981.

Beck, M. Attitudes of parents of pediatric heart patients toward patient care units. *Nursing Research,* 1973, *22,* 334–338.

Bishop, B. A guide to assessing parenting capabilities. *American Journal of Nursing,* 1976, *76,* 1784–1787.

Bloch, D. Attitudes of mothers toward sex education. *American Journal of Public Health,* 1979, *69,* 911–915.

Bowlby, J. *Attachment* (Vol. 1). Attachment and loss series. New York: Basic Books, 1969.

Boyd, S. T. Measurement of paternal attitude toward infant care-taking. *Child Health Care,* 1981, *10,* 66–67.

Brailey, L. J. Mothers have needs too. *The Canadian Nurse,* 1978, *74*(8), 28–31.

Brazelton, T. B. *A neonatal behavioral assessment scale.* Philadelphia: Lippincott, 1973.

Broussard, E. R., & Hartner, M. S. Maternal perception of the neonate as related to development. *Child Psychology and Human Development,* 1970, *1,* 16–25.

Brown, P. W. The use of a descriptive theory in planning nursing intervention. *Maternal-Child Nursing Journal,* 1975, *4,* 171–182.

Bull, M. J. Change in concerns of first-time mothers after one week at home.

Journal of Obstetric, Gynecologic, and Neonatal (JOGN) Nursing, 1981, *10,* 391–394.

Butani, P. Reactions of mothers to the birth of an anomalous infant: A review of the literature. *Maternal-Child Nursing Journal,* 1974, *3,* 59–76.

Cronenwett, L. R. Today's family lifestyles: Tomorrow's parents. *The Michigan Nurse,* 1980, *53*(9), 22–24.

Cronenwett, L. R. Father participation in child care: A critical review. *Research in Nursing and Health,* 1982, *5,* 63–72.

Cronenwett, L. R., & Kunst-Wilson, W. Stress, social support, and the transition to fatherhood. *Nursing Research,* 1981, *30,* 196–201.

Curry, M. A. Maternal attachment behavior and the mother's self-concept: The effect of early skin-to-skin contact. *Nursing Research,* 1982, *31,* 73–78.

D'Antonio, I. J. Mothers' responses to the functioning and behavior of cardiac children in child-rearing situations. *Maternal-Child Nursing Journal,* 1976, *5,* 207–259.

Delvaux, B. L. Husband-wife attitudes toward childrearing. *American Journal of Nursing,* 1978, *78,* 1907. (Abstract)

Donner, G. J. Parenthood as a crisis: A role for the psychiatric nurse. *Perspectives in Psychiatric Care,* 1972, *10,* 84–87.

Edwards, A. L. *Techniques of attitude construction.* New York: Appleton-Century-Crofts, 1957.

Erickson, M. P. Trends in assessing the newborn and his parents. *MCN, The American Journal of Maternal Child Nursing,* 1978, *3,* 99–103.

Erikson, E. H. *Childhood and society.* New York: Norton, 1950.

Erikson, E. H. Identity and the life cycle: Selected papers. *Psychological Issues.* (Vol. 1) New York: International Universities Press, 1959.

Feldman, R. Working mothers: Employed nurses and their children's anxiety levels. *Occupational Health Nursing,* 1978, *26*(7), 16–19.

Fishbein, M., & Ajzen, I. *Belief, attitude, intention, and behavior: An introduction to theory and research.* Reading, Mass.: Addison-Wesley, 1975.

Freiberg, K. H. How parents react when their child is hospitalized. *American Journal of Nursing,* 1972, *72,* 1270–1271.

Galinsky, E. *Between generations: The six stages of parenthood.* New York: Times Books, 1981.

Gilmore, M. Parents of tomorrow. *International Journal of Nursing Studies,* 1966, *3,* 207–217.

Goldfogel, L. Working with the parent of a dying child. *American Journal of Nursing,* 1970, *70,* 1675–1679.

Gordeuk, A. Motherhood and a less than perfect child: A literary review. *Maternal-Child Nursing Journal,* 1976, *5,* 57–68.

Gottlieb, L. Maternal attachment to primiparas. *Journal of Obstetric, Gynecologic, and Neonatal (JOGN) Nursing,* 1978, *7,* 39–44.

Guba, E. G. Criteria for assessing the trustworthiness of naturalistic inquiries. *Educational Communication and Technology: A Journal of Theory, Research and Development,* 1981, *29,* 75–91.

Gudermuth, S. Mothers' reports of early experience of infants with congenital heart disease. *Maternal-Child Nursing Journal,* 1975, *4,* 155–164.

Gutmann, D. Parenthood: A key to the comparative study of the life cycle. In N.

Datan & L. H. Ginsberg (Eds.), *Life-span and developmental psychology.* New York: Academic Press, 1975.

Hall, L. A. Effect of teaching on primiparas' perceptions of their newborn. *Nursing Research*, 1980, *29*, 317–322.

Hanson, S. Single custodial fathers and the parent-child relationship. *Nursing Research*, 1981, *30*, 202–204.

Hines, J. D. Father: The forgotten man. *Nursing Forum*, 1971, *10*, 176–200.

Hobbs, D. F., & Cole, S. B. Transition to parenthood: A decade replication. *Journal of Marriage and the Family*, 1976, *38*, 723–731.

Holaday, B. Maternal response to their chronically ill infants' attachment behavior of crying. *Nursing Research*, 1981, *30*, 343–348.

Horan, M. L. Parental reaction to the birth of an infant with a defect: An attributional approach. *Advances in Nursing Science*, 1982, *4*(1), 57–68.

Hott, J. R. Best laid plans: Pre- and postpartum comparison of self and spouse in primiparous Lamaze couples who share delivery and those who do not. *Nursing Research*, 1980, *29*, 20–27.

Hrobsky, D. M. Transition to parenthood: A balancing of needs. *Nursing Clinics of North America*, 1977, *12*, 457–468.

Humenick, S. S., & Bugen, L. A. Correlates of parent-infant interaction: An exploratory study. *Birth Defects: Original Article Series*, 1981, *17*(6), 181–199.

Hymovich, D. P. Assessing the impact of chronic childhood illness on family and parent coping. *Image*, 1981, *13*, 71–74.

Jarrett, G. E. Childrearing patterns of young mothers: Expectations, knowledge, and practices. *MCN, The American Journal of Maternal Child Nursing*, 1982, *7*, 119–124.

Jones, C. Father to infant attachment: Effects of early contact and characteristics of the infant. *Research in Nursing and Health*, 1981, *4*, 193–200.

Kiernan, B., & Scoloveno, M. A. Fathering. *Nursing Clinics of North America*, 1977, *12*, 481–490.

Klaus, M. H., & Kennell, J. H. *Maternal-infant bonding.* St. Louis: Mosby, 1976.

Knafl, K. A. Parents' views of the response of siblings to a pediatric hospitalization. *Research in Nursing and Health*, 1982, *5*, 13–20.

Knafl, K. A., Deatrick, J. A., & Kodadek, S. How parents manage jobs and a child's hospitalization. *MCN, The American Journal of Maternal Child Nursing*, 1982, *7*, 125–127.

Kunst-Wilson, W., & Cronenwett, L. Nursing care for the emerging family: Promoting paternal behavior. *Research in Nursing and Health*, 1981, *4*, 201–211.

LaRossa, R., & LaRossa, M. M. *Transition to parenthood: How infants change families.* Beverly Hills, Calif.: Sage, 1981.

Lederman, R. P., Raff, B. S., & Carroll, P. (Eds.). *Perinatal parental behavior: Nursing research and implications for newborn health.* New York: Alan R. Liss, 1981.

Lederman, R. P., Weingarten, C. G. T., & Lederman, E. Postpartum self-evaluation questionnaire: Measures of maternal adaptation. *Birth Defects: Original Article Series*, 1981, *17*(6), 201–231.

LeMasters, E. E. Parenthood in crisis. *Marriage and Family Living*, 1957, *19*, 352–355.

Leonard, L. G. Postpartum depression and mothers of infant twins. *Maternal-Child Nursing Journal*, 1981, *10*, 99–109.

Lerner, R. M., & Spanier, G. B. (Eds.). *Child influences on marital and family interactions: A life-span perspective*. New York: Academic Press, 1978.

Lockhart, B. When couples adopt, they too need parenting classes. *MCN, The American Journal of Maternal Child Nursing*, 1982, *7*, 116–118.

Lotas, M. B., & Willging, J. M. Mothers, babies, perception. *Image*, 1979, *11*, 45–51.

Lovell, M. C., & Fiorino, D. L. Combating myth. A conceptual framework for analyzing the stress of motherhood. *Advances in Nursing Science*, 1979, *1*(4), 75–84.

Lowenberg, J. S. The coping behaviors of fatally ill adolescents and their parents. *Nursing Forum*, 1970, *9*, 269–287.

Mann, S. A. Coping with a child's fatal illness: A parent's dilemma. *Nursing Clinics of North America*, 1974, *9*, 81–87.

McAbee, R. Rural parenting classes: Beginning to meet the need. *MCN, The American Journal of Maternal Child Nursing*, 1977, *2*, 315–319.

McBride, A. B. *The growth and development of mothers*. New York: Harper & Row, 1973.

McBride, A. B. Can family life survive? *American Journal of Nursing*, 1975, *75*, 1648–1653.

McBride, A. B. *A married feminist*. New York: Harper & Row, 1976.

McKeever, P. T. Fathering the chronically ill child. *MCN, The American Journal of Maternal Child Nursing*, 1981, *6*, 124–128.

Mercer, R. T. Mothers' responses to their infants with defects. *Nursing Research*, 1974, *23*, 133–137. (a)

Mercer, R. T. Two fathers' early responses to the birth of a daughter with a defect. *Maternal-Child Nursing Journal*, 1974, *3*, 77–86. (b)

Mercer, R. T. Teenage motherhood: The first year. *Journal of Obstetric, Gynecologic, and Neonatal (JOGN) Nursing*, 1980, *9*, 16–27.

Mercer, R. T. Factors impacting on the maternal role the first year of motherhood. *Birth Defects: Original Article Series*, 1981, *17*(6), 233–252. (a)

Mercer, R. T. A theoretical framework for studying the factors that impact on the maternal role. *Nursing Research*, 1981, *30*, 73–77. (b)

Nikolaisen, S. M., & Williams, R. A. Parents' view of support following loss of their infant to sudden infant death syndrome. *Western Journal of Nursing Research*, 1980, *2*, 593–601.

Norbeck, J. S., & Sheiner, M. Sources of social support related to single-parent functioning. *Research in Nursing and Health*, 1982, *5*, 3–12.

Oiler, C. The phenomenological approach in nursing research. *Nursing Research*, 1982, *31*, 178–181.

Palisin, H. The neonatal perception inventory: A review. *Nursing Research*, 1981, *30*, 285–289.

Passo, S. Parents' perceptions, attitudes, and needs regarding sex education for the child with myelomeningocele. *Research in Nursing and Health*, 1978, *1*, 53–59.

Perdue, B. J., Horowitz, J. A., & Herz, F. Mothering. *Nursing Clinics of North America*, 1977, *12*, 491–502.

Rajokovich, M. Meeting the needs of parents with a mentally retarded child. *Journal of Psychiatric Nursing and Mental Health Services*, 1969, *7*, 207–211.

Rapoport, R., Rapoport, R. N., & Strelitz, Z. *Fathers, mothers, and society*. New York: Basic Books, 1977.

Robischon, P., & Scott, D. Role theory and its application to family nursing. *Nursing Outlook*, 1969, *17*(7), 52–57.

Robson, K. M. Mother-baby relationship: "I feel nothing . . ." *Nursing Mirror*, 1982, *154*(25), 24–27.

Rojas, D. Effect of maternal expectations and child-rearing practices on the development of white and Puerto Rican children. *Maternal-Child Nursing Journal*, 1980, *9*, 99–107.

Rossi, A. S. Transition to parenthood. *Journal of Marriage and the Family*, 1968, *30*, 26–34.

Rubin, R. Attainment of the maternal role: Part I. Processes. *Nursing Research*, 1967, *16*, 237–245. (a)

Rubin, R. Attainment of the maternal role: Part II. Models and referrants. *Nursing Research*, 1967, *16*, 342–346. (b)

Shaw, N. R. Teaching young mothers their role. *Nursing Outlook*, 1974, *22*, 695–698.

Snyder, C., Eyres, S. J., & Barnard, K. New findings about mothers' expectations and their relationship to infant development. *MCN, The American Journal of Maternal Child Nursing*, 1979, *4*, 354–357.

Stacey, S. Parents and children growing old. *Australian Nurses Journal*, 1978, *7*(8), 36–39; 42.

Stern, P. N. Affiliating in stepfather families: Teachable strategies leading to stepfather-child friendship. *Western Journal of Nursing Research*, 1982, *4*, 75–89.

Streff, M. B. Examining family growth and development: A theoretical model. *Advances in Nursing Science*, 1981, *3*(4), 61–69.

Sumner, G., & Fritsch, J. Postnatal parental concerns: The first six weeks of life. *Journal of Obstetric, Gynecologic, and Neonatal (JOGN) Nursing*, 1977, *6*, 27–32.

Sweeny, S. L., & Davis, F. B. Transition to parenthood: A group experience. *Maternal-Child Nursing Journal*, 1979, *8*, 59–64.

Swendsen, L. A., Meleis, A. J., & Jones, D. Role supplementation for new parents: A role mastery plan. *MCN, The American Journal of Maternal Child Nursing*, 1978, *3*, 84–91.

Troll, L. E. *Early and middle adulthood: The best is yet to be—maybe*. Monterey Calif.: Brooks/Cole, 1975.

Turner-Woodson, E. Improving parenting practices among adolescents. *MCN, The American Journal of Maternal Child Nursing*, 1982, *7*, 122.

Uphold, C. R., & Susman, E. J. Self-reported climacteric symptoms as a function of the relationships between marital adjustment and childrearing stage. *Nursing Research*, 1981, *30*, 84–88.

Van Steenkiste, S. Adoptive parents need special reassurance. *MCN, The American Journal of Maternal Child Nursing*, 1981, *6*, 122.

Ventura, J. N. Parent coping behaviors, parent functioning, and infant temperament characteristics. *Nursing Research*, 1982, *31*, 269–273.

Walker, L. O. Identifying parents in need: An approach to adoptive parenting. *MCN, The American Journal of Maternal Child Nursing*, 1981, *6*, 118–123.

White, M., & Dawson, C. The impact of the at-risk infant on family solidarity. *Birth Defects: Original Article Series*, 1981, *17*(6), 253–284.

Williams, R. A., & Nikolaisen, S. M. Sudden infant death syndrome: Parents' perceptions and response to the loss of their infant. *Research in Nursing and Health*, 1982, *5*, 55–61.

Woods, N. F. Women's roles and illness episodes: A prospective study. *Research in Nursing and Health*, 1980, *3*, 137–145.

Yanni, M. I. Y. Perception of parents' behavior and children's general fearfulness. *Nursing Research*, 1982, *3*, 79–82.

Zamerowski, S. T. Helping families to cope with handicapped children. *Topics in Clinical Nursing*, 1982, *4*(2), 41–56.

CHAPTER 4

Health Promotion and Illness Prevention

NOLA J. PENDER
SCHOOL OF NURSING
NORTHERN ILLINOIS UNIVERSITY

CONTENTS

During the past decade, health promotion and illness prevention received increased attention in the nursing research literature. While as early as 1859, Florence Nightingale viewed the laws of nursing as synonymous with the laws of health (Reed & Zurakowski, 1983), the primary focus of research in nursing has been on care of persons in illness. Recently, a growing number of nurse investigators focused their research efforts on exploring health processes. This investigative trend in nursing parallels increased public concern about decreasing the cost of medical care and increasing the quality of life through health promotion and illness prevention efforts. Since nurses are the largest group of professionals who provide health services to the public, nurse researchers have major responsibility for generating fundamental knowledge about health and for developing and testing strategies to enhance the health status of individuals, families, and communities.

For this critical review, *health promotion* was defined as activities directed toward developing resources of clients that maintain or enhance well-being and self-actualization. *Illness prevention* was defined as activities aimed at protecting clients from specific or actual health threats and their harmful consequences (Pender, 1982, p. 2). Both health-promoting and health-protecting (preventive) actions were identified as *health behaviors*. This research review covered the period from January 1970 to November 1982. Since many studies fell within the broad purview of health-related investigations, only nursing research with the following emphases was included in this review: measurement of health or health-related concepts; exploration of variables related to promotion of health or prevention of illness; determination of factors affecting the occurrence of health behaviors; and evaluation of nursing interventions for health promotion, primary prevention, and secondary prevention among children and adults.

THEORETICAL FRAMEWORKS

Health has been a dominant theme in theoretical frameworks developed by nurses (Fitzpatrick, 1983; King, 1981; Neuman, 1982; Newman, 1979; Orem, 1971; Parse, 1981). However, few nurse researchers tested the validity of these frameworks for describing health, identifying determinants of health behaviors, or prescribing nursing interventions for health promotion and illness prevention. Only the Orem Self-Care Model was used as a theoretical framework for two of the studies in this review (Denyes, 1980; Kearney & Fleischer, 1979). Further research is needed to determine the utility of the other theoretical frameworks in understanding health and health behaviors.

The Health Belief Model (Becker, 1974; Rosenstock, 1966), developed in the field of public health, was the framework for several studies of preventive behavior described (Brown, Muhlenkamp, Fox, & Osborn,

1983; Hallal, 1982; Sennott, 1980; Stillman, 1977). Since the preventive (avoidance) orientation of the Health Belief Model (Mikhail, 1981; Rosenstock, 1974) limited its potential as a paradigm for explaining health-promoting behaviors without a specific disease referent, Pender (1982) proposed the Health Promotion Model as an explanation of the determinants of health-promoting actions. Cox (1982) described an Interaction Model of Client Health Behavior to explain relationships between client characteristics, the client-provider relationship, and subsequent client health behavior. Studies to test the latter two models are in progress but have not been published to date.

The Theory of Reasoned Action (Ajzen & Fishbein, 1980; Fishbein & Ajzen, 1975) was the framework for two of the studies reviewed (Miller, Wikoff, McMahon, Garrett, & Johnson, 1982; Pender & Pender, Note 1). This value-expectancy model was developed in social psychology to explain attitude-belief-behavior relations. Further testing of all of the above frameworks is essential to determine their potential for explaining the occurrence of health behaviors or prescribing nursing actions that promote health and prevent illness. In addition, new theories that describe fundamental dimensions of human health processes should be developed.

MEASURING HEALTH AND HEALTH-RELEVANT CONCEPTS

Health is a complex concept with physiologic, psychologic, social, spiritual, and environmental dimensions. Little progress was made in operationalizing health so that it could be measured. Nurses focused primarily on developing conceptual definitions of health (Keller, 1981; Smith, 1981), with few attempts to identify empirical referents. While Oelbaum (1974) identified 26 functions of adults in optimum health, this taxonomy of behaviors was not refined further to yield a health index useful in research. In most nursing studies of healthy adults, investigators measured subjective states such as perceived health status (Christiansen, 1981; Pender & Pender, Note 1). Objective criteria for assessing the health status of individuals, families, and communities should be developed before the concept of health can be used meaningfully as a dependent or independent variable in nursing investigations.

Health-related variables that were defined operationally and measured in the nursing studies reviewed include: health attitudes, health locus of control, health values, self-care agency, and health risk. These factors were studied as potential predictors of health behaviors.

Health Attitudes

Few scales were developed to measure attitudes toward health. Those scales reported in nonnursing literature were relatively old (Byrd, Note 2) or specific to college-age populations (Olsen, 1972; Richardson, 1959). Only one instrument, the Miller Health Attitude Scale (Miller et al., 1982), was found in the nursing literature. This scale was developed to assess attitudes of postmyocardial infarction patients toward performance of prescribed behaviors of their medical regimen. Alpha reliabilities ranging from .59 to .70 indicated a high degree of internal consistency among subscale items. Predictive validities of the subscales for adherence behavior were .31 for diet, .46 for activity, .12 for medication, .62 for smoking, and .15 for stress response. The instrument was restricted to measuring attitudes toward adherence behaviors rather than health per se and only in the designated population. General measures of attitudes toward health are needed if the impact of attitudes on health practices is to be studied systematically.

Health Locus of Control

The Multidimensional Health Locus of Control (MHLC) Scale (Wallston, Wallston, & DeVellis, 1978) was used to measure perceptions of control over personal health status. The MHLC consists of three subscales: internality, externality—chance, and externality—powerful others. Two forms of the instrument are available. Reliability of the instrument when only one form was used ranged from .67 to .77, while reliability ranged from .83 to .86 when both forms were administered. Since findings concerning the impact of locus of control on various health practices were inconsistent (Arakelian, 1980), it is possible that the development of more specific scales focused on control of particular dimensions of health (e.g., weight, physical fitness, and stress level) might have better predictive validity (Saltzer, 1978).

Lowery (1981) questioned the assumption of social learning theory that generalized expectancies, such as locus of control, played a significant role in determining health practices. She suggested attribution theory (Har-

vey, Ickes, & Kidd, 1978) as more productive in understanding the determinants of health behavior than the narrower concept, locus of control.
Variables such as ambiguity of the confronting situation, value of reinforcement, alternate behaviors available, and stability of cause (e.g., ability
versus effort, task difficulty versus luck), as well as locus of control may
be important in determining personal health practices. Nurse researchers interested in the relationship between personal control and health
behavior should evaluate attribution theory as a basis for their research
efforts.

Health Values

Wallston, Maides, and Wallston (1976) developed the Health Value Scale
by adapting Rokeach's Terminal Value Survey (1973). The Health Value
Scale was intended to measure the value placed on health in relation to
nine other values (e.g., freedom, happiness, and self-respect). While the
instrument was used in several of the studies reviewed to determine the
importance of health to individuals, the construct validity, reliability,
and susceptibility of the measure to social influence must be investigated further.

Self-Care Agency

Levin, Katz, and Holst (1976) estimated that self-care constitutes at least
75% of personal health care. Self-care was defined as activities that individuals initiated and performed on their own behalf in maintaining life,
health, and well-being. Self-care can be both an ongoing activity and a
personal competence (Orem, 1971, p. 13). Kearney and Fleischer (1979)
developed an instrument to measure self-care agency, after recognizing that
no valid and reliable instrument existed to measure this concept. Items were
generated to reflect five indicants of self-care agency: an attitude of responsibility for self, motivation to care for self, application of knowledge to
self-care, the valuing of health priorities, and high self-esteem. These items
were rated for content validity by a panel of experts. The instrument was
tested for construct validity by correlating self-care agency with scores on
Rotter's (1966) Internal-External Locus of Control Scale and subscores
(e.g., self-confidence, achievement, intraception, abasement, lability) on
the Adjective Check List (Gough & Heilbrun, 1965). No significant correlations were found between self-care agency and internal-external con-

trol. Relationships between self-care agency and the Adjective Check List subscores were significant and in the predicted directions. Test-retest reliability was .77, with split-half reliability ranging from .77 to .81 for the self-care measure. Further evaluation of the tool with nonstudent populations is critical to establish validity.

An instrument to measure self-care agency in adolescents was developed by Denyes (1980). Six dimensions of self-care agency were identified through factor analysis of responses from 161 adolescents to questionnaire items developed by the investigator. The six factors identified were: ego strength and health decision-making capability, valuing of health, health knowledge, physical energy levels, feelings, and attention to health. The final instrument was a Likert-type scale questionnaire containing 35 items related to the six components of self-care agency. Internal consistency of the tool was demonstrated. Further testing of the instrument for concurrent and construct validity is essential prior to its use in nursing research as a measure of self-care agency.

Health Risk

Twenty-nine health risk appraisal formats were described in the monograph *Health Risk Appraisals: An Inventory* (1981). The primary purposes of risk appraisal as delineated here were to identify personal habits that are detrimental to health and to estimate the relative advantage gained from changing such behaviors. Robbins and Hall (1970) developed the first risk appraisal instrument using a normative data base (mortality) from the National Center for Health Statistics. They used an algorithm to estimate the extent to which risk was lowered for a specific illness by behavior change. While theoretical discussions of risk appraisal appeared in the nursing research literature (Doerr & Hutchins, 1981; Goetz & McTyre, 1981), only Stryd (1982) attempted to determine the actual impact of risk appraisal on health practices.

Major methodological problems with regard to health risk appraisals are: accuracy of morbidity and mortality data on which calculations are based, validity of algorithms for weighting risk factors, and applicability of aggregate data to individuals. In addition, there is limited information on the reliability and validity of available risk appraisal tools. In future research, the predictive validity of life expectancy estimates derived from the various appraisals should be determined through longitudinal studies.

STRESSFUL EVENTS AND HEALTH

Since the pioneering work of Holmes and Rahe (1967), nurse researchers have been interested in what could be done to prevent the negative changes in health status that sometimes appeared to follow stressful events. Nuckolls, Cassel, and Kaplan (1972) found that high life change scores in the presence of high psychosocial assets (e.g., ego strength, marital happiness, and confidence in economic or emotional support) resulted in significantly fewer complications of pregnancy than in the context of low psychosocial assets. Nuckolls et al. used the Schedule of Recent Experience developed by Holmes and Rahe (1967) to measure life change. No attempt was made to determine the extent of stress that respondents actually perceived in the life events they experienced. Jordan and Meckler (1982) studied female graduate students to determine if life change, social support, and presence of a confidante affected menstrual discomfort. The investigators found a positive relationship between life change and menstrual distress in both individuals with low social support ($r = .28$) and those with high social support ($r = .41$). However, the highest correlation between life change as measured by the Anderson College Schedule of Recent Experience (Marx, Garrity, & Bowers, 1975) and menstrual distress was exhibited by individuals who reported no confidante ($r = .62$). This study would have been strengthened by controlling other variables that may have affected menstrual discomfort, such as: diet, physical activity, and female role orientation.

Pesznecker and McNeil (1975) examined health habits, psychologic well-being, and social assets as preventive factors that might temper life events, as measured by the Schedule of Recent Experience, and enable individuals to withstand high degrees of life stress without changes in health status. Major health change was correlated with life change ($r = .32$) and health habits ($r = -.12$) at low but significant levels and in the expected directions. Social assets were not correlated significantly with the occurrence of changes in health status. Life change accounted for only 10% of the variance in major health change.

Fuller and Larson (1980) surveyed fifty elderly individuals living in a senior high-rise residence to determine relationships between life change, emotional support, morale, and functional health status. Life change was correlated negatively with functional health status ($r = -.45$) accounting for 20% of the variance. Emotional support was not related to functional health but correlated positively with morale ($r = .28$). Contrary to expectations, higher magnitudes of life change were associated with lower morale (greater agitation) only in conditions of high emotional support. A high level of concern by others, if not appropriately directed, may increase self-concern and resultant agitation in the elderly. Further research is needed to determine if these findings can be replicated.

Bell (1977) compared hospitalized psychiatric patients with mentally healthy adults. She found that the mentally ill individuals experienced a higher degree of life change in the six months prior to hospitalization than the mentally healthy individuals. She also found that hospitalized patients used significantly more short-term than long-term coping methods when compared with healthy adults. It is possible that coping style, rather than life change itself, was the critical variable in the occurrence of illness.

Several instruments were developed to measure life events in children. The Adolescent Life Change Event Scale developed by Yeaworth and associates (Mendez, Yeaworth, York, & Goodwin, 1980; Yeaworth, York, Hussey, Ingle, & Goodwin, 1980) differed from the scale developed previously by Coddington (1972) for this age group. Adolescents themselves weighted the life events rather than teachers, pediatricians, and mental health workers as in the Coddington scale. Yeaworth et al. questioned if weights assigned to life events by adults were a valid reflection of opinions of adolescents. The Adolescent Life Change Event Scale needs further testing for reliability and validity.

Investigators designing studies of the relationship between stressful events and changes in health status should avoid a simplistic approach. Attention should be focused on timing and clustering of events, as well as their emotional impact. Models developed by Rahe and Arthur (1978) and Hyman and Woog (1982) to explain key intervening variables between life change and subsequent symptomatology and disease can facilitate targeted research into possible links between stress and illness. Intervening variables such as coping style and predisposition to psychophysiologic arousal should be studied systematically.

Lack of agreement in the above studies regarding the role of social support in mitigating the negative effects of stressful events may have been due to the weak relationship between life events as currently measured and illness. Variation in health problems explored, differing tools for measuring life change, diverse types of social support assessed, and the lack of reliable and valid tools for measuring social support were also major problems in this investigative area (T. W. Miller, 1981). Norbeck, Lindsey, and Carrieri (1981), as well as Brandt and Weinert (1981), reported on their continuing efforts to develop sound instruments for assessing social support. Future work by these investigators should provide more reliable and valid measures of this psychosocial variable.

DETERMINANTS OF HEALTH BEHAVIOR

With increasing emphasis on health promotion and illness prevention, individuals and families are encouraged to assume personal responsibility for their own health. As a result, there is a critical need to understand the determinants of health behaviors as a basis for effective nursing actions to promote competence of clients in self-care. Of the studies reviewed, only a limited number of nurse investigators focused on this research area.

Utilization of Preventive Services

In early research, Triplett (1970) and Bullough (1974) focused on factors affecting utilization of preventive services. Triplett found that women who were poor users of a well-child clinic were more likely to perceive disparity between expectations of health workers and their own personal resources than good users. Poor users also perceived higher feelings of threat in past interactions with health care professionals, were more likely to be heads of households on welfare assistance, and had more children than good users. In studying low income women, Bullough (1974) found that accessibility to comprehensive neighborhood clinics had little impact on utilization of preventive care services (e.g., postpartum checkups, well-baby checkups, and dental care). Only immunization levels of children were affected positively by accessibility of services. Immunization level was 80% for children in the special clinic area studied versus 67% in the control area.

Stromborg and Nord-Bourque (1979) found that the primary reasons reported by women for attending a cancer detection clinic were: belief in the benefits of preventive checkups (62%), easy access to the clinic (47%), and a friend or relative with suspected cancer (40%). Pender and Pender (1980) identified the best predictors of intention to use prevention and health promotion services provided by nurse practitioners as: expressed interest in preventive and promotive care, education beyond high school, and low life stress. Using a discriminant function that included the above variables, the rate of correct classification of the sample into those intending and not intending to use the services identified was 77%, with 35% of the variance in intent explained.

In future research, efforts should be directed toward identifying incentives that promote increased use of preventive services. Characteristics of client-provider relationships that facilitate consistency in preventive practices also should be explored.

Personal Health Care Practices

Factors that determine use of professional services for prevention and health promotion may differ from factors affecting self-care practices directed toward the same goals. Thus, nursing studies with a focus on preventive or health-promoting self-care behaviors were reviewed. Sennott (1980) explored the effects of perceived seriousness, perceived susceptibility, estimated effectiveness of health actions, importance of health, and difficulty of health practices on intentions to engage in 10 health behaviors (e.g., exercising, limiting salt, and keeping daily stress low). She used the Health Belief Model (Becker, 1974) as the framework for the study. Only difficulty of health practices (barriers) explained a significant amount of the variance in likelihood of taking health actions (92%). Because of the large amount of variance explained by this one factor, instrumentation used to measure difficulty should be refined further and the study replicated with a larger sample. Perceived difficulty of health practices may be a critical area for nursing assessment and intervention in promoting health behaviors.

Christiansen (1981) studied a national probability sample of 378 adults to determine factors that differentiated those who were engaged in preventive and health-promoting activities from those who were not. She found that the following variables accounted for the most variance in reported incidents of health behaviors: importance of health (health value), perceived health status, and comparative health status (in relation to others), as well as the demographic variables of occupation and household size. Importance of health and perceived health status were components of the Health Promotion Model proposed by Pender (1982). The volunteer panel in this study—while selected to be representative of the population of the United States—may have been atypical due to their repetitive participation in surveys as part of a large Consumer Mail Panel. Replication of the study with other population groups is recommended.

Muhlenkamp, Hubbard, and Brown (Note 3) investigated the relationship between social support and positive health practices in a group of elderly individuals attending a senior citizens' center. Level of social support was related positively to health practices ($r = .37$), explaining 14% of the variance. In another study, Brown et al. (1983) investigated the relationship between health locus of control, health values, and positive health practices. Multiple correlation for health locus of control (MHLC) and health values with health practices was .45, explaining 20% of the variation in health behaviors. Of the three health locus of control subscales (Wallston et al., 1978), only chance—externality—correlated (–.37) with health-promoting activities and explained a significant amount of variance (14%). Findings from these studies suggested that social support and self-reliance rather than a chance orientation characterized individuals who engaged in health-promoting behavior. Further refinement and testing of the Personal Lifestyle Activities Questionnaire developed by Brown et al. (1983) could provide a useful tool for measuring health practices. Test-retest reliability of the instrument was .78 and concurrent validity was .83 when compared with Pelletier's (1978) Lifestyle Assessment Questionnaire.

Using the Ajzen and Fishbein Theory of Reasoned Action (1980) as their conceptual framework, Pender and Pender (Note 1) interviewed 377 residents of two northern Illinois communities regarding the impact of attitudes and expectations of others (normative beliefs) on their intentions to exercise regularly, attain or maintain recommended weight, and manage daily stress. Both attitude and normative beliefs were ascertained using the standardized questionnaire format described by Ajzen and Fishbein (1980). Attitude was a significant determinant of intention to engage in all three health behaviors. Only intention to exercise was affected significantly by normative beliefs. Being near ideal weight increased the likelihood of engaging in physical activity and attaining or maintaining ideal weight. Perceiving health status as excellent also increased the likelihood of intention to control weight. Together, these factors explained 13% of the variance in intention to exercise, 18% of the variance in intention to attain or maintain ideal weight, but only 7% of the variance in intention to manage stress. Limitations of the study were measurement of intentions rather than actual behavior and use of single-item as opposed to multi-item measures of behavioral intentions.

One area of prevention that received more attention in the nursing research literature than any other is breast self-examination. Turnbull (1978) investigated the relationship between practice of breast self-examination and frequency of other health-promoting actions (e.g., proper nutrition, weight control, and exercise) among 160 female graduate students. The practice of breast self-examination was related positively to frequency of health actions only in females under 35 years of age. The gamma statistic was 0.3 for graduate students in a health field and 0.5 for those in a nonhealth field. Determining the relationship between frequency of breast self-examination and each of the six individual health behaviors studied would have provided more meaningful information about health behavior patterns.

Stillman (1977) investigated the relationship between factual knowledge about cancer, health beliefs, and breast self-examination. Her findings failed to support the Becker (1974) Health Belief Model. Of the women who perceived themselves to be highly susceptible to breast cancer, less than half (41%) examined their breasts regularly. Only 15% of women who rated benefits as high reported performing monthly examinations. Content validity of the health beliefs instrument used was established by a panel of experts. However, reliability of the instrument was not determined. Using the instrument developed by Stillman (1977), Hallal (1982) studied 207 women to determine factors associated with breast self-examination. She found practice of monthly breast examination was related positively to beliefs in susceptibility to cancer ($r = .15$), perception of health benefits ($r = .29$), and self-esteem ($r = .35$). Practice was related negatively to beliefs in control of health by powerful others ($r = -.17$).

In summary, research conducted to date provided tentative support for the impact of the following variables on the practice of preventive and health-promoting behaviors: health value, perceived health status, self-esteem, perceived control, perceived difficulty, perceived susceptibility, perceived benefits, social support, attitudes, expectations of significant others, and closeness to ideal weight. It is highly probable that the determinants of health actions vary either in type or relative weight depending on the specific behavior being studied. Further research, including replication of studies reported here, is needed before reliable data concerning the determinants of health behavior are available as bases for effective nursing interventions.

HEALTH PROMOTION AND ILLNESS PREVENTION AMONG SCHOOL-AGE CHILDREN

Several nurse investigators focused on school-age children in testing approaches for increasing the incidence of health behaviors. Since health practices are in the formative stages during childhood, they appear more susceptible to influence than they are in the adult years.

Perceptions of Health

In an early study, Aamodt (1972) used ethnographic techniques such as drawings, sentence completion, and stories to determine the views of health and healing of Papago Indian children. The children focused primarily on health problems rather than health per se in their comments. However, Aamodt, through her work, emphasized the importance of exploring cross-cultural differences in health beliefs among children. In a subsequent study, Natapoff (1978) interviewed over 250 first-, fourth-, and seventh-grade children regarding their views of health. The children defined being healthy as eating the right foods, not being sick, exercising, being clean, being in good condition, and being able to do the things that they wanted to do. Findings from these studies could be used as a basis for constructing a tool measuring developmental changes in health beliefs of children.

Health Screening and Instruction Programs

Risk factor screening was conducted in six junior high schools in New York prior to initiation of the Know Your Body program (Williams, Carter, Arnold, & Wynder, 1979). This experimental program was developed by the American Health Foundation and was aimed at teaching children self-care and health decision-making skills (Williams, Carter, & Eng, 1980). Of the students screened, 18% had cholesterol levels of 180 mg or higher, 8% smoked, 2% had blood pressure readings above 140 mm Hg systolic or 90 mm Hg diastolic, and 16% were overweight (at least 120% of ideal weight). Of the total sample, 29% had one risk factor for coronary heart disease, 6% had two risk factors, and 1% had three or more risk factors.

Holder and Hazley (Note 4) screened junior high school students for risk factors prior to initiating the Independence Missouri Health Education Program patterned after the Know Your Body program. They found that 49% of their Missouri sample, as compared to 29% of the New York sample, exhibited at least one risk factor for heart disease. Almost twice as many children in the Missouri group as in the New York group had high serum cholesterol levels. Exploration of differences in eating patterns, exercise, and stress levels between the two groups would provide useful information concerning the precursors of illness risk in adolescents. In addition, long-term follow-up of the students would provide much needed information concerning the predictive validity of risk factors identified in childhood for chronic illness in later years.

Eng, Botvin, Carter, and Williams (1979) studied seventh- and eighth-graders in metropolitan New York to determine the extent to which risk factor screening alone or in combination with a formal curriculum on cancer and cardiovascular diseases increased student knowledge of these diseases. The experimental group received the specialized curriculum while the control group received only screening without educational follow-up. Using a pretest-posttest design, the investigators found that both groups improved significantly in knowledge concerning nutrition, smoking, and blood pressure control. However, the magnitude of change was greater in the screening and curriculum group than in the group that received screening only. Unfortunately, actual changes in health behaviors or risk levels were not analyzed to determine if the program had any positive impact on lifestyle.

Botvin, Cantlon, Carter, and Williams (1979) compared 50 eighth-grade students enrolled in a special 10-week session weight loss program with 69 other students who did not choose to participate. All of the students in the study were 120% or more of ideal weight. The participants in the weight loss program engaged in the following activities: set long- and short-term goals; monitored weight; received instruction in behavior modification, nutrition, and exercise; and spent 10 minutes in moderately strenuous physical activity during each session. Of the students in the program, 51% lost weight compared to 16% of the controls. This difference was significant statistically. With program participants being self-selected, the groups may have differed in level of motivation to lose weight prior to intervention, thus confounding the effects of the experimental program. The permanency of weight loss should have been ascertained in the study given the high rate of recidivism following weight reduction programs.

Botvin, Eng, and Williams (1980) explored the effect of antismoking education on smoking behavior of eighth-, ninth-, and tenth-grade students. The experimental group discussed the nature of social pressures to smoke and learned various techniques for coping with such pressures. The control group was not exposed to the education program. A significantly lower smoking onset rate (4%) among nonsmokers was apparent in the experimental group as compared to the control group (16%). The importance of early antismoking education was demonstrated, as the program was most effective for eighth graders and least effective for tenth graders. Validation with plasma cotinine levels of student self-reports of smoking (Williams, Eng, Botvin, Hill, & Wynder, 1980) was a strength of this study.

In summary, the studies reviewed indicated the positive impact of education programs on health practices of children and adolescents. However, only short-term outcomes were studied. Well-designed, longitudinal studies are needed to ascertain the long-term effects of health instruction interventions. Long-term rather than short-term lifestyle changes appear essential for promoting health, preventing illness, and extending longevity.

HEALTH PROMOTION AND ILLNESS PREVENTION AMONG ADULTS

Few studies in the nursing literature reviewed were focused on health practices of adults or on related nursing interventions. In an early study of health practices, M. A. Miller (1971) investigated the relationship between breakfast-eating habits of 80 office and factory workers and visits to industrial health facilities. Those who used the health facilities were compared to those who did not. Daily basal caloric needs and daily protein requirements were calculated for each individual. Interviews were conducted with each study participant to obtain food recall from the night before until noon of that day. Nutrition was judged to be adequate if one-fourth of the daily caloric and protein requirements was consumed during that time period. Adequate nutrition during the early morning hours was more characteristic of nonusers than users of the health facilities. A major limitation of this study was failure to control for other variables (e.g., hours of sleep and prior health status) that may have influenced the incidence of health facility visits. It is possible that being ill reduced appetite the morning of the interview, resulting in a report of poor nutrition intake which may not be representative of typical eating patterns.

Quaal (1981) explored the relationship between physical fitness activity and cardiovascular risk factors in a group of 50 male office workers. Energy expenditure in leisure time activity was calculated using the Minnesota Metabolic Activity Index (Cooper, 1969). Cardiovascular fitness was determined by calculating estimated maximum oxygen uptake following the Fisher-Fairbanks Walking Test (Fairbanks, 1978/1979). Assays of total cholesterol, triglycerides, high density lipoprotein (HDL), low density lipoprotein (LDL), and very low density lipoprotein (VLDL) were performed on a 12-hour, fasting blood sample. Blood pressure and percentage of body fat also were determined. Individuals with low estimated maximum oxygen uptake had low levels of energy expenditure in leisure time activity. Energy expenditure correlated positively with HDL ($r = .20$) and negatively with diastolic blood pressure ($r = -.33$), triglycerides ($r = -.22$), body fat ($r = -.36$), and weight ($r = -.22$). Thus, it appeared that regular exercise may have decreased cardiovascular risk factors. Errors of recall may have occurred in reporting level of leisure time activity during the previous year. Repeated weekly or monthly measures of energy expenditure during the previous 6 to 12 months could have minimized this source of error.

Sullivan (1979) assessed the impact of nursing care on the health of an elderly population. She compared senior citizens in one high-rise residence where a comprehensive health program was offered by public health nurses and a medical nurse practitioner to residents in two other demographically comparable buildings where fewer services were offered by nurses. A pretest-posttest design was used. In the comprehensive program, traditional home health care was combined with physical evaluation, counseling, teaching, and outreach work. Following one year of program implementation, the greatest improvements in perception of health status, ability to sleep soundly, and use of a reliable source for primary care occurred in residents in the comprehensive program. Replication of the study among other elderly populations is needed to investigate further the impact of nursing services on the quality of life for the elderly.

Edwards (1980) reported a study in which breast self-examination was taught to 130 women attending a cancer screening program in Utah. Four different instructional methods were used: modeling alone, modeling plus guided practice, modeling plus self-monitoring, and modeling plus peer support. The reported reliability was .80 for the Breast Self-examination Knowledge and Practice Inventory developed by the investigator for use in the study. Data collected three and six months after teaching sessions indicated that all groups increased the frequency of examination significantly but no group differences were apparent. It was recommended that modeling be an integral part of breast self-examination. However, as Oberst (1981) observed, this recommendation is not warranted until modeling has been demonstrated to be superior to other forms of instruction that were not evaluated in this study. Since thoroughness, as well as frequency of examination, is important, the quality of breast self-examinations performed by women in this study should have been determined.

Stryd (1982) evaluated the impact of risk assessment and counseling on changes in health behaviors among professional, technical, and office employees. One group received the results of assessment and were counseled personally regarding how they could improve risk status and potential life expectancy. The other group received their risk appraisal by mail with no follow-up contact. At six months, when lifestyle was assessed again, individuals between 20 to 35 years of age had not changed behavior nor increased estimated life expectancy with or without counseling. Among persons 36 to 50 years of age, only those who were counseled increased estimated life expectancy by 3.21 years. Contrary to expectation, the group over 50 years of age whose members were not counseled increased estimated life expectancy, while the counseled group did not. The lack of consistent findings concerning the positive impact of follow-up contact after lifestyle assessment was due possibly to the brief nature (one session) of counseling provided or to age-specific sensitivity to such assessment and counseling activities. In future studies, longer periods of counseling should be provided. In addition, longitudinal studies are needed to evaluate the impact of health risk appraisal on changes in health practices and the effects of these changes on morbidity and longevity.

Further research efforts should be focused on identifying health practices that promote quality of life and productive longevity and on developing nursing interventions that assist adults in adopting these practices as an integral part of lifestyle. While childhood is the ideal time to learn positive health practices, adult health behavior can be altered. With the increasing number of middle-aged and elderly adults in society, these populations must not be overlooked in studies of health promotion and illness prevention.

FUTURE RESEARCH DIRECTIONS

Health promotion and illness prevention are important and challenging investigative areas for nurse researchers. Scientists in nursing have primary responsibility for contributing to basic knowledge of human health processes, as well as developing and testing nursing interventions and health care delivery systems aimed at increasing the incidence of positive health practices among individuals, families, and communities.

Defining health operationally and developing indices for measuring health as a positive state in all its complexity must be a high priority for nurse researchers. Attention should be given to exploring holistic dimensions of health, such as self-care competency, self-actualization, quality of life, productive longevity, and lifestyle patterns. Valid and reliable tools for measuring health and health-related variables should be developed. In addition, improved methods for measuring the effectiveness of health-promoting or health-protecting interventions are essential for assessing future studies.

Collaboration among nurse researchers prepared in the physical and behavioral sciences and in nursing science, as well as cooperation with researchers in other fields, will be critical to understanding health processes throughout the lifespan. Presently, no investigative methods exist by which perspectives of differing disciplines can be combined to obtain knowledge of health as a complex whole (Brown, 1981). Nurse researchers with their diversity of scientific backgrounds and keen interest in holistic phenomena are in an ideal position to develop such integrative research methods. As a beginning, quantitative and qualitative methods should be combined in investigations of health processes. Explication of how hereditary predisposition interacts with lifestyle and environmental conditions to affect health, and ways in which this interaction can be altered to enhance health and prevent illness, will require major interdisciplinary research efforts.

Extant theoretical frameworks in nursing that address human health processes should be tested to determine their heuristic value. While a number of frameworks were proposed, few were tested adequately. These frameworks should be assessed for their usefulness in: differentiating between health promotion and illness prevention orientations to health behavior; explaining the dynamics of competent self-care for health promotion; and prescribing appropriate nursing interventions to improve the health, longevity, and quality of life for diverse populations.

Nurse researchers also should design cross-cultural studies to explore health beliefs and health behavior patterns in various socioeconomic and cultural groups. Barriers that prevent individuals and families from exercising a full range of health-promoting and health-protecting options must be studied systematically. Effective strategies for health promotion extend beyond changing individual and family lifestyles to modifying social policies that are health-damaging for entire societies and populations. The ethical implications of various approaches to health promotion and illness prevention must be assessed as new strategies are developed.

The studies cited in this review are an indication of the substantial contributions that nurse researchers have made to knowledge about health and human health potential. The need for further investigation of the physical and behavioral principles that underlie health and health behaviors will continue to challenge the theoretical creativity and methodological expertise of scientists in nursing.

REFERENCE NOTES

1. Pender, N. J., & Pender, A. R. *Attitudes, normative beliefs, and behavioral intentions concerning exercise, weight loss, and stress management.* Manuscript submitted for publication, 1983.

2. Byrd, O. E. *Byrd Health Attitude Scale*. Palo Alto, Calif.: Stanford University Press, 1940.
3. Muhlenkamp, A., Hubbard, P. E., & Brown, N. J. *Social support and positive health practices among the elderly*. Paper presented at the 16th Annual Communicating Nursing Research Conference, Portland, Oreg., May 1983. *Abstract in Communicating Nursing Research* (Vol. 16). Boulder, Colo.: Western Interstate Commission for Higher Education, 1983.
4. Holder, E. R., & Hazley, B. The *"Know Your Body" project—Comprehensive progress report*. Kansas City, Mo.: American Nurses' Association, 1979.

REFERENCES

Aamodt, A. The child view of health and healing. In M. V. Batey (Ed.), *Communicating Nursing Research* (Vol. 5). Boulder, Colo.: Western Interstate Commission for Higher Education, 1972.

Ajzen, I., & Fishbein, M. *Understanding attitudes and predicting social behavior*. Englewood Cliffs, N.J.: Prentice-Hall, 1980.

Arakelian, M. An assessment and nursing application of the concept of locus of control. *Advances in Nursing Science*, 1980, *3*(1), 25–42.

Becker, M. H. (Ed.). *The health belief model and personal behavior*. Thorofare, N.J.: Charles B. Slack, 1974.

Bell, J. M. Stressful life events and coping methods in mental illness and wellness behaviors. *Nursing Research*, 1977, *26*, 136–141.

Botvin, G. J., Cantlon, A., Carter, B. J., & Williams, C. L. Reducing adolescent obesity through a school-based health program. *Journal of Pediatrics*, 1979, *95*, 1060–1062.

Botvin, G. J., Eng, A., & Williams, C. L. Preventing the onset of cigarette smoking through life skills training. *Preventive Medicine*, 1980, *9*, 135–143.

Brandt, P. A., & Weinert, C. The PRQ—A social support system. *Nursing Research*, 1981, *30*, 277–280.

Brown, N. J., Muhlenkamp, A. F., Fox, L. M., & Osborn, M. The relationship among health beliefs, health values, and health promotion activity. *Western Journal of Nursing Research*, 1983, *5*, 155–163.

Brown, V. A. From sickness to health: An altered focus for health-care research. *Social Science and Medicine*, 1981, *15A*, 195–201.

Bullough, B. The source of ambulatory health services as it relates to preventive care. *American Journal of Public Health*, 1974, *64*, 582–590.

Christiansen, K. E. *The determinants of health promoting behavior*. Unpublished doctoral dissertation, Rush University, 1981.

Coddington, R. D. The significance of life events as etiologic factors in the diseases of children: A survey of professional workers. *Journal of Psychosomatic Research*, 1972, *16*, 7–18.

Cooper, K. H. Quantifying physical activity—How and why: Proceedings of the National Workshop on Exercise in the Prevention, in the Evaluation, and in the Treatment of Heart Disease. *Journal of the South Carolina Medical Association*, 1969, *65* (12, Supplement), 37–40.

Cox, C. L. An interaction model of client health behavior: Theoretical prescription for nursing. *Advances in Nursing Science,* 1982, *5*(1), 41–56.

Denyes, M. J. Development of an instrument to measure self-care agency in adolescents (Doctoral dissertation, The University of Michigan, 1980). *Dissertation Abstracts International,* 1980, *41,* 1716B. (University Microfilms No. 80–25, 672)

Doerr, B. T., & Hutchins, E. B. Health risk appraisal: Process, problems and prospects for nursing practice and research. *Nursing Research,* 1981, *30,* 299–306.

Edwards, V. Changing breast self-examination behavior. *Nursing Research,* 1980, *29,* 301–306.

Eng, A., Botvin, G. J., Carter, B. J., & Williams, C. L. Increasing students' knowledge of cancer and cardiovascular disease prevention through a risk factor education program. *Journal of School Health,* 1979, *49,* 505–507.

Fairbanks, J. G. A submaximal walking test: Prediction of maximum VO_2 and physical fitness in adult males (Doctoral dissertation, Brigham Young University, 1978). *Dissertation Abstracts International,* 1979, *39,* 4121A. (University Microfilms No. 79–01, 588)

Fishbein, M., & Ajzen, I. *Beliefs, attitudes, intention, and behavior: An introduction to theory and research.* Reading, Mass.: Addison-Wesley, 1975.

Fitzpatrick, J. J. A life perspective rhythm model. In J. J. Fitzpatrick & A. L. Whall (Eds.), *Conceptual models of nursing: Analysis and application.* Bowie, Md.: Brady, 1983.

Fuller, S. S., & Larson, S. B. Life events, emotional support, and health of older people. *Research in Nursing and Health,* 1980, *3,* 81–89.

Goetz, A. A., & McTyre, R. B. Health risk appraisal: Some methodologic considerations. *Nursing Research,* 1981, *30,* 307–315.

Gough, H. G., & Heilbrun, A. B. *The adjective check list manual.* Palo Alto, Calif.: Consulting Psychologists Press, 1965.

Hallal, J. C. The relationship of health beliefs, health locus of control, and self-concept to the practice of breast self-examination in adult women. *Nursing Research,* 1982, *31,* 137–142.

Harvey, J. H., Ickes, W. J., & Kidd, R. F. (Eds.). *New directions in attribution research.* Hillsdale, N.J.: Erlbaum Associates, 1978.

Health risk appraisals: An inventory. (United States Public Health Service Publication No. 81–50163) Office of Health Information, Health Promotion and Physical Fitness, and Sports Medicine Monograph. Washington, D.C.: U.S. Government Printing Office, 1981.

Holmes, T., & Rahe, R. The social readjustment rating scale. *Journal of Psychosomatic Research,* 1967, *11,* 213–218.

Hyman, R. B., & Woog, P. Stressful life events and illness inset: A review of crucial variables. *Research in Nursing and Health,* 1982, *5,* 155–163.

Jordan, J., & Meckler, J. R. The relationship between life change events, social support, and dysmenorrhea. *Research in Nursing and Health,* 1982, *5,* 73–79.

Kearney, B. Y., & Fleischer, B. J. Development of an instrument to measure exercise of self-care agency. *Research in Nursing and Health,* 1979, *2,* 25–34.

Keller, M. J. Toward a definition of health. *Advances in Nursing Science,* 1981, *4*(1), 43–64.

King, I. M. *A theory for nursing.* New York: Wiley, 1981.

Levin, L. S., Katz, A. H., & Holst, E. *Self-care: Lay initiatives in health.* New York: Prodist, 1976.

Lowery, B. J. Misconceptions and limitations of locus of control and the I-E scale. *Nursing Research,* 1981, *30,* 294–298.

Marx, M. B., Garrity, T. F., & Bowers, F. R. The influence of recent life experience on the health of college freshmen. *Journal of Psychosomatic Research,* 1975, *19,* 87–98.

Mendez, L. K., Yeaworth, R. C., York, J. A., & Goodwin, T. Factors influencing adolescents' perceptions of life change events. *Nursing Research,* 1980, *29,* 384–388.

Mikhail, B. The health belief model: A review and critical evaluation of the model, research, and practice. *Advances in Nursing Science,* 1981, *4*(1), 65–82.

Miller, M. A. The relationship between employee breakfast-eating habits and visits to industrial health facilities. *Occupational Health Nursing,* 1971, *19*(10), 7–12.

Miller, P., Wikoff, R., McMahon, M., Garrett, M. J., & Johnson, N. Development of a health attitude scale. *Nursing Research,* 1982, *31,* 132–136.

Miller, T. W. Life events scaling: Clinical methodological issues. *Nursing Research,* 1981, *30,* 316–321.

Natapoff, J. N. Children's view of health: A developmental study. *American Journal of Public Health,* 1978, *68,* 995–1000.

Neuman, B. *The Neuman systems model: Application to nursing education and practice.* Norwalk, Conn.: Appleton-Century-Crofts, 1982.

Newman, M. *Theory development in nursing.* Philadelphia, Pa.: F. A. Davis, 1979.

Norbeck, J. S., Lindsey, A. M., & Carrieri, V. L. The development of an instrument to measure social support. *Nursing Research,* 1981, *30,* 264–269.

Nuckolls, K. B., Cassel, J., & Kaplan, B. H. Psychosocial assets, life crises, and the prognosis of pregnancy. *American Journal of Epidemiology,* 1972, *95,* 431–441.

Oberst, M. Testing approaches to teaching breast self-examination. *Cancer Nursing,* 1981, *4,* 246.

Oelbaum, C. H. Hallmarks of adult wellness. *American Journal of Nursing,* 1974, *74,* 1623–1625.

Olsen, L. K. An evaluation instrument for appraising the health related attitudes of college students. *Journal of School Health,* 1972, *42,* 408–411.

Orem, D. E. *Nursing: Concepts of practice.* New York: McGraw-Hill, 1971.

Parse, R. R. *Man—living—health: A theory for nursing.* New York: Wiley, 1981.

Pelletier, K. A conversation with Ken Pelletier. *Medical Self Care,* 1978, *5,* 3–24.

Pender, N. J. *Health promotion in nursing practice.* Norwalk, Conn.: Appleton-Century-Crofts, 1982.

Pender, N. J., & Pender, A. R. Illness prevention and health promotion services provided by nurse practitioners: Predicting potential consumers. *American Journal of Public Health,* 1980, *70,* 798–803.

Pesznecker, B. L., & McNeil, J. Relationship among health habits, social assets, psychologic well-being, life change, and alterations in health status. *Nursing Research,* 1975, *24,* 442–447.

Quaal, S. J. A study of fitness and cardiovascular risk factors in male office workers. *Western Journal of Nursing Research,* 1981, *3,* 9–24.

Rahe, R. H., & Arthur, R. J. Life change and illness studies: Past history and future directions. *Journal of Human Stress*, 1978, *4*(1), 3–15.

Reed, P. G., & Zurakowski, T. L. Nightingale: A visionary model for nursing. In J. J. Fitzpatrick & A. L. Whall (Eds.), *Conceptual models of nursing: Analysis and application*. Bowie, Md.: Brady, 1983.

Richardson, C. E. *Three test instruments measuring health attitudes of college students*. Unpublished doctoral dissertation, University of California, Los Angeles, 1959.

Robbins, L. C., & Hall, J. H. *How to practice prospective medicine*. Indianapolis: Slaymaker Enterprises, 1970.

Rokeach, M. *The nature of human values*. New York: Free Press, 1973.

Rosenstock, I. M. Why people use health services. *Milbank Memorial Fund Quarterly*, 1966, *44* (3, Supplement), 94–127.

Rosenstock, I. M. Historical origins of the health belief model. In M. H. Becker (Ed.), *The health belief model and personal health behavior*. Thorofare, N.J.: Charles B. Slack, 1974.

Rotter, J. B. Generalized expectancies for internal versus external control of reinforcement. *Psychological Monographs*, 1966, *80*(1, Whole No. 609).

Saltzer, E. B. Locus of control and the intention to lose weight. *Health Education Monographs*, 1978, *6*, 118–128.

Sennott, L. L. Value-expectancy theory and health behavior: An exploration of motivating variables (Doctoral dissertation, University of Arizona, 1980). *Dissertation Abstracts International*, 1980, *40*, 6013A. (University Microfilms No. 80–11, 259)

Smith, J. A. The idea of health: A philosophical inquiry. *Advances in Nursing Science*, 1981, *3*(3), 43–50.

Stillman, M. J. Women's beliefs about breast cancer and breast self-examination. *Nursing Research*, 1977, *26*, 121–127.

Stromborg, M. F., & Nord-Bourque, S. A cancer detection clinic: Patient motivation and satisfaction. *Nurse Practitioner*, 1979, *4*(1), 10–11; 51.

Stryd, A. N. Risk appraisal and its effect on lifestyle. *Occupational Health Nursing*, 1982, *30*(11), 19–20.

Sullivan, J. A. Effectiveness of a comprehensive health program for the well-elderly by community health nurses. *Nursing Research*, 1979, *28*, 70–75.

Triplett, J. L. Characteristics and perceptions of low-income women and use of preventive health services. *Nursing Research*, 1970, *19*, 140–146.

Turnbull, E. M. Effects of basic preventive health practices and mass media on the practice of breast self-examination. *Nursing Research*, 1978, *27*, 98–102.

Wallston, K. A., Maides, S., & Wallston, B. S. Health-related information seeking as a function of health-related locus of control and health values. *Journal of Research in Personality*, 1976, *10*, 215–222.

Wallston, K. A., Wallston, B. S., & DeVellis, R. Development of the multidimensional health locus of control (MHLC) scales. *Health Education Monographs*, 1978, *6*, 161–170.

Williams, C. L., Carter, B. J., Arnold, C. B., & Wynder, E. L. Chronic disease risk factors among children: The "Know Your Body" study. *Journal of Chronic Disease*, 1979, *32*, 505–513.

Williams, C. L., Carter, B. J., & Eng, A. The "Know Your Body" program: A developmental approach to health education and disease prevention. *Preventive Medicine*, 1980, *9*, 371–383.

Williams, C. L., Eng, A., Botvin, G. J., Hill, P., & Wynder, E. L. Validation of students' self-reported cigarette smoking status with plasma cotinine levels. *American Journal of Public Health*, 1980, *9*, 1272–1274.

Yeaworth, R. C., York, J., Hussey, M. A., Ingle, M. E., & Goodwin, T. The development of an adolescent life change scale. *Adolescence*, 1980, *15*(57), 91–98.

CHAPTER 5

Coping with Elective Surgery

JEAN E. JOHNSON
SCHOOL OF NURSING
UNIVERSITY OF ROCHESTER

CONTENTS

Historically, the practice of providing surgical patients with information and instruction prior to their operations began with a change in patient management strategies. Instead of confining patients to their beds for many days, surgeons ambulated patients within hours following surgery. Early resumption of physical activities became standard practice because it de-

Preparation of this manuscript was supported in part by Division of Nursing Grant NU 00594 to Jean E. Johnson, Robert Wood Johnson Foundation Grant 7022 to Jean E. Johnson, and National Cancer Institute Grants CA 11198 to Robert A. Cooper, Jr. and CA 33010 to Jean E. Johnson. The assistance of Lillian Nail in the preparation of this chapter is acknowledged gratefully.

creased the frequency of major physical postoperative complications (Leithauser & Bergo, 1941). To reduce patients' fear and to increase their willingness to participate in the beneficial physical activity, nurses and surgeons taught them about the activities they were expected to perform soon after surgery. Even though it was rarely mentioned by investigators, most of the research on preparation of surgical patients stemmed from that major change in methods of management of surgical patients.

This source of stimulation for research on preparatory interventions for surgical patients may have contributed to the emphasis on the empirical versus the theoretical purposes of the research. Investigators of the preparation of surgical patients were interested in finding answers to questions such as *what* can be done to help patients rather than explanations of *why* an intervention helps patients. On the empirical level, the global question of whether or not surgical patients benefit from nonphysical preparatory interventions was addressed in a recently published review that included many of the studies reviewed in this chapter. Using meta-analysis techniques, Mumford, Schlesinger, and Glass (1982) concluded that patients benefit from preparatory interventions. The purpose of the present review is to relate the body of research on preparing patients for surgery to theoretical explanations. Relating the impressive existing empirical base to theoretical perspectives allows that research to serve as a stepping-stone, so that in future research investigators will test, extend, and refine theoretical explanations of coping with surgery.

ORGANIZATION OF THE CHAPTER

Because stress and coping are concepts central to the theories that may explain why patients are helped by preparation for surgery, these concepts are discussed and defined. To achieve the purpose of this review, it was necessary to identify theoretical or explanatory positions referred to by investigators of preparation of surgical patients. Each of the positions is discussed briefly. An attempt was made to include in the review all of the research that met the criteria that are detailed in the section on selection of studies. An apology is offered to authors of reports that may have been overlooked. Because similar methodological flaws occurred throughout the body of research, methodological issues are discussed in general rather than study by study.

Investigators tended to use similar types of interventions in their research on surgical patients. The groups of studies are not mutually exclusive because some investigators used more than one experimental intervention in their studies and others used interventions that were combinations of types of instruction and information. The characteristics of the interventions for each group of studies are described, followed by descriptions of patterns of effects of the interventions on the outcome measures. The outcome measures are grouped according to the sources of the data and the time of data collection (during hospitalization or postdischarge). All of the studies reviewed are listed in Table 5–1. Also shown in the table are types of intervention(s) and outcome measures used in each study.

In the discussion section the pattern of effects identified in the research is related to stress, coping, and theoretical positions. General conclusions are derived from the review of the research. Finally, suggestions for the direction of future research on coping with surgery are offered.

STRESS AND COPING

The concept of stress is so broad that it has limited usefulness as a scientific term. When used as if it has a precise meaning, confusion results. The term has been used to refer to biological, psychological, and social processes which may have little in common with one another. This chapter is focused on psychological stress.

Psychological stress implies that a system or whole organism is taxed with respect to maintaining its usual function. If the taxing circumstances overwhelm the resources available for counteracting the threat, the organisms' usual functions can be disrupted and negative emotional reactions may occur. Viewing stress in this manner emphasizes only usual functions and their disruption, as well as emotional response. This view of psychological stress contrasts with those that emphasize emotional reactions as the indication that a person's resources for coping may be taxed.

Coping refers to psychological processes and behaviors that occur in response to a threat. Psychologists have proposed that coping encompasses two functions: (a) the regulation of emotional response, and (b) the regulation of goal-directed, or problem-solving behaviors (Lazarus & Launier, 1978; Leventhal, 1970). Leventhal hypothesized that the two functions of coping involve different processes and can therefore maintain a degree of independence from each other.

In surgical patients, the threat results from the various aspects of the surgical experience that might tax patients' ability to function in ways that minimize the negative impact on their psychological and physical well-

Table 5-1. Summary of the Research

Studies, type of surgery, and method of subject assignment	Interventions							Outcome Measures																			
								Physiological behavior						Self-report						Provider judgment				Post-discharge			
	Prov./pt. interaction	Physical activity inst.	Relaxation inst.	Positive thinking inst.	Hypnosis	Abstract orient. info.	Concrete orient. info.	Pulse and/or B.P.	Complications	Arterial blood gases	Nausea/vomiting	Pulmonary function	Ambulation	Emotions	Pain	Physical symptoms	Satisfaction	Personal well-being	Coping activity	Medications	Distress or pain	Coping ability	Length of hospital stay	Physical recovery	Return to normal self	Emotions	Usual activities
Dumas & Leonard (1963); Gynecological; NR	X										+			+[a]													
Dumas & Johnson (1972); Gynecological; R	X							0	–		0		0	+[b]						0			0				
Archuleta, Plummer, & Hopkins (1977); Various; NR		X										0								0			0				
Lindeman & Van Aernam (1971); Various; NR		X										+								0			+				

Study												
King & Tarsitano (1982); Abdominal; NR	X							+			0	
Carrieri (1975); Upper Abdominal; R	X			0			+[c]		0	+	0	
Egbert, Battit, Welch, & Bartlett (1964); Abdominal; R	X					0		+	+	+	+	
Wells (1982); Cholecystectomy; R	X					+			0		0	
Field (1974); Orthopedic; R	X	X	0		+	+		+	+	0		
Flaherty & Fitzpatrick (1978); Cholecystectomy, Herniorrhaphy, and Hemorrhoidectomy; NR	X			+		+		+[d]	+[d]			
Bonilla, Quigley, & Bowers (1961); Orthopedic; NR		X						+[d]	+[d]	+	+	
Langer, Janis, & Wolfer (1975); Various; R	X	0					+	+	0	−		
Healy (1968); Various; NR	X	0					+	+[d]	+[d]	+[d]	0	
Fortin & Kirouac (1976); Herniorrhaphy, Cholecystectomy, and Hysterectomy; R	X	+[d]		+	+		+	+	+	0	+	
Felton, Huss, Payne, & Srsic (1976); Various; R	X	0		−		+				+		
	X			−		+				0		

111

Table 5–1. Summary of the Research (continued)

Studies, type of surgery, and method of subject assignment	Prov./pt. interaction	Physical activity inst.	Relaxation inst.	Positive thinking inst.	Hypnosis	Abstract orient. info.	Concrete orient. info.	Pulse and/or B.P.	Complications	Arterial blood gases	Nausea/vomiting	Pulmonary function	Ambulation	Emotions	Pain	Physical symptoms	Satisfaction	Personal well-being	Coping activity	Medications	Distress or pain	Coping ability	Length of hospital stay	Physical recovery	Return to normal self	Emotions	Usual activities
	Interventions							*Outcome Measures*																			
								Physiological behavior						*Self-report*						*Provider judgment*				*Post-discharge*			
Schmitt & Wooldridge (1973); Various; R	X	X				X		+	+		0			+				+		+			+				
Hegyvary & Chamings (1975a, 1975b); Hysterectomy; R																											
Hospital A		X				X			0		0									+			0				
Hospital B		X				X			0		0									0			0				
Johnson, Rice, Fuller, & Endress (1978);		X											0	+[e]	0					0			0				0

Study									
Cholecystectomy; R Herniorrhaphy; R		X			X		0	0	0
			X				+[e]	+	+
				X			+[e]	0	0
							0	0	0
							0	0	0
Johnson, Fuller, Endress, & Rice (1978); Cholecystectomy; NR Herniorrhaphy; NR	X		X				0	0	+
	X		X				+	0	0
Wilson (1981); Hysterectomy and Cholecystectomy; R	X				0		0	+	0
					+		+	+	+
Hill (1982); Cataract; R		X					0	0	0
		X					0	0	0
	X						0	0	+

Note. R = random assignment of patients to intervention groups; NR = no random assignment of patients to intervention groups; X = the intervention was used in the study. The effects of the intervention on outcome measures appear on the same line. Two or more X's on the same line indicate that the intervention was a combination of the individual interventions. + = the intervention had a statistically significant ($p < .05$) effect on the outcome measure; – = the intervention had a statistically significant ($p < .05$) effect on the outcome measure in an undesirable direction; Blank = the outcome measure was not used in the study; 0 = the intervention did not significantly ($p < .05$) effect the outcome measure.

[a] As judged by nurse interaction with patients.
[b] The experimental intervention relieved distress in those with higher distress scores on the pretest.
[c] Effect occurred in only one of three outcome measures.
[d] No inferential statistical tests were used.
[e] Significant effects only for patients above the median score on preoperative fear.

being. The view that coping consists of two functions requires that outcome measures of coping with the experience of surgery reflect both of these functions.

THEORETICAL ORIENTATIONS

Discussions in the nursing literature regarding psychological aspects of surgery often are based on the assumption that the patients' emotional response is an especially important factor in coping with the stress of surgery. Specifically, patients' fear can interfere with the goal-directed functions of coping during the stressful experience. Therefore, interventions that reduce fear are expected to increase patients' psychological comfort and enhance their ability to perform goal-directed behaviors.

In contrast, Janis (1958) proposed that fear may serve a useful function for surgical patients. He hypothesized that a moderate amount of fear before surgery is necessary to motivate patients to worry. Patients use worry to prepare themselves for an operation and to strengthen their abilities to cope with the discomforts and unpleasant experiences that accompany it. Patients who are not fearful need to be given information that arouses some fear so that the work of worry will occur. Extremely frightened patients require interventions to reduce their fear, so that instead of engaging in neurotic worry their worry would be directed toward preparing themselves to cope with the impending experience.

Another rationale for providing patients with preoperative preparation is based on teaching-learning principles. In this context, learning is defined as a relatively permanent change in a behavioral tendency and is the result of reinforced practice (Kimble & Garmezy, 1963, p. 133). Surgical patients who are instructed in and learn behaviors such as deep breathing, coughing, ambulation, and leg exercises preoperatively are expected to perform these behaviors effectively after their surgery. Thus, they reduce the risk of developing postoperative complications. In research based on this rationale investigators emphasize methods of teaching patients the behaviors (e.g., Lindeman & Van Aernam, 1971).

More recently, personal control was offered as an explanation for relationships between preoperative preparatory interventions and postoperative reactions and recovery (e.g., Schmitt & Wooldridge, 1973). Discussions of personal control suggested that patients who have actual control or perceive that they have some control over their experiences during the stressful postoperative recovery period also should have the most positive outcomes when compared to those patients who do not have actual or perceived control. Interventions that provide instruction in (a) activities that enhance physical recovery or (b) coping strategies, could increase patients' sense of personal control over the situation. Descriptions of the experience also could convey a sense of control because such descriptions increase patients' ability to predict their experiences. Investigators of the stress experienced by surgical patients only recently have been concerned with explaining why personal control enhances coping (Schmitt & Wooldridge, 1973).

SELECTION OF STUDIES

This review was limited to studies that were readily available, primarily those published in journals with peer review. No unpublished dissertation research was included. Interventions were considered to have an effect on outcome measures only when alpha levels were .05 or less. Exceptions to these stringent criteria were made when no statistical analyses were reported but the effects of interventions appeared to be strong. Computer literature searches and references listed in research reports were used to identify studies.

Studies were not included if only the time or method of delivering an intervention was manipulated. A true or quasi-experimental design was used in all of the studies reviewed. Main effects of interventions are emphasized, rather than interactions between two types of interventions or between interventions and individual difference variables. This is not to imply that such interactions are not important, but rather that interpretations of interactions are highly speculative when theoretical explanations are in a developmental stage.

All of the subjects of the studies were adults who underwent elective surgical procedures. The practical problems of entering patients undergoing emergency surgery into an experimental preparation study accounted for the lack of research on that population of patients. Studies of patients having surgery in ambulatory settings or cardiac surgery were not included because many of the indicators of response used in that research were unique to those particular situations. For example, mental confusion was frequently used as an indicator of response in studies of cardiac surgical patients, while no study of general surgical patients employed such an indicator. Many of the outcome indicators used in studies of hospitalized patients do not apply in the ambulatory setting. Studies of children undergoing surgery were omitted because of the impact of developmental factors on both the interventions and outcome measures.

Even with these restrictions, there was wide variation in the type of surgical patients included in the studies reviewed. Some samples included patients who did not have surgical incisions (e.g., dilatation of the cervix and curettage of the uterus), as well as those who had abdominal, chest, neurological, or orthopedic surgery.

Twenty-one reports of research were reviewed. Two studies were described in each of two of these reports (Johnson, Fuller, Endress, & Rice, 1978; Johnson, Rice, Fuller, & Endress, 1978). More than one experimental intervention was used in several of the studies (see Table 5–1).

METHODOLOGICAL ISSUES AND PROBLEMS

The major methodological issue in this body of research is its weak connection to both theoretical orientations and to previous research. The effect of the lack of theory was most apparent in some of the reports of replication of earlier studies (e.g., Archuleta, Plummer, & Hopkins, 1977; King & Tarsitano, 1982). Without theory, repetition of the methods and procedures of the original study occurred without improvements in the methods. Repeating a study is not equivalent to an attempt to replicate theoretically predicted relationships. The scientific purposes of replication are to confirm, extend, alter, or reject theory.

A major strength of the research summarized in this review is that in all but nine of the studies, patients were assigned at random to intervention conditions. Random assignment is essential in establishing relationships between interventions and outcomes, although it does not guarantee that groups of patients will be equivalent with regard to factors that could explain variance in outcome.

In the studies, various methods were used for presenting the interventions to patients. With some methods, consistency of content for each patient was insured, while with other methods content was allowed to vary. Interventions that focused on individual needs during provider-patient interaction provided little content consistency (Dumas & Johnson, 1972; Dumas & Leonard, 1963; Felton, Huss, Payne, & Srsic, 1976). Interventions that were structured and delivered in person provided moderate consistency (Egbert, Battit, Welch, & Bartlett, 1964; Felton et al., 1976; Field, 1974; Flaherty & Fitzpatrick, 1978; Fortin & Kirouac, 1976; Healy, 1968; Hegyvary & Chamings, 1975a, 1975b; Langer, Janis, & Wolfer, 1975; Schmitt & Wooldridge, 1973). The use of mechanical recorders for delivery of the interventions insured that each patient received the same content (Archuleta et al., 1977; Hill, 1982; Johnson, Fuller, Endress, & Rice, 1978; Johnson, Rice, Fuller, & Endress, 1978; King & Tarsitano, 1982; Lindeman & Van Aernam, 1971; Wilson, 1981).

In each of the studies, the care received by patients assigned to the nonexperimental intervention control group could have varied. In the most recent studies, the care received by the control group of patients could have included some of the same content as that received by patients in the experimental intervention groups. It may be the case that earlier studies stimulated changes in practice. Although influencing practice is the ultimate purpose of such research, such changes decreased the likelihood of finding differences between experimental and control groups.

In general, investigators did not use designs that allowed identification of the effects of each of the various components of a complex intervention or identification of the effects of interactions between components of the intervention. Some of the interventions consisted of combinations of various types of instruction and information, preventing identification of the component(s) of the intervention that affected the outcome measures (Felton et al., 1976; Field, 1974; Fortin & Kirouac, 1976; Healy, 1968, Hegyvary & Chamings, 1975a, 1975b; Schmitt & Wooldridge, 1973). In addition, patients in all of the experimental intervention groups received more attention from the researchers than the patients in the nonexperimental intervention groups.

The degree of control over the influence of situational variables—such as type of surgery—varied greatly across the studies. In some of the studies, the sample was restricted to patients having one or two types of operations. In others, study groups were equated on type of operation by matching techniques, and in still others, all patients scheduled to go to the operating room were included. The results attributed to interventions in studies in which type of operation varied widely may not be reliable. Differences among study groups on the type of operation patients had undergone could account for the effects, or lack of effects, attributed to the interventions.

Clinically relevant outcome measures were used frequently in studies of preparation of surgical patients. However, the outcome measures rarely were linked to theoretical explanations of coping. The outcome measures used were physiological response, patients' behavior, patients' self-report of reactions, activities that reflect care providers' judgment of patients' progress, and patients' reports of postdischarge activities and reactions. All of the above indicators were vulnerable to the influence of factors extraneous to the primary purpose of the study.

Physiological outcome measures were used infrequently and receive little attention in this review. Outcome measures that reflected physiological processes, such as pulse rate and blood pressure, were especially vulnerable to influence by extraneous variables. Fluctuations within normal ranges of the response had little clinical significance. To a large degree, both length of postoperative hospitalization and pain medication received were subject to influence by situational factors. Consequently, in some of the studies little if any variance in these measures was due to influence by experimental interventions. Patient behavior as measured by pulmonary function tests after surgery could have been influenced by the discomfort caused by such tests. In the study of King and Tarsitano (1982), 51% of the patients refused the postoperative pulmonary function test.

Multiple indicators of effect were used in most of the studies. Investigators tended to use statistical tests repeatedly in order to evaluate the effects of an intervention on each indicator. Such multiple statistical tests may have capitalized on chance results. Some investigators did not include in their statistical analysis designs certain situational variables (e.g., type of surgery and age of patient) that could have explained a significant amount of variance in outcome measures. In some designs, indicators were measured repeatedly over time. Frequently, assumptions about the correlations between data from repeated measures were ignored, or analyses for each occasion of measurement were repeated. Changes in scores from one occasion of measurement to another were also used in analyses. Such scores can be influenced greatly by measurement error (Burckhardt, Goodwin, & Prescott, 1982).

INTERVENTIONS AND THEIR EFFECT ON OUTCOME MEASURES

Provider-Patient Interaction

These interventions were described as interaction with patients for the purpose of identifying the needs of the patient and taking action to meet those needs. No standardized information or instruction was provided to patients. The interventions were highly individualized. In the Schmitt and Wooldridge (1973) study, the interaction occurred in a group situation and was in addition to standardized information and instruction; in the other three studies, the provider interacted with patients individually (Dumas & Johnson, 1972; Dumas & Leonard, 1963; Felton et al., 1976).

In each of the studies, the intervention resulted in a reduction of negative emotions as reported by patients. There was no pattern of effects on other indicators.

Physical Activity Instruction

Interventions in this group consisted of instruction in deep breathing, coughing, ambulation, and leg exercises. Investigators of coping with surgery used this intervention more frequently than any other intervention. Fourteen tests of the intervention were found in the literature (Archuleta et al., 1977; Carrieri, 1975; Felton et al., 1976; Fortin & Kirouac, 1976; Healy, 1968; Hegyvary & Chamings, 1975a, 1975b; Johnson, Fuller, Endress, & Rice, 1978; Johnson, Rice, Fuller, & Endress, 1978; King & Tarsitano, 1982; Lindeman & Van Aernam, 1971; Schmitt & Wooldridge, 1973). In an additional study included in this intervention grouping, one group of cataract patients was instructed in ways to reduce discomfort in the operative eye and in self-care activities (Hill, 1982).

Positive effects of physical activity instruction on self-report outcome measures were reported in five of the eight studies in which those outcome measures were used (Felton et al., 1976; Fortin & Kirouac, 1976; Johnson, Fuller, Endress, & Rice, 1978; Johnson, Rice, Fuller, & Endress, 1978; Schmitt & Wooldridge, 1973). However, the physical activity instruction was combined with orienting information in all but one of the studies in which positive effects on self-report measures were reported (Johnson, Rice, Fuller, & Endress, 1978).

Measures of pulmonary function were used in five studies (Archuleta et al., 1977; Carrieri, 1975; Felton et al., 1976; King & Tarsitano, 1982; Lindeman & Van Aernam, 1971). Positive results were reported in three studies (Carrieri, 1975; King & Tarsitano, 1982; Lindeman & Van Aernam, 1971) and negative results in one (Felton et al., 1976). Methodological flaws were present in each of the studies in which positive effects for pulmonary function tests were reported. In the King and Tarsitano (1982) and Lindeman and Van Aernam (1971) studies, patients were not assigned at random to intervention groups. King and Tarsitano (1982) reported that

51% of the patients were not tested after surgery. Carrieri (1975) reported her concern about the reliability of the results in her study. The expected reduction in the occurrence of postoperative complications was reported in only two of the studies (Healy, 1968; Schmitt & Wooldridge, 1973).

The amount of pain medication patients received was used as an outcome measure in 12 evaluations of the physical activity instruction intervention (Archuleta et al., 1977; Carrieri, 1975; Fortin & Kirouac, 1976; Healy, 1968; Hegyvary & Chamings, 1975a, 1975b; Johnson, Fuller, Endress, & Rice, 1978; Johnson, Rice, Fuller, & Endress, 1978; Lindeman & Van Aernam, 1971; Schmitt & Wooldridge, 1973). A decrease in the use of pain medication was attributed to the intervention in four of the studies (Fortin & Kirouac, 1976; Healy, 1968; Hegyvary & Chamings, 1975a, 1975b; Schmitt & Wooldridge, 1973). In each of the four studies, the intervention consisted of a combination of physical activity instruction and other information.

Length of postoperative hospitalization was used as an outcome measure in each of the 15 evaluations of interventions that included physical activity instructions. Investigators reported a reduction in length of hospitalization in only four studies (Healy, 1968; Johnson, Fuller, Endress, & Rice, 1978; Lindeman & Van Aernam, 1971; Schmitt & Wooldridge, 1973). In three of the four studies, the intervention included elements in addition to instruction in physical activities.

Based on an analysis of the reported effects of physical activity instruction on outcome measures, I conclude that there was no consistent effect of this type of intervention on either tests of pulmonary function or postoperative complications. There was, however, a suggestion of effects on patients' self-reports of their reactions, use of pain medication, and length of hospitalization. These effects occurred most frequently when the physical activity instruction was combined with other content.

Instruction in Coping Strategies

Hypnosis, relaxation, and positive thinking were the coping strategies investigators used in studies of surgical patients. Hypnosis was used by two investigators (Bonilla, Quigley, & Bowers, 1961; Field, 1974). Only Bonilla et al. reported effects for the intervention. Those effects were (a) reduction in use of pain medication, and (b) early return to usual activities. However, patients were not assigned at random to the intervention and no statistical techniques were used for evaluation of the differences between intervention groups.

The relaxation methods studied included total body relaxation (Field, 1974; Wells, 1982; Wilson, 1981) and relaxation of selected muscle groups (Egbert et al., 1964; Flaherty & Fitzpatrick, 1978). Patients' self-report of pain was used as an outcome measure in four of the studies; in three of those studies it was concluded that relaxation reduced reports of pain (Flaherty & Fitzpatrick, 1978; Wells, 1982; Wilson, 1981). Amount of pain medication was an outcome measure used in four of the studies; a reduction in pain medication was reported in two (Egbert et al., 1964; Flaherty & Fitzpatrick, 1978). A reduction in length of postoperative hospitalization was reported in two of the three studies in which this particular indicator was used (Egbert et al., 1964; Wilson, 1981).

The coping strategy of focusing on the positive versus the negative aspects of having surgery (positive thinking) was studied by Langer et al. (1975). Instruction in the strategy was reported to be associated with provider-judged increase in ability to cope and reduction in use of pain medications.

The small number of studies of instruction in coping strategies prevents drawing firm conclusions about patterns of effects of such interventions on outcome measures. The outcome measures that were affected the most consistently were (a) self-report of pain, and (b) use of pain medications.

Abstract Orienting Information

These interventions consisted of descriptions of routines of care, including what will be done to and for patients. The content was selected from textbooks and manuals used by care providers (e.g., Langer et al., 1975). Terms such as recovery room, preoperative medication, skin preparation, and vital signs were included in the descriptions. Because this information did not describe patients' experience in concrete terms, I have referred to this as abstract orienting information.

Nine tests of interventions that consisted of abstract orienting information alone or in combination with instruction in physical activities were found in the literature (Felton et al., 1976; Fortin & Kirouac, 1976; Healy, 1968; Hegyvary & Chamings, 1975a, 1975b; Johnson, Rice, Fuller, & Endress, 1978; Langer et al., 1975; Schmitt & Wooldridge, 1973). Of the five comparisons for which self-report measures were available (Felton et al., 1976; Fortin & Kirouac, 1976; Johnson, Rice, Fuller, & Endress, 1978; Schmitt & Wooldridge, 1973), positive effects were observed for all but one (Johnson, Rice, Fuller, & Endress, 1978). The self-report measures included emotional status, physical symptoms, satisfaction, and personal well-being.

Length of postoperative stay was included as an outcome measure in all nine tests. Investigators reported effects for only two of the tests (Healy, 1968; Schmitt & Wooldridge, 1973). In four of the eight tests with pain medication as an outcome measure, patients who received the intervention required less pain medication than control patients (Fortin & Kirouac, 1976; Healy, 1968; Hegyvary & Chamings, 1975a, 1975b; Schmitt & Wooldridge, 1973). The effects on length of postoperative hospitalization and/or pain medication occurred in studies where the interventions were a combination of abstract orienting information and instruction in physical activities.

In summary, the most consistent effect for abstract orienting information was on patients' self-reports of emotions and other indicators of well-being. The combination of physical activity instruction and abstract orienting information appeared to be more effective than the individual interventions when pain medication and length of hospitalization were outcome measures.

Concrete Orienting Information

Concrete orienting information refers to descriptions of what the patient will experience in specific terms. The descriptions were developed from reports of patients who recently had experienced these events. Such information included descriptions of the physical sensations associated with events, when events will occur, and how long they will last. Terms that describe patients' interpretations of the severity of the sensations were not included. See McHugh, Christman, and Johnson (1982) for a more detailed description.

Concrete orienting information was used for six tests (Hill, 1982; Johnson, Fuller, Endress, & Rice, 1978; Johnson, Rice, Fuller, & Endress, 1978; Wilson, 1981). Two of the tests were the only ones under review that restricted the sample to herniorrhaphy patients. No effects were found for concrete orienting information or any other intervention in the studies of herniorrhaphy patients. Effects of the intervention on measures during hospitalization showed no consistent pattern. A reduction in length of postoperative hospitalization was observed in three of the tests (Johnson, Fuller, Endress, & Rice, 1978; Johnson, Rice, Fuller, & Endress, 1978; Wilson, 1981). The effects of the intervention may have continued after hospital discharge. When patients were followed after discharge, there were positive effects for the intervention on indicators of resuming usual activities in three of five tests (Hill, 1982; Johnson, Fuller, Endress, & Rice, 1978; Johnson, Rice, Fuller, & Endress, 1978). In one of those studies (Hill, 1982), the postdischarge effect was associated with an intervention that consisted of a combination of concrete orienting information and suggestions for self-care.

The pattern of effects of concrete orienting information interventions differed from that of other interventions in the research reviewed. The effects on self-report and behavior measures taken during hospitalization showed little consistency across studies. Length of hospitalization was effected relatively consistently, but the most consistent effect was on indicators of resumption of usual activities after leaving the hospital.

DISCUSSION

Functions of Coping and the Research

A consistent finding in the research was an association between various types of interventions and emotional response. The self-reported indicators of emotional response included emotional state, satisfaction, pain, and personal well-being. Each type of intervention was associated with a reduction in negative emotional response. The data therefore support the conclusion that the coping function focused on regulation of emotional response was enhanced by interventions regardless of the specific composition of these interventions.

Investigators did not identify the indicators that reflected the coping function focused on regulating goal-directed behavior. The lack of links between indicators and the goal-directed function of coping presented obstacles to drawing firm conclusions about the effects of interventions on that component of coping. If it is assumed that the patient's goal is the resumption of usual activities, then length of hospitalization and resumption of usual activities after hospital discharge can be considered to reflect goal-directed behaviors.

I detected no clear pattern of effects of interventions on indicators of resumption of usual life activities. The only investigators who included indicators of resumption of usual activities following hospital discharge in their studies were those who included concrete orienting information interventions as one of several interventions. The investigators reported that *only* the concrete orienting information was associated with indicators of resumption of usual activities.

Length of postoperative hospitalization frequently was used as an outcome measure in the studies reviewed. No pattern of association between specific types of interventions and length of postoperative hospitalization emerged. But there was a pattern of effects associated with the span of years during which the research reports were published. In studies published in 1975 or later, the only interventions associated with reduction in length of hospitalization were concrete orienting information and relaxation. This change in the pattern of results over time could reflect changes in hospital policies and procedures. In the 1970s, hospitals established utilization review committees that impose restrictions on the range of days of hospitalization. Such restrictions may become even more stringent. Thus, length of hospital stay may not be a useful measure of the effects of even powerful preparatory interventions.

The pattern of relationships of interventions to outcome measures provides support for the idea that the two functions of coping can maintain a degree of independence from one another. The finding that interventions had a positive effect on emotional response and not on length of postoperative hospitalization suggests that the coping function of regulating emotional response is not related directly to the coping function of regulating goal-directed behavior. In other words, interventions that help patients control their emotional response may or may not facilitate their goal-directed behavior.

Further support for that conclusion was provided by data collected after patients were discharged from the hospital. Johnson, Rice, Fuller, and Endress (1978) found that interventions associated with low emotional response during hospitalization had no significant effect on indicators of resumption of usual activities after discharge from the hospital.

Relationship between Theory and the Research under Review

The data do not confirm the assumption that emotional reactions are a major problem for most surgical patients. When investigators used mood adjective checklists to quantify elective surgical patients' subjective emotional status, the patients reported low amounts of disturbance (Johnson, Fuller, Endress, & Rice, 1978; Johnson, Rice, Fuller, & Endress, 1978). On scales ranging from none to extreme emotional response, the means of negative mood scores were clustered in the lower third of the scales. This finding was verified by other researchers of surgical patients (Auerbach, 1973; Auerbach & Edinger, 1977; Christopherson & Pfeiffer, 1980; Meikle, Brody, & Pysh, 1977). The preoperative scores for negative emotional response, especially fear, were higher than postoperative scores; but in general, preoperative mean scores were close to the point on the scales labeled "a little."

It is important to take into account the possibility that patients' emotional response to surgery may not be described adequately by measures taken after admission to the hospital. Emotional reactions may be greatest at onset of symptoms or when surgery is recommended. Indecision and uncertainty often elicit emotional response. Once the decision to have surgery is made, uncertainty about the course of action is reduced and tension dissipates. Investigators who track patients' emotional state throughout the time from onset of symptoms through recovery could describe the pattern of response over time and identify if and when emotional response is a significant problem for surgical patients.

Janis' (1958) theoretical position was not tested directly in any of the studies reviewed, although the theory was referred to in reports (Egbert et al., 1964; Langer et al., 1975). A direct test of Janis' theory by Vernon and Bigelow (1974) did not support the theory. In line with the results of the studies reviewed here, Vernon and Bigelow found that patients who were provided with a description of the significant events during hospitalization were more satisfied with the information they received than uninformed patients. However, the informed patients did not differ from uninformed patients on measures of worry. Further, the prediction that patients who did and those who did not engage in problem-oriented worry would differ on postoperative measures of anger and hostility was not supported by the data.

Instruction in physical activities that patients perform to reduce risk of postoperative complications was tested by more investigators than any other intervention. The rationale most often given for the benefits of this intervention for surgical patients emphasized the need for effective teaching to increase the likelihood that patients will perform the activities after surgery (Archuleta et al., 1977; Lindeman & Van Aernam, 1971). Yet cumulative tests of the effects of the intervention on patients' performance of the behaviors and the occurrence of postoperative complications did not support this prediction. Risser (1980) concluded in an article on prevention of pulmonary complications that patient knowledge was not sufficient to assure performance of behaviors to prevent postoperative complications. The investigators who based their research on teaching-learning principles gave inadequate attention to methods of motivating patients to perform activities that cause pain. They also paid little attention to direct measures of patients' performance of the physical activities they were taught. Explanations that were limited to connections between patients' knowledge and behavior did not account for the associations between physical activity interventions and patients' self-reports of emotion and well-being, which some investigators included as outcome measures in their studies.

Each of the interventions used in the research on coping with surgery could have increased patients' feelings of personal control over aspects of the unpleasant or threatening experience. Averill (1973) concluded in a review of the research on personal control that people prefer to have control rather than to have no control. The preference for control could account for the consistent relationship in the research on surgical patients between various interventions and self-reports of emotional status and other indicators of well-being.

However, patients' preference for control did not account for the differences between effects of interventions on indicators during and after hospitalization. In a review of aftereffects of stressful situations, Cohen (1980) concluded that personal control during a stressful experience resulted in increased ability to perform tasks after the experience. The positive aftereffects occurred regardless of the nature of the effects of personal control interventions during the acute phase of a stressful experience. Cohen did not identify the specific processes that caused the positive effect on performance to occur, but the aftereffects appeared to be caused directly or indirectly by the processes used to cope with the stressful situation.

For the elective surgical patient, the time spent in the hospital could be considered the acutely stressful situation and aftereffects could be expected to appear after discharge. Resumption of usual activities could be a measure of aftereffects. If personal control during the acutely stressful experience of undergoing surgery accounts for early resumption of usual activities after hospital discharge, then perhaps interventions that do not have that effect diminish patients' sense of personal control.

Some interventions, such as instructing patients to use specific coping strategies or behaviors, may reduce patients' sense of personal control. When specific directions for means to cope are given to patients, they may feel that their choice of strategies or behaviors is restricted and that they must use only those that have been recommended. Such dictates from providers could undermine patients' confidence in the coping strategies and behaviors they have found to be effective in the past. Although patients who receive such interventions may report satisfaction and a sense of well-being during the acutely stressful phase of the experience, their confidence in their previously existing abilities may be undermined. The lack of confidence may be reflected in their reluctance to resume usual activities after discharge from the hospital.

A consistent result that appeared in the research was that interventions that combined orienting information and instruction in behaviors or strategies to prevent or overcome a problem during hospitalization were more effective than each type of intervention by itself. For patients whose self-confidence might be undermined by specific prescriptions for behaviors or strategies, the orienting information may have reduced that negative effect by also allowing them to rely on existing coping abilities.

The concrete orienting information interventions lessened the postdischarge impact of hospitalization for surgery. The aftereffects of concrete orienting information interventions could have been a result of the types of coping processes used by patients who received such interventions. The descriptions in these interventions allowed patients to predict their postoperative experiences on a sensory level and to predict when events would occur and how long they would last. Additionally, the descriptions could have helped patients to interpret the meaning of their experiences. Patients may have found similarities between the descriptions of present and past experiences. Enhancement of patients' ability to predict and interpret their experiences could have fostered feelings of personal control. Identification of similarities between past experiences and their new experiences could have increased patients' confidence in their existing coping strategies. Coping processes stimulated by feelings of control and confidence in existing coping strategies could explain the early resumption of usual activities by patients who received concrete orienting information interventions.

The above explanations of the ways in which concrete orienting information can ameliorate the aftereffects of hospitalization for surgery were not tested directly. Wilson (1981) reported data that lent some support to the explanations in that all of the patients who received concrete orienting information desired similar information if they were hospitalized again.

The consistent finding of a relationship between various types of interventions and self-reports of satisfaction, well-being, and emotional status implies that many of the interventions shared a common element. Perhaps that common element was personal interest conveyed by researchers who gave individual attention and provided relevant information or instruction. Although investigators have not related their research to the theory of psychological reactance (Brehm, 1966), the theory would predict that relationship. According to Brehm, reactance is experienced when a specific freedom is threatened, and a person experiencing reactance is prone to aggressive behavior. Surgical patients entering the hospital may be concerned about restrictions on their freedom to obtain the information they want or need. When surgical patients are provided with information that they perceive to be relevant to their situation, the threat to the freedom to obtain information could be reduced or eliminated. The reduction of any threats to freedom could minimize negative psychological response in surgical patients.

Conclusions

The following general conclusions are drawn from the research on elective surgical patients.

1. Interventions that provided (a) descriptions of the impending experiences, and/or (b) instruction in coping strategies or behaviors had a positive effect on reactions to and recovery from surgery.
2. Short- and long-term effects of preparatory interventions followed different patterns.
3. Hypotheses based on the assumption that emotional response mediates goal-directed behavior were not supported by the research.
4. Research based on teaching-learning principles contributed little to knowledge of the processes involved in coping with surgery or preventing postoperative complications.
5. The concept of personal control appears to be relevant to coping with surgery, but further research is needed to identify (a) coping processes stimulated by personal control, and (b) the characteristics of interventions that enhance surgical patients' sense of personal control.

SUGGESTIONS FOR FUTURE RESEARCH

More theoretically oriented research is required before a description of the processes of coping with surgery can be developed. The emphasis on theoretical explanations in this review may be useful to the development of such a description. Investigators interested in contributing to the description of coping with surgery should give consideration to the reasons why a particular intervention might be expected to affect a specific coping function. The research contribution will be enhanced when the processes that the intervention is expected to stimulate are assessed. There is also a need for attention to the relationships of outcome measures to the functions of coping. Reliable and valid outcome measures are essential to theory development. Investigators who consider patients' responses after discharge as well as during hospitalization will increase the usefulness and comprehensiveness of their contributions. Clarification of theoretical issues can be enhanced by the use of designs that allow evaluation of the main effects of an intervention, as well as the interactions between interventions.

Individual differences in the population of surgical patients are a fruitful area for investigation. Particularly relevant is research into differences in patients' perceived ability to exert control over aspects of the experience and their need or preference for exerting such control. Differences in the nature of demands made on patients at different stages of the experience of undergoing surgery should also be taken into account.

The research designs should provide straightforward tests of hypotheses or answers to questions. Internal validity of the studies is of great importance. A major threat to the internal validity of future research with surgical patients is the rapidly spreading practice of providing patients with some type of preparatory intervention. It will be difficult to insure that the preparation which the comparison group receives differs in a specific dimension from that given the experimental groups. Although usual practice activities cannot be withheld, researchers can provide the usual practice intervention to control group patients and, in that way, insure that the control and experimental groups differ with regard to the specific dimension of interest. In spite of the problem presented by change in usual practice, productive research still can be done by using theoretically oriented interventions, measures of processes stimulated by interventions, and outcome measures that are both theoretically relevant and sensitive to patients' responses.

Future studies of surgical patients require complex designs that include more than one manipulated variable, measurement of individual differences in personality and demographic factors, and consideration of clinical variables such as type of surgery. Multiple outcome variables, some measured on more than one occasion, probably will continue to be used. Analyses of data from studies with such complex designs will require sophisticated statistical techniques. Multiple regression, multivariate analyses of variance, and time-series analyses are examples of statistical procedures that investigators will find appropriate for the analysis of their data. The use of such appropriate analytical procedures increases confidence in the results of studies, thereby increasing the value of the research.

The first study of a preparatory intervention for surgical patients was published two decades ago (Dumas & Leonard, 1963). Since that time, a sizeable body of research has been generated. For the most part, the investigators presented an atheoretical orientation in their research. This atheoretical approach contributed to the current situation in which there remain many unanswered practical questions about the composition of interventions and their effects on coping with surgery. Since a good theory is very practical, theoretically oriented research has promise for providing answers to many practical questions about the preparation of surgical patients. Confirmed theory about coping with surgery has potential for generalization to other stressful health care experiences. Perhaps this review will stimulate investigators to contribute to the development of a theory of coping with stressful health care experiences, which can be used to guide nursing management of patients in many situations.

REFERENCES

Archuleta, V., Plummer, O. B., & Hopkins, K. D. *A demonstration model for patient education: A model for the project training nurses to improve patient education.* Boulder, Colo.: Western Interstate Commission for Higher Education, 1977.

Auerbach, S. M. Trait-state anxiety and adjustment to surgery. *Journal of Consulting and Clinical Psychology,* 1973, *40,* 264–271.

Auerbach, S. M., & Edinger, J. D. The effects of surgery-induced stress on anxiety as measured by the Haltzman ink blot technique. *Journal of Personality Assessment,* 1977, *41,* 19–24.

Averill, J. R. Personal control over aversive stimuli and its relationship to stress. *Psychological Bulletin,* 1973, *80,* 286–303.

Bonilla, K. B., Quigley, W. F., & Bowers, W. F. Experiences with hypnosis on a surgical service. *Military Medicine,* 1961, *126,* 364–370.

Brehm, J. W. *A theory of psychological reactance.* New York: Academic Press, 1966.

Burckhardt, C. S., Goodwin, L. S., & Prescott, P. A. The measurement of change in nursing research: Statistical considerations. *Nursing Research,* 1982, *31,* 53–55.

Carrieri, V. Effect of an experimental teaching program on postoperative ventilatory capacity. In M. V. Batey (Ed.), *Communicating nursing research: Critical issues in access to data* (Vol. 7). Boulder, Colo.: Western Interstate Commission for Higher Education, 1975.

Christopherson, B., & Pfeiffer, C. Varying the timing of information to alter preoperative anxiety and postoperative recovery in cardiac surgery patients. *Heart and Lung,* 1980, *9,* 854–861.

Cohen, S. Aftereffects of stress on human performance and social behavior: A review of research and theory. *Psychological Bulletin,* 1980, *88,* 82–108.

Dumas, R. G., & Johnson, B. A. Research in nursing practice: A review of five clinical experiments. *International Journal of Nursing Studies*, 1972, *9*, 137–149.

Dumas, R. G., & Leonard, R. C. The effects of nursing on the incidence of postoperative vomiting. *Nursing Research*, 1963, *12*, 12–15.

Egbert, L. D., Battit, G. E., Welch, C. E., & Bartlett, M. K. Reduction of postoperative pain by encouragement and instruction of patients. *The New England Journal of Medicine*, 1964, *270*, 825–827.

Felton, G., Huss, K., Payne, E. A., & Srsic, K. Preoperative nursing intervention with the patient for surgery: Outcomes of three alternative approaches. *International Journal of Nursing Studies*, 1976, *13*, 83–96.

Field, P. B. Effects of tape-recorded hypnotic preparation for surgery. *The International Journal of Clinical and Experimental Hypnosis*, 1974, *22*, 54–61.

Flaherty, G. G., & Fitzpatrick, J. J. Relaxation technique to increase comfort level of postoperative patients: A preliminary study. *Nursing Research*, 1978, *27*, 352–355.

Fortin, F., & Kirouac, S. A randomized controlled trial of preoperative patient education. *International Journal of Nursing Studies*, 1976, *13*, 11–24.

Healy, K. M. Does preoperative instruction make a difference? *American Journal of Nursing*, 1968, *68*, 62–67.

Hegyvary, S. T., & Chamings, P. A. The hospital setting and patient care outcomes. Part 1. *Journal of Nursing Administration*, 1975, *5*(3), 29–32. (a)

Hegyvary, S. T., & Chamings, P. A. The hospital setting and patient care outcomes: Part 2. *Journal of Nursing Administration*, 1975, *5*(4), 36–42. (b)

Hill, B. J. Sensory information, behavioral instructions and coping with sensory alteration surgery. *Nursing Research*, 1982, *31*, 17–21.

Janis, I. J. *Psychological stress*. New York: Wiley, 1958.

Johnson, J. E., Fuller, S. S., Endress, M. P., & Rice, V. H. Altering patients' responses to surgery: An extension and replication. *Research in Nursing and Health*, 1978, *1*, 111–121.

Johnson, J. E., Rice, V. H., Fuller, S. S., & Endress. M. P. Sensory information, instruction in a coping strategy, and recovery from surgery. *Research in Nursing and Health*, 1978, *1*, 4–17.

Kimble, G. A., & Garmezy, N. *Principles of general psychology* (2nd ed.). New York: Ronald Press, 1963.

King, I., & Tarsitano, B. The effect of structured and unstructured preoperative teaching: A replication. *Nursing Research*, 1982, *31*, 324–329.

Langer, E. J., Janis, I. L., & Wolfer, J. A. Reduction of psychological stress in surgical patients. *Journal of Experimental Social Psychology*, 1975, *11*, 155–165.

Lazarus, R. S., & Launier, R. Stress-related transactions between person and environment. In L. A. Pervin & M. Lewis (Eds.), *Perspectives of interactional psychology*. New York: Plenum Press, 1978.

Leithauser, D. J., & Bergo, H. L. Early rising and ambulatory activity after operation: A means of preventing complications. *Archives of Surgery*, 1941, *42*, 1086–1093.

Leventhal, H. Findings and theory in the study of fear communication. In L. Berkowitz (Ed.), *Advances in experimental social psychology* (Vol. 5). New York: Academic Press, 1970.

Lindeman, C. A., & Van Aernam, B. Nursing intervention with the presurgical patient: The effects of structured and unstructured preoperative teaching. *Nursing Research*, 1971, *20*, 319–332.

McHugh, N. G., Christman, N. J., & Johnson, J. E. Preparatory information: What helps and why. *American Journal of Nursing*, 1982, *82*, 780–782.

Meikle, S., Brody, H., & Pysh, F. An investigation into the psychological effects of hysterectomy. *The Journal of Nervous and Mental Disease*, 1977, *164*, 36–41.

Mumford, E., Schlesinger, H. J., & Glass, G. V. The effects of psychological intervention on recovery from surgery and heart attacks: An analysis of the literature. *American Journal of Public Health*, 1982, *72*, 141–151.

Risser, N. L. Preoperative and postoperative care to prevent pulmonary complications. *Heart and Lung*, 1980, *9*, 57–67.

Schmitt, F. E., & Wooldridge, P. J. Psychological preparation of surgical patients. *Nursing Research*, 1973, *22*, 108–115.

Vernon, T. A., & Bigelow, D. A. Effect of information about a potentially stressful situation on responses to stress impact. *Journal of Personality and Social Psychology*, 1974, *29*, 50–59.

Wells, N. The effect of relaxation on postoperative muscle tension and pain. *Nursing Research*, 1982, *31*, 236–238.

Wilson, J. F. Behavioral preparation for surgery: Benefit or harm? *Journal of Behavioral Medicine*, 1981, *4*, 79–102.

PART II

Research on Nursing Care Delivery

CHAPTER 6

Assessment of Quality
of Nursing Care

Norma M. Lang
AND
Jacqueline F. Clinton
School of Nursing
University of Wisconsin-Milwaukee

CONTENTS

There has been formal interest in the assessment and assurance of the quality of nursing care since Florence Nightingale (1858) used a set of standards to assess the care provided during the Crimean War. By comparing mortality experience in the British armed forces during the Crimean War with experience in civilian populations, Nightingale (1858) forcefully

The authors wish to acknowledge Susan J. Hanus, for editorial assistance, and graduate students Marge Balzer, Linda Walters, Jane Maskrey, Marian Hein, Marynell Heier, and Bruce Schmidt from the University of Wisconsin–Milwaukee Center for Nursing Research and Evaluation for their assistance in coding of articles.

135

brought to the attention of the government and the public the atrocious standards of care for military personnel. Although by today's standards the data were crude, the report was instrumental in bringing about substantial reforms in the living standards and health services for the armed forces.

Objective and systematic evaluation of nursing care has continued to be a priority within the nursing profession. Reports of such studies have increased during the past decade. Among the stimuli for this priority were the public's concern about the quality and spiraling cost of health services, nursing's commitment to direct accountability to the public, its evolution as a scientific discipline, and nurses' increasing involvement in shaping both public as well as individual health agency policies.

In the first part of this critical review chapter, the authors describe a few selected early studies. These references were selected on the basis of being representative of the state of the art for that period of time and on the basis that each was referenced frequently in subsequent publications. For a more extensive review of the literature, the reader is referred to Lang's (1980) Nurse Planning Series Volume 12, *Quality Assurance in Nursing: A Selected Bibliography* which contains 367 abstracts classified according to types of foci of the studies. The second part of this chapter includes a critical review of empirical work from 1974 to 1982 designed to assess the quality of nursing care. Finally, the chapter contains a summary and overall recommendations for future research.

EARLY STUDIES

Standards for nursing practice long have been sought and are still in the process of evolution. From 1950 to 1954, Reiter and Kakosh (Note 1) conducted a study in which they attempted to establish reliable, valid, objective, and usable criteria for the appraisal of nursing care. Criteria were expected to be useful to hospital nursing administrators, nurse educators, and nurse practitioners because of the description of ongoing patient care and indications given of possible and desirable goals toward which the nursing profession might direct its attention. Although the Reiter and Kakosh pioneering study was done in the early 1950s, it was not widely adopted nor replicated.

Another early effort in developing criteria for nursing care was undertaken by Aydelotte and Tener (Note 2) who identified specific behavioral and physical characteristics of patients as indicators of patient welfare. The investigators established outcome criteria in terms of patient welfare statements and structure criteria in terms of a staffing pattern and staff development; they tested the relationship between the two sets of criteria. The findings of the study did not support a significant relationship between structural variables and patient outcomes.

The need to develop outcome criterion measures to assess the effect of nursing practice on patients' progress was emphasized by Abdellah (1961), Brodt and Anderson (1967), Diers (1973), Hagen (1972), and Zimmer (1974). Lindeman (1975) considered the determination of reliable and valid indicators of quality nursing care as the first priority for investigating nursing impact on patient welfare. The measurement of the quality of care was established as the priority for targeted research efforts of the Western Interstate Commission for Higher Education (WICHE) Regional Program for Nursing Research Development (Krueger, 1980).

The Nursing Audit, after a long period of development, was published by Phaneuf (1976); it has been in use for over 20 years. The audit tool, based upon seven legal functions of nursing, measures the quality of nursing care received by a patient after a cycle of care was completed and the patient was discharged. Records of patients are used and the retrospective audit is conducted by peer professional nurses.

The Slater Nursing Competencies Rating Scale (Wandelt & Stewart, 1975) was developed for measuring the competencies displayed by a nurse when delivering care. The instrument is used by professional peer nurses in direct observation of nurses delivering nursing care.

The Quality Patient Care Scale (QualPac) is an instrument consisting of 68 items developed by Wandelt and Ager (1974) to measure the quality of nursing care received by a patient while care is ongoing. Peer professional nurses use direct observation of the care received by patients. The QualPac instrument measures the following aspects of nursing care: Psychosocial Individual (15 items), Psychosocial Group (8 items), Physical (15 items), General (15 items), Communication (8 items), and Professional Implications (7 items).

The Rush-Medicus System (Haussmann, Hegyvary, Newman, & Bishop, 1974; Hegyvary & Haussmann, 1976a; Jelinek, Haussmann, Hegyvary, & Newman, 1974) instrument consists of 257 items applicable to medical, surgical, and pediatric units, as well as to normal newborn nurseries and recovery rooms. There are 205 patient-specific items; the remaining 52 items are unit-specific. The items were grouped into homogenous clusters to define these six nursing objectives: Plan of Care is

Formulated (30 items), Physical Needs are Attended (69 items), Nonphysical Needs are Attended (46 items), Achievement of Objectives is Evaluated (11 items), Unit Procedures are Followed for the Protection of All Patients (8 items), and Delivery of Nursing Care is Facilitated by Administrative and Managerial Services (43 items). These six objectives were further delineated into 28 subobjectives. Each individual subobjective was considered an independent characteristic for which a performance measure can be obtained. Patients were classified as types I, II, III, or IV according to their level of self-sufficiency. Each item used was coded according to the type of patient to which it was most applicable.

EMPIRICAL STUDIES, 1974 TO 1982

The authors undertook a survey of the literature to determine the scope of empirical works that were published from 1974 to 1982. The survey involved literature search, abstracting, and critique. Studies were identified by computer and manual searches of literature in nursing and other health-related fields. Computer sources included Medline, National Health Standards and Quality Information Clearinghouse, Lockheed System's DIALOG, the Division of Nursing's National Health Planning Information Center, and the National Technical Information Service. Manual searches included the *Cumulative Nursing Index* and the *International Nursing Index*.

Criteria for inclusion of a study in the survey were that reports must: (a) be systematic, (b) involve data collection, (c) present findings, and (d) be written or translated into English. Purely theoretical manuscripts or ones limited to reporting research in progress were not included. The publications that were excluded numbered well over a thousand.

A content analysis tool was developed to code the characteristics of each empirical study. Items were designed to capture the various structure, process, and outcome elements measured or manipulated in a study; type of design and analyses; clinical area(s) where study was conducted; and factors identified as promoting or impeding quality of nursing care. Inter-rater reliability was established early in the study by having all raters code the same random sample of studies. The overall average for interrater reliability across all coders and all items reported herein was 93.5% agreement and ranged from 84.4% to 100% agreement.

GENERAL FINDINGS

A total of 164 research reports assessing quality of nursing care published since 1974 met the criteria for inclusion in this review. The majority of studies (82%) were conducted in the United States. The remainder originated from Canada, Europe, Australia, Israel, and Haiti. While nurse investigators carried out most of these nursing studies (78%), a substantial proportion (22%) were done by nonnurses.

The distribution of studies by type of research design was as follows: descriptive survey (48%), quasi-experimental (24%), experimental (10%), and tool development (18%). This distribution was relatively comparable across all clinical specialty areas including parent-child nursing, community health nursing, psychiatric/mental health nursing, gerontological nursing, and nursing of the adult. A detailed review of nursing quality assurance research specific to each clinical specialty is available in Lang and Clinton (1983). Descriptive surveys on a single group of subjects were predominant. There were few comparative studies. In the studies devoted solely to instrument development and testing, almost half (45%) of the investigators used existing tools for measuring quality of nursing care or additional quality indicators developed in other disciplines. What this reflects is that researchers actively are using and accumulating further knowledge on tools for assessing quality of nursing care developed in the 1960s and early 1970s by pioneers like Aydelotte and Tener (Note 2), Phaneuf (1976), Wandelt and Ager (1974), and Haussman et al. (1974). A small proportion of the studies can be considered true experiments in that randomization and successful control of confounding variables were achieved. Although the vast majority of studies contained quantified data, only half of the investigators (51%) submitted data to inferential testing as a basis for conclusions and recommendations.

The extent to which investigators tested the instruments they used for reliability and validity was coded. Investigators differed markedly in these two dimensions. Some made no mention of reliability or validity. Others assumed that tools developed and tested on one population would be reliable and valid for a different population. Still others conducted rigorous testing such as is found in those studies conducted by Ventura, Hageman, Slakter, and Fox (1980, 1982) on numerous quality of nursing care indices and in those done by Hinshaw and Atwood (1982) on patient satisfaction.

In the following sections, studies are reviewed according to seven single and multifocused categories: (a) structure, (b) process, (c) outcome,

(d) structure-process, (e) structure-outcome, (f) process-outcome, and (g) structure-process-outcome. Major variables for each category are described.

Structure Studies

Of all the studies in which researchers focused on structure, those in which investigators measured financial resources or cost (17%) are most eagerly sought by nurses and health policymakers. Table 6–1 shows the specific cost analyses done and the studies in which they were reported. In all but three studies, the investigators demonstrated that health care costs can be reduced while quality of care is improved or maintained. It is interesting to note that Fagin (1982) reached similar conclusions when she documented the economic value of nursing research.

Researchers primarily concerned with other structural aspects of quality assurance focused on variables such as profit and ownership status, human and hardware resources and utilization, level of nursing care requirements for different patient populations, interdisciplinary collaboration, program implementation, clinician competency, and clinician perceptions of nursing practice and quality assurance. Profit status and ownership of nursing homes were investigated by Greene and Monahan (1981) who found that for-profit and distantly headquartered chain operations provided lower levels of care than nonprofit, locally owned nursing homes. The use of contracts with temporary nurse employment agencies and orientation standards for registry nurses reported by Sheridan, Bronstein, and Walker (1982) insured competency and resulted in cost savings. Jacoby and Kindig (1975) developed a task analysis methodology for nurses and physicians which was useful in improving personnel management in clinics. The use of nurse practitioners in clinics combined with an interactive video communication system for physician consultation was found feasible and economically efficient by Sanders, Sasmor, and Natiello (1976). Kane, Rubenstein, Brook, Van Ryzin, Masthay, Schoenrich, and Harrell (1981) found that a tool for measuring level of nursing care requirements in nursing homes was highly reliable and useful in reducing workload demands for skilled professional judgment. Using the Automatic Interactive Detection program developed by Sonquist (Note 3), Trivedi (1979) found that only a few patient classification variables were necessary for distinguishing between various levels of nursing care time requirements in the hospital setting. Furthermore, different sets of patient classification variables were essential for different shifts on the same nursing unit.

Table 6–1. Investigators Assessing Quality of Nursing Care That Included Cost Analysis: 1974 to 1982

Cost Factor Measured	Studies
Health Care Agency Expenditures	
salaries	Feldman, Taller, Garfield, Collen, Richart, Cella, & Sender, 1977
	DeAngelis & McHugh, 1977
	Soghikian, 1978
	Hastings, Vick, Lee, Sasmor, Natiello, & Sanders, 1980
	Salkever, Skinner, Steinwachs, & Katz, 1982
nurse absenteeism and turnover	Droessler & Maibusch, 1979
	Fairbanks, 1981
unscheduled overtime and sick pay	Roberts, 1980
temporary nursing personnel	Sheridan, Bronstein, & Walker, 1982
supplies	Droessler & Maibusch, 1979
patient care episode costs	King, Fougere, Webb, Berggren, & Berggren, 1978
	Hastings, Vick, Lee, Sasmor, Natiello, & Sanders, 1980
patient day costs	Felton, 1975
administrative expenditures	Greene & Monahan, 1981
audit costs	Trussell & Strand, 1978
patient education costs	Crabtree, 1978
Health Services Utilization Costs	
length of stay	Fujimoto, Fareau, Forsman, & Wilson, 1978
hospitalization rate	Ginsberg & Marks, 1977
	Fujimoto, Fareau, Forsman, & Wilson, 1978
emergency room use	Fujimoto, Fareau, Forsman, & Wilson, 1978
clinic visit costs	Feldman, Taller, Garfield, Collen, Richart, Cella, & Sender, 1977
	Soghikian, 1978
	Salkever, Skinner, Steinwachs, & Katz, 1982

Quality benefits derived from interdisciplinary collaboration were documented by Vaughan and Large (1976) and Robertson, McDonnell, and Scott (1976). Quality assurance program implementation strategies in the mental health setting were outlined by Forquer and Anderson (1982) based on their survey of clinicians' concerns about what quality assurance would mean for their job tasks and impact on patients. Tools for measuring clinical competency in nurses were developed and tested by Ibrahim, Wagner, Williams, Greenberg, and Kleinbaum (1978) and McLaughlin, Carr, and Delucchi (1979). Role strain experienced by nurses was a major deterrent to high quality nursing care in the hospital setting where nurses' views of nursing practice conflicted with views of patients and physicians (Hinshaw & Oakes, 1977). Finally, a national survey of perceived quality assurance needs in public health nursing revealed differences related to type and size of agency and methods in use for assessing quality of care (Januska, Engle, & Wood, 1976).

It is noteworthy that no investigators assessing quality of nursing care used nursing diagnosis to classify patients. Because the theoretical emphasis on nursing diagnosis has increased dramatically, empirical studies structured around nursing diagnosis should be expected to increase. The relationship between other patient classifications and quality assessment also requires attention. At a minimum, accuracy of diagnosis or classification should be examined. In addition, the relationship of nursing interventions to the specific classification and the resulting outcomes are important topics for study.

Process Studies

Instrument development and testing was the predominant theme of studies in which investigators addressed solely the process component of quality nursing care. A major example was the Rush-Medicus Nursing Process Monitoring Methodology (Hegyvary, Haussmann, Kronman, & Burke, 1979) which was described previously. Extensive reliability and predictive validity testing of several process measures was conducted by Ventura, Hageman, Slakter, and Fox (1982) using different patient populations. The need for routine interrater reliability testing prior to data collection was demonstrated for both the Rush-Medicus and QualPacs instruments (Ventura et al., 1980). A solution to interrater reliability issues with QualPacs was tested by Ventura and Crosby (1978), who developed an instruction program for increasing nurse competencies in administering the tool. Concurrent application of the Rush-Medicus and QualPacs instruments revealed no association between their physical and psychosocial subscales, which suggested that the tools measured different dimensions of quality of the nursing process (Ventura, Hageman, Slakter, & Fox, 1982). A lack of association also was found between QualPacs data and Phaneuf audit data from the same sample that reflected differences between retrospective and concurrent data sources (Ventura, 1980).

Weinstein (1976) developed the Selected Attribute Variable Evaluator (SAVE) for pediatric units based on QualPacs. Schwirian (1978) tested a self-administered nurse performance scale that included six dimensions: leadership, critical care, teaching and collaboration, planning and evaluation, interpersonal communication, and professional development. Aldhizer, Solle, and Bohrer (1979) created a multidisciplinary audit tool for evaluating care and treatment of diabetics in both inpatient and ambulatory settings. The Doncaster Nursing Management Audit, the first to be developed in Great Britain (Huczynski, 1977), included multiple indicators of nursing practice and clinical teaching.

A second theme of process-only research was evaluation of more specific indicators of care. Galton and Reilly (1977) evaluated six areas of nursing care provided to terminally ill cancer patients and found that the lowest scores were achieved in the category of patient comfort. Goodman and Perrin (1978) reported that nurse practitioners can manage acute illnesses competently over the telephone.

Outcome Studies

Considerable research effort was devoted to generating nursing outcome measures, that is, patient indices thought to be amenable to nursing influence. A major focus of these studies was patient health knowledge, related behaviors, and self-care skills. Horn and Swain (1978) developed 539 outcome criterion measures reflecting 8 universal and 10 health deviation self-care demand categories. In addition, 414 of these measures were tested with adult, medical-surgical, hospitalized patients. Of these measurements, 328 were related to the universal demands for air, food, elimination, water, rest/activity/sleep, solitude and social interaction, and normality. The health deviation section of the instrument included descriptions of intravenous and wound observations, patients' knowledge and self-care abilities relative to their health problems, their medications, therapeutic diet and fluid intake, prescribed rehabilitative exercises, restrictions on physical activity, skin and wound care, the use of special appliances, and recommended rest. The objective of the research was to develop, refine, and validate measures of the quality of nursing care. The validated measurement items and an instrument for matching observer techniques to particular patients were included in the investigators' final report. This extensive Horn-Swain instrument should be given serious consideration by researchers attempting to measure outcomes of patient care.

Gallant and McLane (1979) tested the Patient Self-Rating Scale for use by patients and nurses to assess patients' health knowledge and self-care skills. Self-care outcomes for use in residents of extended care facilities were created by Howe, Coulton, Almon and Sandrick (1980).

Another focus in the development of patient outcomes was measurement of nurse-influenced iatrogenesis from disease and medical treatment. For example, the Sickness Impact Profile (Gilson, Gilson, Bergner, Bobbitt, Kressel, Pollard, & Vesselago, 1975) incorporates both professional and lay perspectives of the disabling effects of illness. Derdiarian (1977) tested measures of independence/dependence among adults experiencing stress from illness and hospitalization. The Patient Indicators of Nursing Care (PINC) instrument developed by Majesky, Brester, and Nishio (1978) contained physiological measures of complications in hospitalized samples. Lewis, Firsich, and Parsell (1979) presented a tool measuring physical, psychological, and functional outcomes for adult cancer patients receiving extended chemotherapy treatment in inpatient and outpatient settings. A tool for measuring medication-taking behavior of the elderly was developed by Lundin (1978). Measures of parenting skills, coping, and couples' perceptions of pregnancy were tested by Blair, Hauf, Loveridge, Murphy, and Roth (1978).

Affective and behavioral status was another category of patient outcomes explored by nurse researchers. Measures of morale and behavior were developed for use with patients on a home dialysis program (MacElveen, 1977). A Goal Attainment Scale which contained measures of affective, cognitive, and behavioral functioning was applied in the inpatient psychiatric setting by Guy and Moore (1982). Ward and Lindeman (1978) compiled a collection of data-gathering devices measuring various patient indices including affective, cognitive, and physical status. In the area of patient satisfaction, Hinshaw and Atwood (1982) reported a summary of extensive testing of their Patient Satisfaction Instrument containing three factors: technical-professional care, trust, and patient education.

Among the numerous studies in which investigators included outcome measures, only Carey and Posavec (1978) applied repeated measures methodology. They reported the results of a time-series study testing the usefulness of the LORS (Level of Rehabilitation Scale) for monitoring progress of stroke victims. Because the nature of nursing is continuous over time in most settings, the monitoring of outcome achievement over time increasingly should become a part of nursing quality assessment research, regardless of the criterion measures being applied. We also recommend that researchers be more specific in documenting critical points in time when outcomes are measured and the rationale used in making such decisions. Both of these recommendations are geared toward maximizing the potential for documenting nursing's impact on patient welfare.

Structure-Process Studies

The most comprehensive study of the relationship between structural characteristics and the process of nursing care in the hospital setting was done by Hegyvary and Haussmann (1976b). Structural measures included five components: facility characteristics, unit organization structure, unit staff perceptions and attitudes, supervisor perceptions and expectations, and nursing staff education. Using the Rush-Medicus instrument (Hegyvary et al., 1979) for measuring quality of nursing care provided, they found that quality of nursing care was correlated positively with primary nursing, extensive coordination of services, flexible and sensitive leadership, clinical orientation of staff, acceptance of change by supervisors, and higher level of education among registered nurses. Quality of care was associated negatively with unit size, average census, licensed practical nurse and nurse aide hours per patient day, and level of satisfaction among supervisory staff.

Implementation and evaluation of standards for nursing practice was a major theme of studies in which researchers examined structure and process. Dyer, Monson, and Cope (1975) found that quality of nursing care provided to psychiatric patients was associated positively with overall ward atmosphere but unrelated to a career counseling protocol used to assist nurses in their jobs. The implementation of criteria for personalizing nursing care in the hospital setting resulted in more personalized care planning (Joyce, 1977). Dunn (1977) demonstrated that the use of standardized care plans in the hospital setting resulted in better documentation of nursing care. An audit tool developed by Huczynski (1977) for self-assessment of nursing performance helped nurses improve their own care. Inservice education on documentation of care and patient teaching for nurses resulted in better utilization of care plans (Distel, 1981b; Girouard, 1978; Kass, 1981). Mackley, Heslop, and McAllister (1979) made observations of the nursing time required by hospitalized patients experiencing varying degrees of helplessness which led to the generation of standards for basic nursing procedures. Rothman and Saunders (1982) developed standards that improved care to dying patients in a psychiatric facility. Mech (1980) surveyed long-term care facilities and showed that patients with similar nursing care requirements received care that was uneven in quality. The implementation of criteria for hospital discharge and standards for discharge planning increased the number and quality of nurse referrals (Dake, 1981). Criteria for early screening, diagnosis, and treatment in well-child clinics led to better case management by nurses (Nassif, Garfink, & Greenfield, 1982).

Organization of nursing care at the unit level constituted another category of studies in which structure and process were linked. Evaluation of primary nursing on a pediatric unit by Felton (1975) resulted in higher quality of care received by patients and increased clinical competency among nurses at lower cost per patient day. Eichhorn and Frevert (1979) conducted a longitudinal study of primary nursing in four surgical units which yielded mixed findings: quality of care did not change in pediatric units but did improve on a burn unit. In a comparison of team and primary nursing, Shukla (1981) found no differences in quality of care given to patients or in nurse competencies. Hamera and O'Connell (1981) found no differences in nurturance, patient involvement, and frequency of nurse-patient contact between primary and team nursing. Harman (1975) found that quality of nursing care provided to patients was no different in units with an all-registered nurse (RN) staff compared to those staffed with both RNs and nurse aides. Montgomery and Kelly (1979) established a relationship between patient care quality and difficulty of patient care assignments that was useful in determining staffing needs.

Conflicting findings on the effects of shift length of nurses on quality of care were reported. Eaton and Gottselig (1980) found no differences in quality of care (measured by the Phaneuf audit) on units with 8-hour versus 12-hour shifts. A later study by Vik and MacKay (1982) showed that quality of nursing care (measured with QualPacs) was significantly higher on units with 8-hour shifts compared to those with 12-hour shifts.

The relationship between health care provider characteristics and setting (both elements of structure) and quality of care process also was investigated. The quality of care delivered by nurses was measured by several investigators who utilized medical criteria. Moscovice (1978) examined the influence of educational levels and practice settings on nurses' medical management of patients with otitis media and urinary tract infection and found no differences in quality of medical management of otitis media between family nurse practitioners and RNs without advanced education. Differences were found in the treatment of urinary tract infection; registered nurses were more inclined to use antibiotics without laboratory tests. Patterns of care were influenced significantly by the practice setting in both groups. In a study of five family practice settings before and after attachment of a family practice nurse, Chambers, Burke, Ross, and Cantwell (1978) detected no nursing influence on the quality of medical management. In each of the studies, however, the quality of nursing care was not assessed. The lack of nursing criteria and their measurement is a severe limitation in most evaluation studies of nurse practitioners.

Prescott and Driscoll (1980) discussed concerns about studies in which investigators did not measure nursing explicitly. In their analysis of nurse practitioner studies, they concluded that investigators commonly compared nurse practitioners' performance with physicians' performance rather than using explicit nursing criteria. This approach implied that physician practice was generally an adequate and acceptable standard against which to compare nurse performance. Two problems were inherent in this type of study. One problem was illustrated by Brook as reported in Prescott and Driscoll (1980). Brook concluded that of nearly 1,100 studies of physician performance, virtually all detected basic problems in the level of quality delivered. When nurse performance was compared with a questionable physician standard of performance, Prescott and Driscoll (1980) questioned the validity of the study. The second problem was the need for explicit standards and criteria that reflect nursing process and outcome variables.

In a study of the quality of care measured by medical criteria, Goldberg and Jolly (1980) found that the same quality of care can be achieved by primary nurse practitioners and physicians' assistants. Elhai (1981) reported that lay paramedics do as good a job at history taking and routine gynecological examination as nurse practitioners. The influence of demographic and professional characteristics of nurses on quality of job performance was investigated by DiMarco and Hilliard (1978) and Koerner (1981).

Other researchers looking at the relationship between structure and process reported improvements in nursing care and documentation resulting from the implementation of standards and mechanisms for monitoring quality of care (Ayer, 1978; Feuerstein, 1978; Mast, 1978). Trussell and Strand (1978) determined that concurrent audit of nursing care quality cost twice as much as retrospective audit.

Structure-Outcome Studies

The majority of researchers examining the relationship between structure and outcome evaluated patient responses and human resource requirements that occurred when changes were made in how nursing care was delivered or how health personnel and programs were organized. Evaluation of nursing assignment patterns was one theme dominated by comparisons of team and primary nursing. Jones (1975) documented that primary nursing decreased physical complications and length of hospital stay in renal transplant patients. McCarthy and Schifalacqua (1978) found that patients' opinions about quality of nursing care were significantly more positive with primary nursing than with team nursing and that nurse turnover decreased with the implementation of primary nursing. Equal levels of patient satisfaction with team and primary nursing were reported by Ventura, Fox, Corley, and Mercurio (1982), as well as Roberts (1980), who also documented a higher level of nurse satisfaction, increased continuity of care, and no additional staffing requirements for primary nursing units. Simultaneous implementation of a unit management system and clinical nurse specialist resulted in more positive patient opinions of quality nursing care (Hardy, 1977).

   In another group of structure-outcome studies researchers evaluated the impact of the nurse practitioner. Introduction of nurse practitioners in ambulatory medical clinics resulted in comparable patient and physician satisfaction with care and improved nurse satisfaction (Garfield, Collen, Feldman, Soghikian, Richart, & Duncan, 1976). Counseling of neurotics by nurse psychotherapists resulted in a decrease in psychopathology, use of health services, costs for extra help to manage the home, and time missed from work by relatives while improving ability to maintain employment and engage in leisure activities (Ginsberg & Marks, 1977). In Israel, the use of nurse practitioners in primary medical clinics resulted in significant increases in patient reliance on nursing judgments (Yodfat, Fidel, & Eliakim, 1977). Chambers and West (1978) found that patients treated by family nurse practitioners had a higher physical functioning status and equal levels of emotional and social functioning compared to those treated by family practice physicians. In another comparison of nurse practitioner and physician performance, Soghikian (1978) found that blood pressure reduction in hypertensives and patient satisfaction were equal in both groups. Zikmund and Miller (1979) surveyed patient attitudes toward nurse practitioner competency and concluded that competency generally was accepted by patients, but the nurse practitioner's ability to diagnose correctly was doubted.

   In a third category of studies, researchers investigating structure-outcome variables evaluated the impact of health programs involving the coordination of nursing care or multidisciplinary services. Polliack and Shavitt (1977) determined that physician-nurse teamwork which was coordinated with social and community services reduced the need for hospitalization in the elderly. Home visits to discharged psychiatric patients by visiting nurses proved successful in reducing recidivism and medication errors while improving employment status of patients (Vincent & Price, 1977). In Haiti, locating maternal-child services in buildings with cooking equipment typical of areas served, coupled with formal and informal teaching, improved child-care practices and the nutritional status of children (King, Fougere, Webb, Berggren, & Berggren, 1978). Use of a comprehensive, multidisciplinary clinic service for patients with Down's syndrome decreased illness episodes and hospitalization rates (Fujimoto, Fareau, Forsman, & Wilson, 1978). Decker, Stevens, Vancini, and Wedeking (1979) demonstrated that a statewide inservice program in quality assurance led to higher levels of patient outcomes in community health nursing.

Weekly care from a nonjudgmental interdisciplinary team situated in schools improved health practices and physical status of pregnant adolescents (Berg, Taylor, Edwards, & Hakanson, 1979). Coordination of services from public health nurses and a medical nurse practitioner resulted in improved functional and mental health status of residents in an elderly high-rise apartment (Sullivan & Armignacco, 1979). Lower incidences of ketoacidosis, amputation, and hospitalization rates were found for diabetics in nurse-operated decentralized clinics as compared to traditional hospital clinics (Runyan, VanderZwaag, Joyner, & Miller, 1980).

The remaining studies in which structure and outcomes were linked represented a wide variety of research problems. Several researchers investigated patient classification systems (not including nursing diagnosis classifications). Using Diagnostic Related Group (DRG) criteria and a severity of illness index, Kreitzer, Loebner, and Roveti (1982) discovered considerable variation in the relationships among severity of illness, length of hospital stay, and changes among patients with the same diagnosis. Newman (1982) demonstrated the usefulness of a chronicity classification and functional baseline scale to quality assurance methodology. Measurement of severity of patient problem status coupled with problem-oriented records improved functional and mental health status in psychiatric patients using outpatient services (Allen, 1982). Other investigators, including Linn, Linn, and Gurel (1977), documented that patient survival in a nursing home was related positively to the number of RN hours per patient. Wood (1977) found that sensory disturbances in hospitalized patients were correlated inversely with the number of beds occupied in a room. Shanahan and Walker (1975) tested an audit tool for evaluating nurse competency that helped verify the impact of nursing care on patient outcomes. Blake, Cheatle, and Mack (1980) found that retrospective audit was as effective as prospective audit in detecting nosocomial infections.

Process-Outcome Studies

Studies in which researchers examined the relationship between process and outcome elements were concentrated primarily on evaluating the impact of patient education programs and use of clinical judgment. Patient education by nurses improved the health status of subjects with chronic cardiovascular disease (Shanahan, 1976). Postoperative respiratory status was improved in patients taught by the nurse in groups compared to individual instruction (Crabtree, 1978). Nurse counseling in a family practice clinic increased patient compliance with recommended treatment regimes (Talkington, 1978). Structured teaching in conjunction with nurses' encouragement to patients to be involved in care decisions successfully improved self-esteem and knowledge in subjects receiving chemotherapy (Lum, Chase, Cole, Johnson, & Johnson, 1978). In one of the first studies in which the Horn/Swain tool was applied, Hageman and Ventura (1981) developed a teaching program that improved surgical subjects' knowledge about self-care. Provision of education and role supplementation by nurses with expectant couples decreased anxiety and depression and enhanced couples' responsiveness to the newborn (Meleis & Swendsen, 1977). Providing structured information to parents of hospitalized children proved useful in their participation and contribution to their children's care (Roskies, Mongeon, & Gagnon-Lefebvre, 1978). Home visits by nurses for educating adolescent mothers about infant development and stimulation had a significant and positive impact on infant growth and development rates and mothers' attitudes toward child-rearing (Field, Widmayer, Stringer, & Ignatoff, 1981). One of the first attempts to link cultural differences and quality assurance was the development of culture-specific patient education materials and models for use in preoperative teaching (Archuleta, Plummer, Hopkins, & Bender, 1977). However, no improvement in patient health status resulted from using these instruction aids.

Relative to clinician judgment and performance, Given, Given, and Simoni (1979) documented that the quality of provider-related processes of diagnostic and therapeutic approaches had a significant and favorable impact on patients' cognitive, perceptual, and physical health status. Clinical decision making of nurse practitioners in caring for hypertensive clients compared favorably with that of physicians (Hill & Reichgott, 1979). Cuddihy (1979) demonstrated that both nursing process and outcomes improved when quality of care data were shared with nurses who had given the care.

In the most comprehensive examination of the association between process and outcomes of nursing care in the hospital setting, Hegyvary and

Haussmann (1976b) found that the relationship varied with different patient populations. Shannon (1976) also reported the relationship to be inconsistent in assessing care given to elderly populations.

Structure-Process-Outcome Studies

Implementation and evaluation of standards for nursing practice was one type of research in which the relationships among structure, process, and outcome were investigated. Standardization of birth control clinic visits and records followed by inservice education for staff improved clinician documentation and efficiency, as well as increased patient return rates (Grover & Greenberg, 1976). Use of a standardized surveillance system for monitoring patients' conditions improved clinicians' documentation and patients' health status (Kaszuba & Gibson, 1977). Introduction of standards and criteria for teaching hospitalized diabetics resulted in improved, more uniform care; higher levels of patient knowledge; and better self-care skills in adults (Distel, 1981a) and children (Hurwitz & Kohler, 1981). Standardized classification of pressure sores and criteria for nursing care were helpful in improving care, decreasing the incidence of ulcers, and accelerating the healing rate of prehospital admission sores (Distel, 1982; Droessler & Maibusch, 1979). Knight (1980) indicated that the use of standard criteria for preventive care in well-child clinics enhanced documentation and execution of care and increased patient return rates. In the area of mental health, Sinclair and Frankel (1982) documented that the implementation of standards for client involvement in decision making and participation of clinicians in quality assurance activities improved clinician skills in normalization, the mental health status of clients, and their satisfaction with care.

Some researchers examining all three components of quality assurance focused on nursing assignment patterns or selected elements of nursing assignment patterns. In a comparison of functional and primary nursing, Hegedus (1979) found higher quality of nursing care and lower levels of patient stress on primary nursing units. Fairbanks (1981) found that the implementation of primary nursing led to increased nurse professionalism, increased involvement of patients in their own care, a 47% reduction in nurse turnover, a higher level of patient satisfaction, and feelings that the care received was more personalized. Williams, Holloway, Winn, Wolanin, and Lawler (1979) found that greater continuity in nursing personnel for the hospitalized elderly yielded better assessment and planning by nurses, and improved mental health status of patients.

Structure-process-outcome research also included evaluation of the impact of nurses in expanded roles. In the area of child health, no differences were found between nurse practitioners and physicians in terms of quality of medical management and patient health status in two studies (DeAngelis & McHugh, 1977; Salkever, Skinner, Steinwachs, & Katz, 1982). However, Graham (1978) reported that pediatric nurse practitioners achieved significantly higher scores than pediatricians in all areas of documentation, care-giving, and patient satisfaction. In the area of adult health, nurse practitioner performance of medical protocols, referral, and resulting patient satisfaction were comparable to those of physicians (Feldman, Taller, Garfield, Collen, Richart, Cella, & Sender, 1977). Wagener and Carter (1978) found that gynecological patients expressed a decided preference for nurse practitioners over physicians, particularly because of the quality of patient education. An evaluation of nurse performance in a hypertensive clinic showed that nurses could manage effectively a large population of hypertensives (Hogan, Wallin, Kelly, Baer, & Barzyk, 1978). In a review of 21 studies of care given by nurse practitioners and physicians' assistants, Sox (1979) concluded that health care given by these two groups of practitioners was comparable in quality. In a recent study on nurse practitioners in a jailhouse setting, Hastings, Vick, Lee, Sasmor, Natiello, and Sanders (1980) documented that introduction of nurse practitioners resulted in technical care equal to that of medical residents, increased patient satisfaction, and a significant decrease in suicide attempts among inmates.

For the future, we recommend a greater emphasis on research that includes all three quality components simultaneously. Clinicians and administrators rarely perceive or experience these components in isolation. The goal for researchers is to create a more accurate fit between scientific inquiry in nursing quality assessment and the realities of clinical practice, organizational resources, and policy development.

SUMMARY AND OVERALL RECOMMENDATIONS FOR FUTURE RESEARCH

Most of the publications about the assessment of quality assurance were at the conceptual level, the development of models and standards, instrument development, and the single case or institution or noncomparative study. Few comparative studies were identified. The very large number of conceptual and development type of publications were not included in this review.

We believe that a very large but unknown number of research and evaluation projects to assess the quality of nursing care were never published. Of those studies published, few were found in other than nursing publications. Few nursing studies were referred to in health and medical care literature. We strongly encourage an increase in the publication of studies on the assessment of the quality of nursing care in both nursing and health literature. It is essential that findings of such studies be used in the development of health and nursing policy.

Future studies should not be limited to any single focus or methodology but should include the development of models, qualitative and quantitative descriptive studies, experimental or controlled clinical trials, and historical archiving of quality assurance in nursing studies and activities. Modeling should continue to provide answers to the questions of definitions of quality, quality assessment, quality assurance, standards, criteria, measurement, and resulting actions. Modeling should provide frameworks or road maps for the overall direction of the assessment of quality of nursing care.

A primary need is for descriptive studies. What are the prevalent patterns of nursing care? What are the structure, process, and outcome criteria that describe current nursing care? What are the norms for these criteria? How are patients or clients classified and diagnosed relative to nursing? What are the interventions or processes, including client-nurse relationships? What are the outcomes? Data banks of descriptions or norms of nursing practice would be most useful as a first step in the process of scientific inquiry. Such descriptive studies should be encouraged. These elements of nursing care must be considered parts of minimum data sets for health care information systems. The computerization of health care data systems will make this goal possible.

Secondly, there is need for comparative studies. Many evaluation studies have been done in response to political pressures to produce information to meet the decision needs of particular programs without sufficient longer-range attention to the need for comparative data. Prescott (1978, p. 73) summarized the problem well: "The results of such short range focus and reliance on single program evaluation have led to a large body of evaluation research with little or no generalizability. What is needed is a greater emphasis on comparative studies." These comparative studies would answer the question about existing relationships among the criterion variables of structure, process, and outcome. The authors agree with Donabedian (1982, p. 373) who suggested two domains for studies of causal validity; he advocated studying aspects of causal validity under quality assessment, leaving the core issues to be settled by clinical researchers. His preference, and ours, is to leave research on the validity of clinical procedures in the hands of the clinical researchers.

The responsibility of those who formulate the criteria of quality assessment is to find and use the information that clinical research generates. The task of quality assessment is to contribute to clinical research by pointing out gaps in present knowledge. It also should bring to the attention of clinical researchers gaps and issues that may not be readily apparent to them. Relationships among structure, process, and outcomes—especially in terms of the monetary costs—are representative of concerns that are more apparent to quality assessment researchers than clinical researchers. We recommend that cost-benefit measures become a part of all nursing quality assessment research.

Phaneuf and Wandelt (1981) identified obstacles to progress in the assessment of the quality of nursing care. These obstacles were prevailing emphasis on locally developed criteria and standards; the movement toward combining medical and nursing evaluation, specifically audits; the increasing focus on problems; and longstanding conflicts over whether structure, process, or outcomes of care should be measured. Research on the assessment of the quality of nursing care will be critiqued increasingly for its impact on nursing care or the assurance of care. Emphasis has been given to assessment and measurement of the quality of care. Emphasis also must be given to the assurance aspect of the quality of care. Luke, Krueger, and Modrow (1983) suggested that quality assurance activities should be linked to authority structure of health care institutions and health policymakers. Also needed for further understanding of quality control and improvement is an infusion of organizational theory, management science, change theory, and decision-making models.

Regardless of design, there is a need for more rigor in submitting data to inferential testing. This includes continued reliability and validity testing of instruments as they are applied to different populations or in different settings. Investigation of the complex relationships among structure, process, and outcome components, as well as the relationships among the numerous elements within each of these components, requires the use of statistical technologies designed specifically to analyze such complexities. With the recent advances in statistical theory and computer technologies, integrative, multivariate approaches can and should be applied to quality assessment research in nursing.

To assess the quality of nursing care one must first determine the meaning of quality. Given the large number of variables and ambiguities associated with nursing, it is not surprising that the quality of nursing care is perceived, defined, and measured in many ways. In this chapter, we utilized a structure-process-outcome framework to review published empirical studies on the assessment of the quality of nursing care. The framework and the actual selection of studies may prove to be too limiting for a full discussion of the quality of nursing care. However, this chapter represents a beginning in a search for understanding of the assessment of the quality of nursing care.

REFERENCE NOTES

1. Reiter, F., & Kakosh, M. E. *Quality of nursing care: A report of a field study to establish criteria: 1950–1954*. New York: New York Medical College, Graduate School of Nursing, 1963.
2. Aydelotte, M. K., & Tener, M. E. *An investigation of the relation between nursing activity and patient welfare*. Iowa City, Iowa: University of Iowa, 1960.
3. Sonquist, J. A. *Multivariate model building: The validation of a search strategy*. Ann Arbor, Mich.: University of Michigan, Institute for Social Research, 1971.

REFERENCES

Abdellah, F. G. Criterion measures in nursing. *Nursing Research*, 1961, *10*, 21–25.

Aldhizer, T., Solle, M., & Bohrer, R. A multidisciplinary audit of diabetes mellitus. *Journal of Family Practice*, 1979, *8*, 947–951.

Allen, R. H. Use of the problem-oriented record to evaluate treatment in a chronic psychiatric population. *Quality Review Bulletin*, 1982, *8*(3), 13–16.

Archuleta, V., Plummer, O., Hopkins, K., & Bender, N. *Demonstration model for patient education: A model for the project training nurses to improve patient education*. Boulder, Colo.: Western Interstate Commission for Higher Education, June 1977. (NTIS No. HRP-0900550/5ST)

Ayer, G. M. Is nursing audit affecting patient care? *Association of Operating Room Nurses Journal*, 1978, *28*, 114–115; 118–126.

Berg, M., Taylor, B., Edwards, L., & Hakanson, E. Prenatal care for pregnant adolescents in a public high school. *American Journal of Public Health*, 1979, *49*, 32–35.

Blair, E., Hauf, B., Loveridge, C., Murphy, J., & Roth, M. Instrument development: Measuring quality outcomes in ambulatory maternal-child nursing. *Nursing Administration Quarterly*, 1978, *2*(4), 81–93.

Blake, S., Cheatle, E., & Mack, B. Surveillance: Retrospective versus prospective. *American Journal of Infection Control*, 1980, *8*, 75–78.

Brodt, D. E., & Anderson, E. H. Validation of a patient welfare evaluation instrument. *Nursing Research*, 1967, *16*, 167–169.

Carey, R., & Posavec, E. Program evaluation of a physical medicine and rehabilitative unit: A new approach. *Archives of Physical Medicine and Rehabilitation*, 1978, *59*, 330–337.

Chambers, L., Burke, M., Ross, J., & Cantwell, R. Quantitative assessment of the quality of medical care provided in five practices before and after attachment of a family practice nurse. *Canadian Medical Association Journal*, 1978, *118*, 1060–1064.

Chambers, L. W., & West, A. E. St. John's randomized trial of the family practice nurse: Health outcomes of patients. *International Journal of Epidemiology*, 1978, *7*, 153–161.

Crabtree, M. Application of cost-benefit analysis to clinical nursing practice: A comparison of individual and group preoperative teaching. *The Journal of Nursing Administration*, 1978, *8*(12), 11–16.

Cuddihy, J. Clinical research: Translation into nursing practice. *International Journal of Nursing Studies*, 1979, *16*, 65–72.

Dake, N. Nursing responsibilities for discharge planning in a community hospital. *Quality Review Bulletin*, 1981, *7*(10), 26–31.

DeAngelis, C., & McHugh, M. The effectiveness of various health personnel as triage agents. *Journal of Community Health*, 1977, *2*, 268–277.

Decker, F., Stevens, L., Vancini, M., & Wedeking, L. Using patient outcomes to evaluate community health nursing. *Nursing Outlook*, 1979, *27*, 278–282.

Derdiarian, A. Analysis of dependence, independence behavior variables in surgical patients with emphasis on trait and state dependence. In M. V. Batey (Ed.), *Communicating Nursing Research* (Vol. 8). Boulder, Colo.: Western Interstate Commission for Higher Education, 1977.

Diers, D. Research for nursing. *The Journal of Nursing Administration*, 1973, *3*(1), 8, 11.

DiMarco, N., & Hilliard, M. Comparisons of associate, diploma and baccalaureate degree nurses' state board, quality of patient care, competency rating, supervisor rating, subordinates' satisfaction with supervision and self-report job satisfaction scores. *International Journal of Nursing Studies*, 1978, *15*, 163–170.

Distel, L. Diabetic teaching. *Quality Review Bulletin*, 1981, *7*(6), 8–12. (a)

Distel, L. More than chart review: A new problem-oriented nursing quality assurance program. *Quality Review Bulletin*, 1981, *7*(1), 26–29. (b)

Distel, L. A nursing quality assurance investigation of orthopedic patient care. *Quality Review Bulletin*, 1982, *8*(10), 20–22.

Donabedian, A. *The criteria and standards of quality: Explorations in quality assessment and monitoring* (Vol. 2). Ann Arbor, Mich.: Health Administration Press, 1982.

Droessler, D., & Maibusch, R. M. Development of a nursing care plan for healing and preventing decubiti. *Quality Review Bulletin*, 1979, *5*(8), 10–14.

Dunn, M. G. *A study of the effect of standard nursing care plans on nurses' documentation on individualized care plans and patient medical records*. San Francisco, Calif.: Veterans Administration Hospital, February 1977. (NTIS No. PB82–135229)

Dyer, E. D., Monson, M. A., & Cope, M. J. Increasing the quality of patient care through performance counseling and written goal setting. *Nursing Research,* 1975, *24,* 138–144.

Eaton, P., & Gottselig, S. Effects of longer hours, shorter week for intensive care nurses. *Dimensions in Health Services,* 1980, *57*(8), 25–27.

Eichhorn, M. L., & Frevert, E. I. Evaluation of a primary nursing system using the quality patient care scale. *The Journal of Nursing Administration,* 1979, *9*(10), 11–15.

Elhai, L. S. The quality of medical care delivered by lay practitioners in a feminist clinic. *American Journal of Public Health,* 1981, *71,* 853–855.

Fagin, C. M. The economic value of nursing research. *American Journal of Nursing,* 1982, *82,* 1844–1849.

Fairbanks, J. E. Primary nursing: More data. *Nursing Administration Quarterly,* 1981, *5*(3), 51–62.

Feldman, R., Taller, S. L., Garfield, S. R., Collen, M. F., Richart, R. H., Cella, R., & Sender, A. J. Nurse practitioner multiphasic health checkups. *Preventive Medicine,* 1977, *6,* 391–403.

Felton, G. Increasing the quality of nursing care by introducing the concept of primary nursing: A model project. *Nursing Research,* 1975, *24,* 27–32.

Feuerstein, M. T. Evaluation—By the people. *International Nursing Review,* 1978, *25,* 146–153.

Field, T. M., Widmayer, S. M., Stringer, S., & Ignatoff, E. Teenage, lower-class, black mothers and their preterm infants: An intervention and developmental follow-up. In H. E. Freeman & M. A. Solomon (Eds.), *Evaluation Studies Review Annual* (Vol. 6). Beverly Hills, Calif.: Sage Publications, 1981.

Forquer, S. L., & Anderson, T. B. A concerns-based approach to the implementation of quality assurance system. *Quality Review Bulletin,* 1982, *8*(4), 14–19.

Fujimoto, A., Fareau, G. E., Forsman, I., & Wilson, M. G. An evaluation of comprehensive health care in the management of Down's syndrome. *American Journal of Public Health,* 1978, *68,* 406–408.

Gallant, B., & McLane, A. Outcome criteria: A process for validation at the unit level. *The Journal of Nursing Administration,* 1979, *9*(1), 14–20.

Galton, M., & Reilly, M. Evaluation of nursing care through a nursing audit. *Australian Nurses' Journal,* 1977, *6*(11), 34–36.

Garfield, S. R., Collen, M. F., Feldman, R., Soghikian, K., Richart, R. H., & Duncan, J. H. Evaluation of an ambulatory medical-care delivery system. *The New England Journal of Medicine,* 1976, *294,* 426–431.

Gilson, B. S., Gilson, J. S., Bergner, M., Bobbitt, R. A., Kressel, S., Pollard, W. E., & Vesselago, M. The sickness impact profile: Development of an outcome measure of health care. *American Journal of Public Health,* 1975, *65,* 1304–1310.

Ginsberg, G., & Marks, I. Costs and benefits of behavioral psychotherapy: A pilot study of neurotics treated by nurse-therapists. *Psychological Medicine,* 1977, *7,* 685–700.

Girouard, S. Role of the clinical specialist as change agent: An experiment in preoperative teaching. *International Journal of Nursing Studies,* 1978, *15,* 57–65.

Given, B., Given, C. W., & Simoni, L. E. Relationships of processes of care to patient outcomes. *Nursing Research*, 1979, *28*, 85–93.

Goldberg, G. A., & Jolly, D. G. *Quality of care provided by physician's extenders in Air Force primary medicine clinics*. Santa Monica, Calif.: Rand Corporation, January 1980. (NTIS No. AD–AO82 491/2)

Goodman, H. C., & Perrin, E. C. Evening telephone call management by nurse practitioners and physicians. *Nursing Research*, 1978, *27*, 233–237.

Graham, N. A quality of care assessment: Pediatricians and pediatric nurse practitioners. *Image*, 1978, *10*, 41–48.

Greene, V., & Monahan, D. Structural and operational factors affecting quality of patient care in nursing homes. *Public Policy*, 1981, *29*, 399–415.

Grover, M., & Greenberg, T. Quality of care given to first time birth control patients at a free clinic. *American Journal of Public Health*, 1976, *66*, 986–989.

Guy, M. E., & Moore, L. S. The goal attainment scale for psychiatric inpatients: Development and use of a quality assurance tool. *Quality Review Bulletin*, 1982, *8*(6), 19–29.

Hageman, P. T., & Ventura, M. R. Utilizing patient outcome criteria to measure the effects of a medication teaching regimen. *Western Journal of Nursing Research*, 1981, *3*, 25–33.

Hagen, E. Appraisal of quality in nursing care. In *American Nurses' Association Eighth Nursing Research Conference*. Kansas City, Mo.: American Nurses' Association, 1972.

Hamera, E., & O'Connell, K. A. Patient-centered variables in primary and team nursing. *Research in Nursing and Health*, 1981, *4*, 183–192.

Hardy, M. Implementation of unit management and clinical nurse specialists: Patients' perceptions of the quality of general hospital care and nursing care. In M. V. Batey (Ed.), *Communicating Nursing Research* (Vol. 8). Boulder, Colo.: Western Interstate Commission for Higher Education, 1977.

Harman, R. Does an all R.N. staff provide better quality care? *Hospital Administration in Canada*, 1975, *12*(4), 35–38.

Hastings, G. E., Vick, L., Lee, G., Sasmor, L., Natiello, T. A., & Sanders, J. H.Nurse practitioners in a jailhouse clinic. *Medical Care*, 1980, *18*, 731–744.

Haussmann, R. D., Hegyvary, S. T., Newman, J. F., & Bishop, A. C. Monitoring quality of nursing care. *Health Services Research*, 1974, *9*, 135–148.

Hegedus, K. S. A patient outcome criterion measure. *Supervisor Nurse*, 1979, *10*(1), 40–45.

Hegyvary, S. T., & Haussmann, R. D. Correlates of the quality of nursing care. *The Journal of Nursing Administration*, 1976, *6*(9), 22–27. (a)

Hegyvary, S. T., & Haussmann, R. D. Relationship of nursing process and patient outcomes. *The Journal of Nursing Administration*, 1976, *6*(9), 18–21. (b)

Hegyvary, S. T., Haussmann, R. D., Kronman, B., & Burke, M. *Users' manual for Rush-Medicus nursing process monitoring methodology*. Chicago, Ill.: Medicus Systems Corporation, April 1979. (NTIS No. HRP-0900638/8)

Hill, M. N., & Reichgott, M. J. Achievement of standards for quality care of hypertension by physicians and nurses. *Clinical and Experimental Hypertension*, 1979, *1*, 665–684.

Hinshaw, A. S., & Atwood, J. R. A patient satisfaction instrument: Precision by replication. *Nursing Research*, 1982, *31*, 170–175.

Hinshaw, A. S., & Oakes, D. L. Theoretical model-testing: Patients', nurses', and physicians' expectations for quality nursing care. In M. V. Batey (Ed.), *Communicating Nurse Research* (Vol. 10). Boulder, Colo.: Western Interstate Commission for Higher Education, 1977.

Hogan, M. J., Wallin, J. D., Kelly, M. R., Baer, R., & Barzyk, P. Computerized paramedical approach to the outpatient management of essential hypertension. *Military Medicine*, 1978, *143*, 771–775.

Horn, B. J., & Swain, M. A. *Criterion measures of nursing care quality* (Final Report). Hyattsville, Md.: National Center for Health Services Research, U.S. Department of Health, Education, and Welfare, 1978. (NTIS No. PB-287 449/3GA)

Howe, M. J., Coulton, M. R., Almon, G. M., & Sandrick, K. M. Developing scaled outcome criteria for a target patient population. *Quality Review Bulletin*, 1980, *6*(3), 17–22.

Huczynski, A. Nursing management audit: The reaction of users. *Journal of Advanced Nursing*, 1977, *2*, 521–531.

Hurwitz, L. S., & Kohler, E. The benefits of evaluating care provided to children hospitalized with insulin dependent diabetes mellitus. *Quality Review Bulletin*, 1981, *7*(6), 13–21.

Ibrahim, M. A., Wagner, E. H., Williams, C. A., Greenberg, R. A., & Kleinbaum, D. G. *Assessing the clinical skills of nurse practitioners.* Hyattsville, Md.: U.S. Public Health Service, Division of Nursing, June 1978. (NTIS No. HRP-0900601/6)

Jacoby, I., & Kindig, D. Task analysis in national health service corps field stations: A methodological evaluation. *Medical Care*, 1975, *13*, 308–317.

Januska, C., Engle, J., & Wood, J. *Status of quality assurance in public health nursing.* Washington, D.C.: American Public Health Association, 1976.

Jelinek, R. C., Haussmann, R. D., Hegyvary, S. T., & Newman, J. F. *A methodology for monitoring quality of nursing care* (DHEW Publication No. 76–25). Washington, D.C.: U.S. Government Printing Office, 1974.

Jones, K. Study documents effects of primary nursing on renal transplant patients. *Hospitals*, 1975, *49*(24), 85–89.

Joyce, A. Systematic review: You can afford it. *Supervisor Nurse*, 1977, *8*(9), 13–18.

Kane, R. L., Rubenstein, L. Z., Brook, R. H., Van Ryzin, J., Masthay, P., Schoenrich, E., & Harrell, B. Utilization review in nursing homes: Making implicit level-of-care judgments explicit. *Medical Care*, 1981, *19*, 3–13.

Kass, E. J. *A process to integrate a new patient care plan into the medical record.* Washington, D.C.: Veterans Administration, January 1981. (NTIS No. GRAI 8207)

Kaszuba, A. L., & Gibson, G. Hospital emergency department surveillance system: A data base for patient care, management, research and teaching. *Journal of the American College of Emergency Physicians*, 1977, *6*, 304–307.

King, K. W., Fougere, W., Webb, R. E. Berggren, G., & Berggren, W. L. Preventive and therapeutic benefits in relation to cost-performance over 10 years of mothercraft centers in Haiti. *American Journal of Clinical Nutrition*, 1978, *31*, 679–690.

Knight, J. Community health care: Assuring the quality of preventive care. *Quality Review Bulletin*, 1980, *6*(3), 6–11.

Koerner, B. L. Selected correlates of job performance of community health nurses. *Nursing Research*, 1981, *30*, 43–48.

Kreitzer, S., Loebner, E., & Roveti, G. Severity of illness: The DRG's missing link? *Quality Review Bulletin*, 1982, *8*(5), 21–34.

Krueger, J. C. Establishing priorities for evaluation and evaluation research: A nursing perspective. *Nursing Research*, 1980, *29*, 115–118.

Lang, N. M. *Quality assurance in nursing: A selected bibliography* (Nurse Planning and Information Series No. 12, United States Department of Health, Education and Welfare Publication No. HRA 80–30 HRP–0501301). Washington, D.C.: U.S. Government Printing Office, 1980.

Lang, N. M. & Clinton, J. Assessment and assurance of the quality of nursing care: A selected overview. *Evaluation and the Health Professions*, 1983, *6*, 211–231.

Lewis, F. M., Firsich, S. C., & Parsell, S. Clinical tool development for adult chemotherapy patients: Process and content. *Cancer Nursing*, 1979, *2*, 99–108.

Lindeman, C. Delphi survey of priorities in clinical nursing research. *Nursing Research*, 1975, *24*, 434–444.

Linn, M. W., Linn, B. S., & Gurel, L. Patient outcome as a measure of quality of nursing home. *American Journal of Public Health*, 1977, *67*, 337–344.

Luke, R. D., Krueger, J.C. & Modrow, E.R.(Eds.). *Organization and change in health care quality assurance*. Rockville, Md.: Aspen Systems, 1983.

Lum, J. L., Chase, M., Cole, S. M., Johnson, A., & Johnson, J. A. Nursing care of oncology patients receiving chemotherapy. *Nursing Research*, 1978, *27*, 340–346.

Lundin, D. V. Medication taking behavior of the elderly. *Drug Intelligence and Clinical Pharmacy*, 1978, *12*, 518–521.

MacElveen, P. A. Observational measure of patient morale: The behavior-morale scale. In M. V. Batey (Ed.), *Communicating Nursing Research* (Vol. 9). Boulder, Colo.: Western Interstate Commission for Higher Education, 1977.

Mackley, B., Heslop, T., & McAllister, D. Aberdeen formula: Evaluation on the larger scale. *Nursing Times*, 1979, *75*, 33–36.

Majesky, S. J., Brester, M. H., & Nishio, K. T. Development of a research tool: Patient indicators of nursing care. *Nursing Research*, 1978, *27*, 365–371.

Mast, F. L. Monitoring statewide maternal and child health program activities. *MCN, The American Journal of Maternal Child Nursing*, 1978, *3*, 139–140; 142.

McCarthy, D., & Schifalacqua, M. M. Primary nursing: Its implementation and six month outcome. *The Journal of Nursing Administration*, 1978, *8*(5), 29–32.

McLaughlin, F. E., Carr, J. W., & Delucchi, K. L. *Primary care judgments of nurses and physicians. Volume 4. Reliability and validity research report*. San Francisco, Calif.: Veterans Administration, July 1979. (NTIS No. HRP–0900623/0)

Mech, A. B. Evaluating the process of nursing care in long term care facilities. *Quality Review Bulletin*, 1980, *6*(3), 24–30.

Meleis, A. I., & Swendsen, L. Does nursing intervention make a difference—A test of role supplementation. In M. V. Batey (Ed.), *Communicating Nursing Research* (Vol. 8). Boulder, Colo.: Western Interstate Commission for Higher Education, 1977.

Montgomery, J. E., & Kelly, M. *Assignment element difficulty as a basis for nursing personnel staffing at naval hospitals. Phase 1. Project Report.* Bethesda, Md.: Naval School of Health Sciences, September 1979. (NTIS No. AD–A078 584/0)

Moscovice, I. Influence of training level and practice setting on patterns of primary care provided by nursing personnel. *Journal of Community Health,* 1978, *4,* 4–14.

Nassif, D., Garfink, C., & Greenfield, C. Does continuity equal quality in the assessment of well-child care? *Quality Review Bulletin,* 1982, *8*(6), 11–18.

Newman, F. Outcome evaluation and quality assurance in mental health. *Quality Review Bulletin,* 1982, *8*(4), 27–31.

Nightingale, F. *Notes on matters affecting the health, efficiency, and hospital administration of the British army.* London: Harrison & Sons, 1858.

Phaneuf, M. C. *The nursing audit and self-regulation in nursing practice.* New York: Appleton-Century-Crofts, 1976.

Phaneuf, M. C., & Wandelt, M. A. Obstacles to and potentials for nursing quality appraisal. *Quality Review Bulletin,* 1981, *7*(4), 2–5.

Polliack, M. R., & Shavitt, N. Utilization of hospital in-patient services by the elderly. *Journal of the American Geriatric Society,* 1977, *25,* 364–367.

Prescott, P. A. Evaluation research: Issues in evaluation of nursing programs. *Nursing Administration Quarterly,* 1978, *2*(4), 63–80.

Prescott, P. A., & Driscoll, L. Evaluating nurse practitioner performance. *The Nurse Practitioner,* 1980, *5*(4), 28–32.

Roberts, L. E. Primary nursing? Do patients like it—Are nurses satisfied—Does it cost more? *The Canadian Nurse,* 1980, *76*(11), 20–23.

Robertson, L. H., McDonnell, K., & Scott, J. Nursing health assessment of preschool children in Perth County. *Canadian Journal of Public Health,* 1976, *67,* 300–304.

Roskies, E., Mongeon, M., & Gagnon-Lefebvre, B. Increasing maternal participation in the hospitalization of young children. *Medical Care,* 1978, *16,* 765–777.

Rothman, G., & Saunders, J. M. Thanatology review in a psychiatric facility. *Quality Review Bulletin,* 1982, *8*(10), 5–10.

Runyan, J. W., VanderZwaag, R., Joyner, M. B., & Miller, S. T. The Memphis diabetes continuing care program. *Diabetes Care,* 1980, *3,* 382–386.

Salkever, D. S., Skinner, E. A., Steinwachs, D. M., & Katz, H. Episode-based efficiency comparisons for physicians and nurse practitioners. *Medical Care,* 1982, *20,* 143–153.

Sanders, J. H., Sasmor, L., & Natiello, T. A. *An evaluation of the impact of communication technology and improved medical protocol on health care delivery in penal institutions* (Vol. 4). Washington, D.C.: National Science Foundation, Engineering and Applied Science, December 1976. (NTIS No. PB 80–105893)

Schwirian, P. M. Evaluating the performance of nurses: A multidimensional approach. *Nursing Research*, 1978, *27*, 347–351.

Shanahan, M. Wrap session: Critique of a nursing audit of pulmonary embolism and infarction. *Quality Review Bulletin*, 1976, *2*(5), 7–11.

Shanahan, M., & Walker, P. A silent illness: Clinical basis and comparative analysis of nursing audit criteria for essential hypertension. *Quality Review Bulletin*, 1975, *1*(5–7), 15–25.

Shannon, M. Measure of the fulfillment of health needs. *International Journal of Aging and Human Development*, 1976, *7*, 353–377.

Sheridan, D. R., Bronstein, J. E., & Walker, D. D. Using registry nurses: Coping with cost and quality issues. *The Journal of Nursing Administration*, 1982, *11*(10), 26–34.

Shukla, R. K. Structure vs. people in primary nursing: An inquiry. *Nursing Research*, 1981, *30*, 236–241.

Sinclair, C., & Frankel, M. The effect of quality assurance activities on the quality of mental health services. *Quality Review Bulletin*, 1982, *8*(7), 7–15.

Soghikian, K. Role of nurse practitioners in hypertension care. *Clinical Science and Molecular Medicine*, 1978, *55*, 345–348.

Sox, H. C. Quality of patient care by nurse practitioners and physician assistants: A ten-year perspective. *Annals of Internal Medicine*, 1979, *91*, 459–468.

Sullivan, J. A., & Armignacco, F. Effectiveness of a comprehensive health program for the well-elderly: By community health nurses. *Nursing Research*, 1979, *28*, 70–75.

Talkington, D. R. Maximizing patient compliance by shaping attitudes of self-directed health care. *Journal of Family Practice*, 1978, *6*, 591–595.

Trivedi, V. M. Nursing judgment in selection of patient classification variables. *Research in Nursing and Health*, 1979, *2*, 109–118.

Trussell, P. M., & Strand, N. A comparison of concurrent and retrospective audit on the same patients. *The Journal of Nursing Administration*, 1978, *8*(5), 33–38.

Vaughan, V. C., & Large, J. T. *A study of professional relationships among physicians, nurses and social workers in a medical center for children. Phase 1, Identification of factors that influence professional practice.* Philadelphia, Pa.: Christopher's Hospital for Children, 1976. (NTIS No. HRP–0019417/5ST)

Ventura, M. R. Correlations between the quality patient care scale and the Phaneuf audit. *International Journal of Nursing Studies*, 1980, *17*, 155–162.

Ventura, M., & Crosby, F. Preparing the nurse observer to use the quality patient care scale: A modular approach. *Journal of Continuing Education in Nursing*, 1978, *9*(6), 37–40.

Ventura, M. R., Fox, R. N., Corley, M. C., & Mercurio, S. M. A patient satisfaction measure as a criterion to evaluate primary nursing. *Nursing Research*, 1982, *31*, 226–230.

Ventura, M. R., Hageman, P. T., Slakter, M. J., & Fox, R. N. Interrater reliabilities for two measures of nursing care quality. *Research in Nursing and Health*, 1980, *3*, 25–32.

Ventura, M. R., Hageman, P. T., Slakter, M. J., & Fox, R. N. Correlations of two quality of nursing care measures. *Research in Nursing and Health*, 1982, *5*, 37–43.

Vik, A. G., & MacKay, R. C. How does the 12-hour shift affect patient care? *The Journal of Nursing Administration*, 1982, *12*(1), 11–14.

Vincent, P., & Price, J. R. Evaluation of a VNA mental health project. *Nursing Research*, 1977, *26*, 361–367.

Wagener, J. M., & Carter, G. Patient's evaluations of gynecologic services provided by nurse practitioners. *Journal of the American College Health Association*, 1978, *27*, 98–100.

Wandelt, M., & Ager, J. W. *Quality patient care scale.* New York: Appleton-Century-Crofts, 1974.

Wandelt, M. A., & Stewart, D. S. *Slater nursing competencies rating scale.* New York: Appleton-Century-Crofts, 1975.

Ward, J., & Lindeman, C. A. *Instruments for measuring nursing practice and other health care variables* (2 vols.). Hyattsville, Md.: Public Health Service, Division of Nursing, 1978. (NTIS No. HRP–0900610/7)

Weinstein, E. Developing a measure of the quality of nursing care. *The Journal of Nursing Administration*, 1976, *6*(6), 1–3.

Williams, M. A., Holloway, J. R., Winn, M. C., Wolanin, M. O., & Lawler, M. L. Nursing activities and acute confusional states in elderly hip-fractured patients. *Nursing Research*, 1979, *28*, 25–35.

Wood, M. J. Clinical sensory deprivation: A comparative study of patients in single care and two-bed rooms. *The Journal of Nursing Administration*, 1977, *7*(10), 28–32.

Yodfat, Y., Fidel, J., & Eliakim, M. Analysis of the work of nurse-practitioners in family practice and its effect on the physicians' activities. *Journal of Family Practice*, 1977, *4*, 345–350.

Zikmund, W. G., & Miller, S. J. Factor analysis of attitudes of rural health care consumers toward nurse practitioners. *Research in Nursing and Health*, 1979, *2*, 85–90.

Zimmer, M. (Ed.). Symposium on quality assurance. *Nursing Clinics of North America*, 1974, *9*, 303–380.

CHAPTER 7

Public Health Nursing Evaluation, Education, and Professional Issues: 1977 to 1981

Marion E. Highriter
Department of Public Health Nursing
School of Public Health
University of North Carolina at Chapel Hill

CONTENTS

The research included in this review is focused on public health nurses—evaluative studies of their practice and education, in addition to selected professional issues. The author did a prior review of community health nursing studies for 1972 to 1976 (Highriter, 1977). The present review is an update for the 1977 to 1981 period, using a more rigorous definition of research and excluding categories of studies in areas that are scheduled for separate review chapters in the *Annual Review of Nursing Research* series. For analysis, studies were divided into three categories: (a) evaluation of public health nursing practice; (b) education for public health nursing practice; and (c) delivery system and professional issues. Selection of these categories permitted comparisons with the groups of studies in the preceding five-year review in order to determine trends. Although some investigators made distinctions, in studies reviewed for this chapter the terms public health nursing and community health nursing are used interchangeably here, with general use assigned to the former but employing the latter when it is used frequently in studies on a given topic.

The major difficulty in study retrieval and in determining the scope of this review was related to controversy within the field with regard to the definition of public health or community health nursing. The recent definitions of this practice area published by the American Nurses' Association (ANA, 1980) and the American Public Health Association (APHA, Note 1) have many features in common. Their differences are the source of the controversy. At risk of oversimplification, the APHA definition includes emphasis on population groups rather than individuals as the focus of services; it does not emphasize the setting as the characteristic feature of public health nursing practice. The ANA definition emphasizes primary care in outpatient settings as the characterizing feature, but also includes a population-focused approach. Study *retrieval* was guided by the more inclusive ANA definition because library cataloging seemed to be largely by setting. Study *review,* on the other hand, was guided more by the APHA definition since its population focus emphasizes delivery system issues. However, strict adherence to this definition was not feasible because too few studies would have been available for review.

Computer programs employed for initial study retrieval in the 1977 to 1981 MEDLARS search were essentially the same as those used for the preceding five-year review. Public health nursing was defined as "any nursing other than inpatient care" and equated the terms of public health, community health, home health, and district nurse, as well as health visitor. The specialty branches of occupational health and community mental health nursing were included in the definition. School nursing, discharge planning, and nurse-midwifery studies were recovered but excluded, because a chapter on school nursing is planned for the next volume in this series, and the latter two are often not considered part of public health nursing. Likewise, most of the clinically oriented primary-care or nurse practitioner studies were eliminated as not fitting the APHA definition of public health nursing and also were likely to be reviewed elsewhere.

In the computer searches the terms for public health nursing were linked with broadly defined research terms that included: health surveys, health services research, evaluation studies, epidemiologic methods, questionnaires, health-status indicators, effectiveness, and quality assurance. To provide as much of a worldwide perspective as possible, all studies were sought, although review had to be restricted to those in English. The searches produced approximately 800 references that were reduced to less than 50 when definitions for public health nursing research were applied strictly. In the practice evaluation section, investigations were ruled out when the activities of a public health nurse were not the subject of study. Thus, large bodies of research relevant to public health nursing practice (e.g., basic research in client behavior) were excluded. Likewise, community assessments of the need for public health nursing services, although an integral part of population-focused nursing, were ruled out due to a planned Annual Review chapter in Volume 3 on health needs assessment in communities. The types of articles included in the prior review under service description studies were eliminated as not rigorous enough to be considered research.

Even with the large number of studies retrieved in the computer search, a primary limitation of this review may be retrieval failures, since many relevant nursing studies may not have been cataloged under any of the terms used for public health nursing. This was offset to some extent by manual searches that produced approximately 15 of the 56 studies reviewed here. Although research published other than in journals was not purposely excluded, the focus was on the more accessible journal articles.

EVALUATIVE STUDIES OF PUBLIC HEALTH NURSING

Public health programs are often multidisciplinary efforts at goal attainment in which it is not possible to isolate the results of nursing care. The 26 studies in this section included 15 in which the interventions evaluated were almost entirely nursing efforts and 11 in which public health nurses and other team members all were working toward the outcomes measured. Eleven studies were conducted in the United States, eight in England, three in Finland, and two each in Canada and Scotland. Nine were authored only by nurses, 10 by multidisciplinary groups usually including a nurse, five by physicians alone, one by health educators, and one by an osteopath.

All but two studies in this area contained evaluations of public health nursing practice based on progress toward desired client outcomes ranging from primary prevention to peaceful death. Outcomes included detection of defects, control and resolution of health problems, client satisfaction, and attainment of goals at a reduced cost. Rigor of study design varied; there were 10 experimental or quasi-experimental designs involving control groups, two before-and-after studies, and 14 descriptive studies generally basing evaluation on after-only descriptions of goal attainment. The studies are summarized below according to the client groups with which interventions occurred.

Interventions with Mothers and Young Children

The eight studies of mothers and young children included some of the first to show the effectiveness of comprehensive child health supervisory activities. Four were primarily multidisciplinary efforts that involved the public health nurse, and four were focused primarily on nursing activities. The most comprehensive effort was a six-year follow-up of 47 normal first-born black infants born to unmarried schoolgirls living near Children's Hospital in Washington, D.C. (Gutelius, Kirsch, MacDonald, Brooks, & McErlean, 1977). The intervention was extensive counseling and anticipatory guidance by a pediatrician-public-health-nurse team. During the first three years of the child's life, they provided 38 hour-long individual visits supplemented by group sessions. On 32 out of 300 indicators, study infants showed significantly better performance than infants randomly allocated to a control group that received regular well-baby clinic supervision.

In Finland (Lauri, 1981), a much less intensive public health nursing intervention than that conducted in the Washington, D.C. study did not show dramatic results. The Finnish study group of 119 children was exposed to a systematic nursing process in five nursing contacts that included one home visit during the second year of life. In contrast, the matched control group averaged three ordinary clinic visits during the same time period. The study children showed better outcomes than their controls on only a few of the many variables studied. Their mothers more frequently acknowledged the practical value of public health nursing guidance; the children showed a higher developmental level than their controls in some areas. Subjectivity of measurements by service personnel, however, cannot be discounted in this pilot work where intervention and evaluation were managed without increase in overall service costs. In a third study in Montreal, Canada (Thibaudeau & Reidy, 1977), mothers' knowledge of and compliance with prescribed treatment regimes for upper respiratory infections in their young children were used as indicators of the effectiveness of experimental person-focused nursing care for 84 mother-child dyads. This care was significantly more effective than the illness-focused control care.

The health visitor's effectiveness in dealing with specific child health problems was shown in two British studies. In London (Sanger, Weir, & Churchill, 1981), a child psychiatrist gave health visitors group instruction and support in the use of behavioral modification techniques to assist parents with their children's sleep problems. Improvement was demonstrated in 13 out of 16 children. In Edinburgh (Houston & Howie, 1981), 28 mothers were given extra home support through a planned visit every two weeks by the same nurse. They showed significantly higher rates of breast-feeding continuation (100% at 12 weeks) than their 52 matched controls who received the usual care. The prenatal education studies in this time period illustrated how difficult it is to set the boundaries of public health nursing. They were conducted in the hospital clinic setting and did not fit the criteria for inclusion, although one was conducted by a public health nurse (Petrowski, 1981).

In a series of three articles in *Health Visitor,* Robertson (1981a, 1981b, 1981c) outlined an epidemiologic approach to the evaluation of screening programs and aptly illustrated it with data from her own efforts in preschool vision screening. Screening activities and an emphasis on cost-effectiveness were linked in a multidisciplinary study in Manchester, England (Komrower, Sardharwalla, Fowler, & Bridge, 1979), where health visitors played an important role in the screening and follow-up of children with phenylketonuria (PKU). There were no false-negative results and program costs compared to costs for long-term care of untreated PKU children were dramatically lower. Cost-effectiveness was also demonstrated in a multidisciplinary health education program in New York City that produced savings as a result of reduced morbidity and mortality from children's falls out of tenement windows (Spiegel & Lindaman, 1977).

Studies Emphasizing Home-Care Cost Savings, Primarily in Care of the Dying

In the last decade, home care services for persons who prefer to die at home were promoted first as a humane approach to improvement of the quality of the last days of life. However, research in this area reflected society's pressure to demonstrate cost-effectiveness of such a new service. The cost-saving theme continued in the seven studies where services equally or more desirable than hospital services were provided in the home at lesser cost. In a series of articles, Martinson described systematically pioneering efforts in supportive nursing services, cost savings, and favorable outcomes for 63 Minnesota families who cared for their dying child at home (Martinson, Armstrong, Geis, Anglim, Gronseth, MacInnis, Nesbit, & Kersey, 1978; Martinson, Armstrong, Geis, Anglim, Gronseth, MacInnis, Kersey, & Nesbit, 1978; Moldow & Martinson, 1980). In the early phases of the project, 24-hour nursing coverage was provided entirely by the research nurses, but in later stages the arrangements included local public health nursing agencies.

In Vermont, 22 patients received home care in a multidisciplinary rural outreach program that involved oncology nurse practitioners and local public health nursing services. Their care was contrasted to the care of 49 patients in nursing homes and hospitals during the last month of life (Kassakian, Bailey, Rinker, Stewart, & Yates, 1979). The home-care patients experienced dramatic cost savings and more independence and participation in hobbies and physical activities than their institutionalized counterparts. In Ohio, the cost-effectiveness of home care (at $65 per day), as compared to a hospital room ($126 per day), was shown for the last 42 days of life for 70 90%-satisfied patients of the Hospice of Columbus (Creek, 1982). Their nursing services were provided by city and county health departments supplemented by volunteer nurses.

In Edinburgh, discharging 117 hernia and varicose vein patients on the afternoon of their surgery to receive home care by community nursing sisters resulted in cost savings, nursing and client satisfaction, and recovery rates similar to patients with the usual hospital stay (Ruckley, Garraway, Cuthbertson, Fenwick, & Prescott, 1980). In a study of mostly elderly London residents, Martin and Ishino (1981) reported large cost savings as well as satisfied clients and staff, when domiciliary night nursing services enabled 242 clients (65 with terminal cancer) to remain in their homes. In analysis of data from all the health centers in Finland, Kekki (1980) found the number of public health nurses working in a health center area inversely related to the number of days of hospital care required by health center clients.

Edwards (1980) compared the effectiveness of instructional methodologies for teaching breast self-examination. Cost savings could result from her finding that the more time-consuming experimental methods, involving return demonstrations and other forms of follow-up, were no more effective than the less costly control ones. However, further research to determine whether increased teaching time could promote longer-term behavior change was recommended.

Interventions with Chronically Ill Clients

Public health nursing participation was effective in four medically directed hypertension control programs. The two large-scale programs described had different purposes and utilized nurses in different roles. In North Karelia, Finland, where the aim was to demonstrate community-wide control without the use of extra resources, existing community nurses were specially trained to play the primary role in detection, individual client instruction, and monitoring. Community hypertension control, based on five indicators, was significantly better in North Karelia than in a matched reference area (Nissinen, Tuomilehto, Elo, Salonen, & Puska, 1981). In England, the Medical Research Council is conducting a large clinical trial of drug therapy for mild hypertensives. The role of six research nurse trainers in the standardization of blood pressure measurement was described in the only article that appeared regarding this important study (Barnes, 1981).

In two smaller studies, investigators found nurses were more effective than physicians in maintaining hypertension control. Among 206 hypertensives followed at the workplace by specially trained nurses in Toronto, Canada, control was significantly better than in those randomly allocated to family-doctor care after nurse screening at work (Logan, Milne, Achber, Campbell, & Haynes, 1979). In Minnesota, 120 hypertensives who elected to be followed for a year by nurses from a free, nurse-practitioner-run, community clinic showed greater decreases in blood pressure than those electing care by the private physicians who supported the clinic (Brennan, Krishan, Nobrega, Labarthe, Timm, McGrath, Sheps, & Hunt, 1979). In the nurse-run clinic, 48% of the men and 67% of the women had diastolic blood pressures less than 90 mm Hg at 24 months, even though weight control had been unsuccessful.

Two health visitors attached to the rehabilitation unit of a hospital in Leeds, England, facilitated the use of community resources and kept from 50% to 80% of 196 chronically ill patients at home with decreasing needs for services (Firth, Chamberlain, Fligg, Wright, & Wright, 1978). In 1963, maintenance of stroke rehabilitation gains by 33 rehabilitants discharged from a hospital rehabilitation unit at the University of Minnesota was facilitated by involving public health nurses; however, in 1973—when family training by the rehabilitation team was substituted for home nursing—the training was equally successful with 79 rehabilitants (Anderson, Anderson, & Kottke, 1977). In Cleveland, Ohio, the minimal nature of the support that could be afforded for 75 discharged psychiatric patients (an average of 2.3 visiting-nurse visits per month for six months) and sampling difficulties may explain why findings were statistically insignificant. The patients showed better outcomes on some variables than did those patients randomly assigned to the control group (Vincent & Price, 1977).

Interventions with the Elderly

Three studies of public health nursing services for the elderly were largely descriptive without tight measures of service effectiveness. As part of a larger study (Luker, 1981), a hundred elderly Scottish women who lived alone were asked five open-ended questions to elicit their views about four visits at monthly intervals by a health visitor. Most of the clients enjoyed and valued the visits, which were a new experience; half of them wished to have visits continued. Utilization of three health visitor counseling and referral clinics for persons over 50 in London resulted in referrals for 145 of the 198 clients seen in the first six months of operation (Figgins, 1979). In Rochester, New York, extensive public health nursing services for the well-elderly were associated only with increases in positive perceptions of their own health, effective responses to dental screening programs, and frequent arrangements for primary care among many variables investigated in the 195 public housing residents studied (Sullivan & Armignacco, 1979). Descriptions of the characteristics and needs of the residents provided valuable information about this population.

In Miami, Florida, a geriatric nurse practitioner and a social worker (Brower & Tanner, 1979) provided instruction, a film, and discussion on human sexuality for low-income elderly volunteers at a neighborhood center. Both the need for sexual information and the difficulties of providing and evaluating such programs were demonstrated. Many participants were upset by the explicit discussion and failed to complete the posttest. The only other studies of the elderly were service need assessments in both the United States and South Africa (Franck, 1979; Newman, 1977; Pender & Pender, 1980).

Discussion

Only 26 practice evaluation studies were located in this five-year review period, compared to 44 in the preceding five years (Highriter, 1977). It should be noted, however, that utilization of the criteria for inclusion of studies in the present review would have reduced the prior total almost to the present number. Likewise, the authorship pattern, the proportion of quasi-experimental designs, and the great variety of subject matter covered was similar. New themes that emerged in the second five-year period were cost issues and care of the dying.

Research in the community setting where investigators have little control is difficult at best. Design considerations affecting internal validity and generalizibility of findings, discussed in the prior review (Highriter, 1977), merited continued vigilance. However, it appears some strengthening of research designs in the areas of sample adequacy and equivalent control groups may have occurred. Of the studies reviewed here, half had intervention-group sample sizes over 50 and eight of these were over 100. Although only three groups of investigators were able to engage in systematic or random assignment of subjects to experimental and control groups (Gutelius et al., 1977; Thibaudeau & Reidy, 1977; Vincent & Price, 1977), none of those with quasi-experimental designs noted major differences between the characteristics of these groups. This design-tightening may have been rewarded, for out of nine experimental or quasi-experimental program evaluation studies in each review period, significant positive results were found in only three (Epstein, Avni, Hopp, & Flug, 1973; Long, Whitman, Johansson, Williams, & Tuthill, 1975; Shah, Wagh, Kulkarni, & Shah, 1975) of the nine earlier studies but in six of the present set. Since most of the experimental or quasi-experimental studies with positive findings involved substantial amounts of nursing time, the larger nature of the interventions may have contributed as much to the positive findings as did the design rigor.

Nurses are understandably eager to demonstrate their effectiveness. Thus, it is gratifying that in both periods approximately 75% of the nursing activities reported were successful by at least some of the criteria used. Reasons for lack of success were generally discussed by their authors. Two of the studies with negative findings for the research questions asked, nevertheless, included documentation of successful nursing interventions (Anderson et al., 1977; Edwards, 1980). Methodological difficulties were cited by the investigators in the only two studies with no statistically significant findings (Brower & Tanner, 1979; Vincent & Price, 1977). These were quasi-experimental studies, as were two others that provided only weak support for their quite minimal nursing interventions (Lauri, 1981; Sullivan & Armignacco, 1979). The primary value of these last four studies lies in the useful descriptive information provided about the programs and populations served. The difficulties of demonstrating nursing effectiveness through quasi-experimental studies were illustrated by these four studies.

Investigators in the present group of studies, like those in the prior review, provided reasonably clear descriptions of the nursing interventions under study and generally selected measurable indicators of successful intervention. Bias due to subjective measurement techniques and data collection by service personnel is an ever present hazard when resources are limited and the concepts difficult to measure (e.g., Lauri, 1981; Luker, 1981; Vincent & Price, 1977). However, on the whole, this group of investigators seemed quite successful in selecting measurable indicators without making major validity compromises. In future multidisciplinary studies, nurse investigators might try to include more indicators that focus on the kind of client outcomes likely to result from nursing's contribution to the intervention.

PUBLIC HEALTH NURSING EDUCATION STUDIES

The controversy with regard to the scope and focus of public health nursing in a changing world (Anderson, 1983; Kelly, 1982) was reflected in both the choice of topics and the findings of the studies of education in this area. Further, although United States and British nursing curricula have different structures and historical developments, some of the same themes and concerns appeared in both countries. There were 13 studies for review—six conducted in the United States, four in England, and one each in Canada, Nigeria, and Switzerland. Methods were generally descriptive with surveys predominating, although two evaluation studies had quasi-experimental designs with matched control groups (Hauf, 1977; Owen, 1977). All of the studies dealt with educational effectiveness, frequently judged by relevance for practice; those with subject matter in areas of greater current concern were reviewed in slightly more detail. Only two studies did not include nurse authors (Dellar, 1981; Kostas, 1980).

Description of Studies

A study of master's level education in Massachusetts based evaluation on relevance of the program to subsequent service delivery. The majority of 24 former students felt that the program did not prepare them for the realities of community health nursing. Needs were expressed for more preparation in two areas: (a) management, planning, and budgeting; and (b) physical and emotional assessment (Ulin, 1978). This investigator also addressed another timely concern in public health nursing education, namely, whether management and expert clinical skills should be expected in the same person. An, as yet, uncompleted study involving the alumnae of a number of graduate programs, sparked by the Association of Graduate Faculty in Community Health/Public Health Nursing, is presently in the data analysis stage at Indiana University School of Nursing (Flynn, Note 2). When published, findings should provide a broader perspective on the same important subjects addressed by Ulin. In the only other study of master's education, Ostrand and Willis (1978) responded to concerns regarding the adequacy of school of public health Master's of Public Health (MPH) preparation for teaching in schools of nursing. They surveyed 142 graduates of schools of public health serving as community health nursing faculty in schools of nursing and 52 deans and chairpersons in National League for Nursing (NLN) accredited schools of nursing; response rate was only 51%. Deans and faculty agreed that the strengths of MPH preparation were in public health content and dealing with community agencies, while the weaknesses lay in curriculum planning and evaluation.

Concern about whether United States baccalaureate curricula were preparing graduates adequately to meet the needs of public health agency clients was one of the primary factors that led to a national survey by educators and administrators in the Public Health Nursing Section of the American Public Health Association. Approximately half of NLN-accredited programs and a comprehensive sample including persons from nearly 4,000 agencies responded to questions regarding (a) the nature of baccalaureate community health nursing education, (b) major concerns of educators and administrators, and (c) collaboration mechanisms (White, Knollmueller, & Yaksich, 1980). The data showed that the majority of students had a block field placement in the senior year, even though they were in so-called integrated curricula. Placement was most likely in a traditional public health agency although many site innovations were being tried. Faculty from many schools expressed concern about the difficulty of locating sites. Although the majority of agencies and schools were satisfied with their collaboration, there were many suggestions for better planning and collaboration, especially from the agencies.

Utilization of nontraditional sites for baccalaureate community health nursing field experience was described systematically in several articles, but only one study on this subject was found. In Montana, course outcomes for students serving a married student population were not significantly different from those of a matched control group having the traditional field experience (Hauf, 1977). Detailed anecdotal comments from graduate nurses in a 6-month public health nursing certificate program in Geneva,

Switzerland, showed the anxieties that had to be overcome in forming an extended, nonjudgmental, therapeutic relationship with families who did not require any technical nursing services (Chafetz & Gaillard, 1978).

Integration of community health into the basic nursing curriculum, a much-discussed if not investigated topic in the United States, was the subject of an English study of six educational programs that for the past 10 years had combined one year of health visitor training with the three-year state registered nurse (SRN) curriculum (Owen, 1977). These courses were in different types of educational institutions, only two of which granted a baccalaureate degree for the program. Graduates of the integrated curriculum were compared to a matched control group of same-year graduates of the separate one-year health visitor training. For integrated curriculum graduates, expectations of the ideal job more frequently involved adventure and opportunities to help others. They perceived health visiting as coming closer to meeting these expectations than did general nursing, and, in fact, a high proportion became health visitors. Commonly expressed expectations for graduates of the integrated curriculum—that they would have a broad perspective on patient care, retain curiosity, and seek the cause of problems, but also would lack confidence—sound like expressions about baccalaureate graduates in the United States. A survey of the employers of English integrated-curriculum graduates confirmed these expectations to a large extent but also raised questions regarding whether they might result from a self-fulfilling prophecy (Owen, 1977).

Other English concerns involved preparing hospital nurses to appreciate the community component of health care and selecting students for health visitor training. Davies (1977) found that 831 Nottingham SRN-course students over a six-year period provided generally high evaluations of 1- to 13-week community care courses. These courses involved a variety of field placements, both near the beginning and end of their basic course. On returning to the hospital, a high proportion of a subsample of 29 claimed attitude change toward patients, their relatives, and community nursing staff (Davies, 1977). Investigations of the relationship between possible selection criteria for health visitor training and student performance were conducted in Gloucestershire (Dellar, 1981) and in Surry (Jarvis & Gibson, 1981). No reliable predictors were found in records of past academic performance, standard educational performance examinations, personality tests, or interview data. Further systematic investigation of all areas was recommended since selection for training controls entrance into the profession.

Two continuing education studies based on small samples were the only ones in which investigators demonstrated the impact of education on subsequent nursing practice. In Iowa, public health nursing supervisors reported improved attitudes and competence in maternal child health care eight months after a 12-day course on the childbearing family (Heick, 1981). Knowledge retention and use of teaching materials continued two years after a hypertensive diet education program for nurses working with hypertensive residents in public housing in New Orleans (Kostas, 1980). The educational needs of practicing nurses and students were assessed in two studies: one in Ontario, Canada, in which nurses felt the need for additional preparation to provide contraceptive services to youth (Herold & Thomas, 1977), and the other in Nigeria, where it was found that screening for handicaps in children was not being taught in the nursing schools and not taking place in community health centers (Okunade, 1980).

Discussion

The studies reviewed in this area dealt with a wide variety of educational programs and issues. The number (13) did not increase much from the preceding five years (Highriter, 1977), but the recent studies more frequently dealt with broad basic issues than did those in the preceding five years, and more were authored by nurses. Studies tended to be descriptive, using opinion surveys and small samples. There is need for a concerted effort to address educational issues in depth by studying them in several similar education programs; the researchers who started this trend are to be commended (Owen, 1977; White et al., 1980). More studies with experimental or quasi-experimental designs and evaluations based on subsequent performance would increase confidence in the research findings. The relevance of curricula to public health nursing practice should be a subject of ongoing study by both individual schools and groups of schools; investigation should not await complaints from unhappy alumnae and their employers.

STUDIES OF DELIVERY SYSTEM AND PROFESSIONAL ISSUES

Of the 17 studies of delivery system and professional issues, 11 were conducted in the United States, four in Canada, and one each in England and Scotland. They fall into two main areas: (a) development of quality assurance methodology; and (b) nursing role, teamwork, and attitudes o perceptions of public health nurses compared to hospital nurses. Thirteen o the studies were nurse-authored.

Quality Assurance Methodology

Using a tested, record-audit tool based on the 1975 ANA standards o quality care, Koerner (1981) employed a multiple regression analysis to study the correlates of supervisor-rated job performance scores of 32 nurse volunteers from the Visiting Nurse Association of Hartford, Connecticut Only 38% of the variation in these scores was explained by experience knowledge, and environmental variables. The investigator questioned whether record audits reflected the true quality of care rendered or merely other factors that influenced charting. Engle and Barkauskas (1979) de scribed the development and testing, within the Chicago Department o Health, of a performance evaluation tool that used record review, observation, and interview to evaluate patient and family care given by individual nurses. They were satisfied with the tool's content validity and interna consistency, but not with interrater reliability or score ranges.

In California, investigators found implementation of a diagnosis specific type of care standard, the Oncology Nursing Society Outcome Standard on Nutrition, both feasible and desirable (Singer, Baker, Valencius, Packard, Herlt, Brainerd, Thomas, & Browning, 1981). In three type of agencies, documentation with regard to five of the standard's six outcome criteria showed high compliance with the standard. However, the documentation time required for each diagnosis-specific standard would force an agency to focus on frequently occurring indicator diagnoses rather than making a total caseload review. This might be adequate if fitted within an overall evaluation scheme like the Key Factor Analysis described by Hauf (1981).

Different evaluation approaches that were applicable across caseloads of varying medical diagnoses were taken by three other agencies. Although not reported as research, the Visiting Nurse Association of New Haven developed a patient classification scheme based on client rehabilitation potential that provided outcome criteria for each of five levels from full recovery to death (Daubert, 1979). In Hartford, the Visiting Nurse Association is testing a scheme, also based on client self-management, that permits measurement of levels of progress toward independence in five areas, including knowledge and activities of daily living (Torpey, Note 3). Feasibility and utility of these systems were demonstrated and they could be subjected to reliability testing. Investigators from the Visiting Nurse Association of Omaha and three other agencies conducted a methodological study to test their scheme for categorizing the client problems with which public health nurses deal. This category system provided the foundation for an overall evaluation scheme that is being developed based on expected client outcomes for each of 38 listed problems. Nurses found the list exhaustive for their use in the testing agencies (Martin, 1982; Simmons, 1980).

In the final study in this group, Ford and Lake (1979) described an audit system, based on general process-oriented criteria, that was developed for nursing under very special circumstances, those of preflight and inflight nursing service provided by the Aeromedical Evacuation System of the United States Air Force (Air Evac). The method of evaluating criteria validity and measurability was described as was the extent to which criteria were met on the first audit. In a second article about the Air Evac audit, Hansen (1980) described the addition of a diagnosis-specific audit and compared findings from follow-up audits to those from the initial general audit.

The status of methodological development in quality assurance is at a higher level in hospitals than in public health agencies. Staff in these agencies are now beginning to recognize the limitations of relying solely on the convenience of record audits (Koerner, 1981), but in attempts to broaden the approach they have not attained desired standards of reliability (Engle & Barkauskas, 1979). These studies reflected beginning concern for the importance of measurement issues in an area where many practitioners are using any feasible method and seem unaware of the need for input from researchers. The studies also contained some sound conceptual bases for future evaluation studies. Both diagnosis-specific and more general approaches to program and performance evaluation were tested with utilization of both process and outcome indicators. Much more work is needed both on measurement and on the advantages and disadvantages of the different approaches to conceptualization.

Role, Teamwork, and Attitude Studies

While United States studies dominated the quality assurance arena, Canadian and British investigators focused on issues affecting the functioning of public health teams. There were seven studies in this area. Morale, defined in terms of group compatibility, was associated significantly with intrateam professional communication for 55 members of seven multidisciplinary teams studied by Warren (1978) in two Ontario health centers. In another Ontario study, Bass, Warren, and Mumby (1980) explored advantages and disadvantages in the attachment of 106 public health nurses to the practices of both urban and rural family physicians. The attached nurses had better communications and more referrals from physicians than nonattached nurses; they spent more time on counseling activities and more time with patients over 65 and with patients having psychosocial problems. Initially, it was difficult for nurses to try attachments to physician practices; and there was also the possibility of failure to reach those clients who did not seek physician care, especially babies. In a study in Scotland, 16 students from each of four primary care disciplines (general medical practice, health visiting, district nursing, and social work) tended to define their own roles broadly and the roles of other team members narrowly and stereotypically. The potential for overlap conflicts in practice was believed to be great unless modifications were made in training for team practice (Milne, 1980).

In contrast, the integration of male nurses into district nursing teams in England seemed to present little difficulty. A three-part study by Chung (1981) showed that most of 60 female nurse respondents had experience with male nurses and favorable attitudes toward them. Only four of the 14 divisional nursing officers surveyed felt that male nurses could be employed only selectively with female patients. When Chung himself spent a day visiting female patients at home with another male district nurse, patients gave them universally favorable receptions.

The likely effects of environmental and situational factors on public health nursing role behavior were shown in three United States studies in the primary care arena. Fiske and Munroe (1981) found that 27 public health nurses engaged in screening programs functioned like physician-extenders and collected little information beyond that required on an agency-provided health history and physical examination form. When interviewed, only a fourth of them provided any information about health behaviors, risk factors, or family problems of the clients. Moscovice (1977) found that patterns of management for otitis media (antibiotic, throat culture, follow-up visit, or combination) within the Frontier Nursing Service apparently were influenced by whether care was given in the district or hospital and by provider skill level. High skill levels and hospital practice were associated with expensive care patterns. High skill levels were also associated with increased job satisfaction for 50 licensed vocational nurses, 47 registered nurses, and 14 nurse practitioners in a health maintenance organization (Smith, 1981).

In two United States and two Canadian studies, investigators explored public health nurses' attitudes and perceptions that might influence their performance; the same factors were studied in hospital nurses and comparisons were made. In the first study, decision-making processes in the selection of living situations for the elderly were compared for 26 hospital nurses, 21 visiting nurse association nurses, and 16 elderly people (Grier, 1977a, 1977b). When a quantitative decision-making process was used with regard to a written patient situation, all three groups agreed that the patient's needs were most likely to be met in a nursing home. However, when using an intuitive decision-making process, visiting nurses generally disagreed with the other two groups and with their own quantitative decision making.

Looking at the stress levels of 26 hospice nurses in New Jersey, Barstow (1980) found no between-group differences in the relatively low anxiety levels of both inpatient and home care nurses in two hospices. However, the groups differed on the sources of stress, with home care nurses more likely to report difficulty managing medications and respiratory problems. They also had difficulty coping with depressed patients, childhood deaths, and the death of patients with whom they strongly identified. In Ontario, little difference in attitude toward care of the dying was found between 88 public health nurses from both official and voluntary agencies and nurses in chronic and acute care institutions (Gow & Williams, 1977). Nurses over 40 had more positive attitudes and less anxiety in care of the dying than younger nurses. Nearly a third of all nurses found care of the dying frustrating, with those in chronic-care institutions most likely to find it rewarding.

In a final attitude study, also conducted in Ontario, Rosenbaum (1977) examined the attitudes of 10 public health nurses toward 41 alcohol abusers. Significant positive correlations were found between nonmoralistic nursing attitudes, optimism regarding prognosis, and a disease-oriented view of alcohol abuse.

Discussion

The findings of the descriptive studies in this area suggested the importance of situational factors, as well as personality characteristics and nurses' life experiences in influencing their practice of public health nursing. Since the public health nurses studied were, in most instances, from a single agency and some sample sizes were quite small, replication seems especially important. With the difficulty of inferring causality from correlation and the low level of most of the associations noted, extreme caution must be used in predicting individual nurses' behavior.

TRENDS, IMPLICATIONS, AND RESEARCH RECOMMENDATIONS

Comparison of studies in the recent and immediately preceding five-year periods revealed many more similarities than differences. This leads one to conclude that the status of public health and community health nursing research did not change substantially. For those categories of studies reviewed in both the present and preceding five-year periods, the total number published was still only about 10 per year. Over half the studies had nurses as the primary author, while a fourth included no nurses in the group of authors. The proportion conducted in the United States decreased from 65% to 50%, but this may have been a function of retrieval difficulties with United States studies. Investigators from Great Britain and Canada were the other primary contributors to publications in English, and Japan investigators to the group of studies published in other languages.

In both periods, most studies were descriptive, with experimental or quasi-experimental designs employed in just under a fourth of the studies. Most studies were confined to a single or small number of agencies; sample sizes, although perhaps increasing, still were relatively small (under 100). Great variation in subject matter within a similar range of topics was characteristic of studies in both periods; there were only a few studies on the same subject and no replications were reported. During the latter time period topics on which several studies were conducted included: effectiveness of child health supervision and hypertension control activities, evaluation of screening programs, care of the dying, cost-effectiveness of home care, development of quality assurance methodology, factors affecting multidisciplinary team functioning, major curricular issues in basic nursing education such as integration, and the nature of field placements in the community. All but the first two represented new emphases.

Evaluation was the predominant theme of the 56 studies reviewed in this chapter; 45 of the studies were directly concerned with evaluating the delivery of either service or education, or with the development of methodology for such evaluations (the quality assurance studies). The basis for evaluation was the attainment of desired outcomes that might be physiological, behavioral or cognitive changes, client or student satisfaction, or cost savings. In the remaining 11 studies, situational, environmental, and nurse variables that might be expected to influence practice were investigated. These variables affect attainment of the kinds of outcomes sought in evaluation studies and are therefore related to the evaluation process.

Most of the studies were pragmatic in nature and dealt with current practice and educational concerns. A desire to document effectiveness and control costs probably provided the motivation for most of the practice studies. Theory discussion was almost nonexistent except for discussion of the theoretical foundations of some of the interventions. Perhaps this was due to the fact that public health nursing is a hybrid discipline with foundations in both public health and nursing science, and the synthesis of these two had not as yet been conceptualized fully. Present nursing theories pertain most directly to one-to-one relationships with clients or small groups, while public health nursing is committed to a population focus. Public health science provides epidemiological theory and various applications of administrative, educational, and social science theories to public health problems, but it does not provide an integrated practice theory. Current work on the definition of public health or community health nursing by major professional organizations (American Nurses' Association, 1980; American Public Health Association, Note 1) and recent publications (Archer, 1982; Crow, 1981; Goeppinger, Lassiter, & Wilcox, 1982; Shamansky & Pesznecker, 1981; White, 1982; Williams, 1977) may represent the beginnings of such theory development. If so, a theoretical framework may emerge that will serve as a means of drawing together studies that currently seem very diverse, since the health problems and human responses with which public health nurses deal are diverse. The knowledge base required for public health nursing practice is much broader than the studies included in this review would lead one to believe, because much basic research about the biomedical, psychosocial, and cultural nature of human beings is relevant to practice, whether or not nursing interventions themselves were studied.

Research is of little value to clients unless nurses utilize it in their practice. Krueger (1982) reported the results of a survey of research utilization in community health nursing agencies. She noted that 67% of these nurses felt they had a favorable climate for utilization, and 24% identified a person or position with specific responsibility for identifying scientific knowledge ready for use. In examining nursing content used in community health agencies, Krueger used the protocols prepared for nursing research utilization through the Conduct and Utilization of Research in Nursing (CURN) project in Michigan (Horsley, Crane, & Bingle, 1978). This was research dealing with nursing practice problems irrespective of practice setting where, in the judgment of project staff, sufficient replication had taken place to recommend use of the findings in practice. Two issues became apparent to this reviewer: (a) much nursing research not conducted in community settings is nevertheless applicable to community nursing practice; and (b) much of the research reviewed in this chapter has not been replicated and is therefore not ready for use except in settings where replication (with or without modification or extension) is possible. General nursing research indexed by client problems is much easier to retrieve than community health nursing research, which now can be found only by setting specifications (that may or may not reflect a type of nursing). Hopefully, further conceptual development in the public health or community health nursing area will facilitate both retrieval and replication of this research.

At the end of the first five-year review of community health nursing research (Highriter, 1977), recommendations were made with regard to the need for improving measurement and control techniques and providing for increased research preparation and activity in the field; all still apply. Doctoral preparation of nurse-researchers was documented in many of the articles reviewed in this chapter, while preparation was frequently unspecified in articles of the former review. This and the fact that six of the quasi-experimental studies in the practice evaluation section of this review documented public health nursing effectiveness indicate that public health nursing research is moving in the desired direction. The activities recommended for emphasis as a result of the present review are: (a) development of a theoretical framework for public health nursing practice, based on synthesis of frameworks from nursing and public health; (b) examination of public health nursing activities within this framework; (c) utilization of experimental and quasi-experimental designs where possible to test practice elements; (d) building on previous studies with replication of appropriate aspects; (e) focusing on major practice problems common in health nursing and engaging in both basic and applied research needed to improve practice; and (f) planning ongoing educational research that involves groups of schools.

REFERENCE NOTES

1. American Public Health Association (APHA). *The definition and role of public health nursing in the delivery of health care: A statement of the Public Health Nursing Section* (A mimeographed booklet). Author, November 1980. (Address: 1015 Fifteenth Street, N. W., Washington, D.C., 20005)
2. Flynn, B. C., contact person for the consortium of graduate faculty in public health nursing, July, 1983. Department of Community Health Nursing. (Address: Indiana University School of Nursing, Indianapolis, Ind. 46223)
3. Torpey, J. A., Personal Communication, June 2, 1983. (Quality Assurance Specialist, Visiting Nurse and Home Care, Inc., 167 New Britain Avenue, Plainville, Conn. 06062)

REFERENCES

American Nurses' Association, Division on Community Health Nursing. *A conceptual model of community health nursing* (ANA Publication Code CH-10 2M 5/80). Kansas City, Mo.: Author, 1980.

Anderson, E. T. Community focus in public health nursing: Whose responsibility? *Nursing Outlook,* 1983, *31,* 44–48.

Anderson, E., Anderson, T. P., & Kottke, F. J. Stroke rehabilitation: Maintenance of achieved gains. *Archives of Physical Medicine and Rehabilitation,* 1977, *58,* 345–352.

Archer, S. A. Synthesis of public health science and nursing science. *Nursing Outlook,* 1982, *30,* 442–446.

Barnes, G. The nurse's contribution to the Medical Research Council's trial for mild hypertension. *Nursing Times,* 1981, *77,* 1240–1245.

Barstow, J. Stress variance in hospice nursing. *Nursing Outlook,* 1980, *28,* 751–754.

Bass, M., Warren, S., & Mumby, D. Some observations on a program attaching public health nurses to family physicians' offices. *Journal of Community Health,* 1980, *5,* 194–203.

Brennan, L. A., Krishan, I., Nobrega, F. T., Labarthe, D. R., Timm, M. E., McGrath, J. V., Sheps, S. G., & Hunt, J. C. The Mayo three-community hypertension control program: III. Outcome in a community-based hypertension clinic. *Mayo Clinic Proceedings,* 1979, *54,* 307–312.

Brower, H. T., & Tanner, L. A. A study of older adults attending a program on human sexuality: A pilot study. *Nursing Research,* 1979, *28,* 36–39.

Chafetz, L., & Gaillard, J. The impact of a therapeutic nurse-family relationship on post graduate public health nursing students. *International Journal of Nursing Studies,* 1978, *15,* 37–49.

Chung, D. The gentle touch—could we—should we? A project which looked at the deployment of male nurses in the district. *Nursing Times,* 1981, *77,* 287–290.

Creek, L. V. A homecare hospice profile: Description, evaluation, and cost analyses. *The Journal of Family Practice,* 1982, *14,* 53–58.

Crow, R. Theories and concepts are important when planning research into health visiting practice. *Nursing Times,* 1981, *77,* 284–286.

Daubert, E. A. Patient classification system and outcome criteria. *Nursing Outlook,* 1979, *27,* 450–454.

Davies, J. M. A 6-year survey of community care courses for basic nursing students. *Journal of Advanced Nursing,* 1977, *2,* 597–608.

Dellar, C. J. The selection of students for health visitor training courses. *Journal of Advanced Nursing,* 1981, *6,* 111–115.

Edwards, V. Changing breast self-examination behavior. *Nursing Research,* 1980, *29,* 301–306.

Engle, J., & Barkauskas, J. E. The evolution of a public health nursing performance evaluation tool. *Journal of Nursing Administration,* 1979, *9*(4), 8–16.

Epstein, L. M., Avni, A., Hopp, C., & Flug, D. Evaluation of a program of aftercare for patients discharged from the hospital. *Medical Care,* 1973, *11,* 320–327.

Figgins, P. Screen now—Benefit later. *Nursing Mirror*, 1979, *149*(9), 24–25.

Firth, D., Chamberlain, M. A., Fligg, H., Wright, J., & Wright, V. Health visitors in a rehabilitation unit. *Nursing Times*, 1978, *74*, 249–250.

Fiske, M., & Munroe, D. Are PHN skills used in screening clinics? *Nursing and Health Care*, 1981, *2*, 196–199.

Ford, M. L., & Lake, L. R. Establishing an audit system for Air Evac. *Aviation, Space, and Environmental Medicine*, 1979, *50*, 284–289.

Franck, P. A survey of health needs of older adults in northwest Johnston County, Iowa. *Nursing Research*, 1979, *28*, 360–364.

Goeppinger, J., Lassiter, P. G., & Wilcox, B. Community health is community competence. *Nursing Outlook*, 1982, *30*, 464–467.

Gow, C., & Williams, J. I. Nurses' attitudes toward death and dying: A causal interpretation. *Social Science and Medicine*, 1977, *11*, 191–198.

Grier, M. R. Choosing living arrangements for the elderly. *International Journal of Nursing Studies*, 1977, *14*, 69–76. (a)

Grier, M. R. Living arrangements for the elderly. *Journal of Gerontological Nursing*, 1977, *3*(4), 19–22. (b)

Gutelius, M. F., Kirsch, A. D., MacDonald, S., Brooks, M. R., & McErlean, T. Controlled study of child health supervision: Behavioral results. *Pediatrics*, 1977, *60*, 294–304.

Hansen, P. J. A look at quality assurance through the audit process. *Aviation, Space, and Environmental Medicine*, 1980, *51*, 937–938.

Hauf, B. J. An evaluative study of a nursing center for community health nursing student experiences. *Journal of Nursing Education*, 1977, *16*(8), 7–11.

Hauf, B. J. Program evaluation in nursing utilizing key factor analysis. *Nursing Leadership*, 1981, *4*(3), 6–13.

Heick, M. A. Continuing education impact evaluation. *The Journal of Continuing Education in Nursing*, 1981, *12*(4), 15–23.

Herold, E. S., & Thomas, E. R. Attitudes of nurses to providing contraceptive services for youth. *Canadian Journal of Public Health*, 1977, *68*, 307–310.

Highriter, M. E. The status of community health nursing research. *Nursing Research*, 1977, *28*, 183–192.

Horsley, J. A., Crane, J., & Bingle, J. D. Research utilization as an organizational process. *Journal of Nursing Administration*, 1978, *8*(7), 4–6.

Houston, M. J., & Howie, P. W. Home support for the breast feeding mother. *Midwife, Health-visitor and Community Nurse*, 1981, *17*, 378–382.

Jarvis, P., & Gibson, S. J. An investigation into the validity of specifying 5 'O' levels in the General Certificate of Education as an entry requirement for the education and training of district nurses. *Journal of Advanced Nursing*, 1981, *6*, 471–482.

Kassakian, M. G., Bailey, L. R., Rinker, M., Stewart, C. A., & Yates, J. W. The cost and quality of dying: A comparison of home and hospital. *Nurse Practitioner*, 1979, *4*(1), 18–23.

Kekki, P. Analyses of relationships between the availability of resources and the use of health services in Finland. *Medical Care*, 1980, *18*, 1228–1240.

Kelly, L. S. Crossroads in public health nursing. *Nursing Outlook*, 1982, *30*, 503. (Editorial)

Koerner, B. L. Selected correlates of job performance of community health nurses. *Nursing Research,* 1981, *30,* 43–48.

Komrower, G. M., Sardharwalla, I. B., Fowler, B., & Bridge, C. The Manchester regional screening programme: A 10-year exercise in patient and family care. *British Medical Journal,* 1979, *2,* 635–638.

Kostas, G. Evaluation and follow-up of a hypertension diet education program. *Journal of the American Dietetic Association,* 1980, *77,* 574–576.

Krueger, J. C. Using research in practice: A survey of research utilization in community health nursing. *Western Journal of Nursing Research,* 1982, *4,* 244–248.

Lauri, S. The public health nurse as a guide in infant child-care and education. *Journal of Advanced Nursing,* 1981, *6,* 297–303.

Logan, A. G., Milne, B. J., Achber, C., Campbell, W. P., & Haynes, R. B. Work-site treatment of hypertension by specially trained nurses. *The Lancet,* 1979, *2,* 1175–1178.

Long, G. V., Whitman, C., Johansson, M. S., Williams, C. A., & Tuthill, R. W. Evaluation of a school health program directed to children with history of high absence. *American Journal of Public Health,* 1975, *65,* 388–393.

Luker, K. Elderly women's opinions about the benefits of health visitor visits. *Nursing Times,* 1981, *77*(12, March 19), 33–36. (Occasional Paper No. 9)

Martin, K. A client classification system adaptable for computerization. *Nursing Outlook,* 1982, *30,* 515–517.

Martin, M. H., & Ishino, M. Domiciliary night nursing service: Luxury or necessity? *British Medical Journal,* 1981, *282,* 883–885.

Martinson, I. M., Armstrong, G. D., Geis, D. P., Anglim, M. A., Gronseth, E. C., MacInnis, H., Kersey, J. H., & Nesbit, M. E. Home care for children dying of cancer. *Pediatraics,* 1978, *62,* 106–113.

Martinson, I. M., Armstrong, G. D., Geis, D. P., Anglim, M. A., Gronseth, E. C., MacInnis, H., Nesbit, M. E., & Kersey, J. H. Facilitating home care for children dying of cancer. *Cancer Nursing,* 1978, *1,* 41–45.

Milne, M. A. Training for team care. *Journal of Advanced Nursing,* 1980, *5,* 579–589.

Moldow, D. G., & Martinson, I. M. From research to reality—Home care for the dying child. *Maternal Child Nursing,* 1980, *5,* 159–166.

Moscovice, I. A method for analyzing resource use in ambulatory care settings. *Medical Care,* 1977, *15,* 1024–1044.

Newman, T. F., The setting up of a geriatric screening clinic in Cape Town. *South African Medical Journal,* 1977, *51,* 427–430.

Nissinen, A., Tuomilehto, J., Elo, J., Salonen, J., & Puska, P. Implementation of a hypertension control program in the County of North Karelia, Finland. *Public Health Reports,* 1981, *96,* 503–513.

Okunade, A. O. Screening for handicaps in children: Are Nigerian nurses equipped? *International Journal of Nursing Studies,* 1980, *17,* 181–187.

Ostrand, L., & Willis, W. Faculty preparation: An MPH or MSN degree? *Nursing Outlook,* 1978, *26,* 637–640.

Owen, G. M. Curriculum integration in nursing education: A concept or a way of life? A study of six courses integrating basic nursing education and health visiting in a single course. *Journal of Advanced Nursing*, 1977, *2*, 443–460.

Pender, N. J., & Pender, A. R. Illness prevention and health promotion services provided by nurse practitioners: Predicting potential consumers. *American Journal of Public Health*, 1980, *70*, 798–803.

Petrowski, D. D. Effectiveness of prenatal and postpartum instruction in postpartum care. *Journal of Obstetric, Gynecologic, and Neonatal (JOGN) Nursing*, 1981, *10*, 386–389.

Robertson, C. Evaluation and screening: An epidemiological approach. 1. Measuring the effectiveness of health visitors. *Health Visitor*, 1981, *54*, 20–21. (a)

Robertson, C. Evaluation and screening: An epidemiological approach. 2. A review of vision screening in pre-school children. *Health Visitor*, 1981, *54*, 52–57. (b)

Robertson, C. Evaluation and screening: An epidemiological approach. 3. Monitoring pre-school screening of visual acuity by health visitors—A feasibility study. *Health Visitor*, 1981, *54*, 104–105. (c)

Rosenbaum, P. D. Public health nurses in the treatment of alcohol abusers. *Canadian Journal of Public Health*, 1977, *68*, 503–508.

Ruckley, C. V., Garraway, W. M., Cuthbertson, C., Fenwick, N., & Prescott, R. J., The community nurse and day surgery. *Nursing Times*, 1980, *76*, 255–256.

Sanger, S., Weir, K., & Churchill, E. Treatment of sleep problems: The use of behavioural modification techniques by health visitors. *Health Visitor*, 1981, *54*, 421–424.

Shah, P. M., Wagh, K. K., Kulkarni, P. V., & Shah, B. The impact of hospital and domiciliary nutrition rehabilitation on diet of the child and other young children in the family and in neighbourhood. *Indian Pediatrics*, 1975, *12*, 95–98.

Shamansky, S. L., & Pesznecker, B. A community is . . . *Nursing Outlook*, 1981, *29*, 182–185.

Simmons, D. *A classification scheme for client problems in community health nursing* (DHHS Publication No. HRA 80–16). Hyattsville, Md.: Division of Nursing, Health Resources Administration, U.S. Department of Health and Human Services, June 1980. (NTIS No. HRP–0501501)

Singer, M., Baker, V., Valencius, J., Packard, R., Herlt, L., Brainerd, C., Thomas, C., & Browning, B. Implementation of one standard of care in a variety of patient care agencies. *Cancer Nursing*, 1981, *4*, 293–297.

Smith, H. L. Nurses' quality of working life in an HMO: A comparative study. *Nursing Research*, 1981, *30*, 54–58.

Spiegel, M. A., & Lindaman, F. C. Children can't fly: A program to prevent childhood morbidity and mortality from window falls. *American Journal of Public Health*, 1977, *67*, 1143–1147.

Sullivan, J. A., & Armignacco, F. Effectiveness of a comprehensive health program for the well-elderly by community health nurses. *Nursing Research*, 1979, *28*, 70–75.

Thibaudeau, M. F., & Reidy, M. M. Nursing makes a difference: A comparative study of the health behavior of mothers in three primary care agencies. *International Journal of Nursing Studies*, 1977, *14*, 97–107.

Ulin, P. R. What master's students want to know. *Nursing Outlook*, 1978, *26*, 629–632.

Vincent, P., & Price, J. R. Evaluation of a VNA mental health project. *Nursing Research*, 1977, *26*, 361–367.

Warren, S. The relationship between morale and communication among health center team members. *Canadian Journal of Public Health*, 1978, *69*, 133–138.

White, C., Knollmueller, R., & Yaksich, S. Preparation for community health nursing: Issues and problems. *Nursing Outlook*, 1980, *28*, 617–623.

White, M. S. Construct for public health nursing. *Nursing Outlook*, 1982, *30*, 527–530.

Williams, C. A. Community health nursing—What is it? *Nursing Outlook*, 1977, *25*, 250–254.

PART III

Research on
Nursing Education

CHAPTER 8

Research on the Teaching-Learning Process in Nursing Education

RHEBA DE TORNYAY

SCHOOL OF NURSING

UNIVERSITY OF WASHINGTON

CONTENTS

During the past thirty years nursing education has become an accepted part of higher education and a focus of inquiry for nurses. However, nursing educational research has varied in quantity and quality. This chapter includes a review of research on one aspect of nursing education: the teaching-learning process.

EDUCATION RESEARCH: HISTORICAL PERSPECTIVE

In considering the research on teaching-learning in nursing education, studies appearing in the literature from 1971 to 1982 were reviewed. The major reason for limiting the review to this period is because teaching-learning research during the 1960s usually was focused on the effects of what was termed the "new media." In the early 1960s, educators highly proclaimed the efficiency derived from television, programmed instruction, and other innovations to help students learn. In much of this research, investigators compared results obtained in courses using two or more media. By the end of the decade, the researchers found that educators could use these media effectively but not for all purposes (Trent & Cohen, 1973). Educational technology joined the textbook as a teaching tool available to both educator and student. In some studies reported in this chapter, investigators attempted to compare one teaching strategy with another; generally such studies are no longer considered a fruitful field for inquiry.

There were other changes during the 1960s that influenced the decision to limit the studies reviewed. During the 1960s, institutional and federal financial support permitted curriculum and teaching research in nursing to be approached with a commitment not known previously nor subsequently. New curricula and new ways of approaching teaching and learning were tested erratically. Often evaluations were made after the point when change could take place. In vogue at the time were process-oriented curricula, integrated curricula, and others that were added to teachers' vocabularies, but without clear definition. Such curricula and accompanying teaching methods rarely described replicable procedures.

During the 1970s, investigators addressed to a greater degree the core problems pertaining to the science of instruction or the process by which individual students learn. The objective of the research was to increase teachers' power to understand, predict, and control those events central to teaching and learning through observational or experimental data.

Definitions and Method

In this chapter, teaching is viewed as an interpersonal influence aimed at changing the ways in which other persons can or will behave. Learning is defined as a change in behavior due to experience. Researchers in teaching-learning examine how the teacher influences students, as well as the behavior change that results from learning experiences. The literature included in this review is limited to empirical studies. These studies were focused on teachers' behaviors such as lecturing, questioning, and testing, as well as teachers' influence on learner characteristics. The characteristics of learners included cognitive styles, achievement of knowledge, personality, and motivation. Historically, the determination of educational objectives and consideration of instructional goals has been the concern of curriculum development. Although it is an artificial separation to isolate teaching-learning problems in nursing education from curriculum outcomes, there is a need to emphasize the particular problems inherent in teaching-learning research.

Studies selected for review included only those where students were in a formal course of study in a basic nursing curriculum or graduate study in nursing. Of the 37 studies selected, subjects in 25 studies were nursing students in baccalaureate programs; six studies had students in graduate nursing programs; and in six studies, subjects were divided equally between hospital diploma nursing schools or associate degree programs in nursing.

ORGANIZATION FOR REVIEW

Thirty-seven investigations of the teaching-learning process in nursing education were found through a review of published nursing literature from 1971 through 1982. In this chapter these empirical studies are divided into four major groupings: effect of specific teaching strategies on student achievement of educational objectives; teaching-learning effects on the development of attitudes and values; teaching-learning effects on the development of clinical skills, including clinical decision making and psychomotor skills; and evaluation of student performance.

It is interesting to note the characteristics of authors whose studies were reviewed. Of the 37 senior authors, all but two were nurses. The educational backgrounds of the nurse authors were: 14 held the PhD; 4 an EdD; 15 a master's degree; and 2 either a BS or a nonacademic certificate. Twenty-nine of the studies were presented by senior authors who were faculty members in college or university schools of nursing. At the time of publication, the authors' academic ranks were: 2 professors, 6 associate professors, 16 assistant professors, and 3 instructors. The academic rank of two authors was not stated. The eight remaining authors held positions in community colleges, diploma schools, or schools other than nursing. One conclusion that could be drawn from this profile is that research in this area has not received much attention from senior faculty members.

Effect of Teaching Strategies on Student Achievement

Fifteen studies were categorized into this group where the investigator(s) wanted to study the effect(s) of a specific teaching strategy or strategies on student achievement of educational objectives. These objectives included both knowledge of content and student satisfaction in the learning process.

In 11 studies (Blatchley, Herzog, & Russell, 1978; Huckabay, 1978; Huckabay, Anderson, Holm, & Lee, 1979; Kirchhoff & Holzemer, 1979; Kissinger & Munjas, 1981; Mackie, 1973; Moser & Kondracki, 1977; Pensivy, 1977; Stein, Steele, Fuller, & Langhoff, 1972; Thompson, 1972; White & Chavigny, 1975) investigators attempted to examine the effectiveness of a specific teaching strategy on learning outcomes. Comparing one method of teacher or media presentation to another was emphasized. In the majority of the studies the investigators performed both methods used, thus raising questions of bias that will be discussed later in this chapter. In these studies, investigators compared "traditional" teaching methods—like lecture-discussion—to the use of learning modules, television (black and white compared to color), multimedia autotutorial approaches, and computer-assisted instruction. The dependent variables included cognitive learning, attitudes about the subject, transfer of learning, and student satisfaction.

Kirchhoff and Holzemer (1979) examined the effectiveness of computer-assisted instructional programs in an attempt to examine the relationship between students' learning preference styles, attitudes, and performance. They suggested that different learning styles do not penalize students' learning in a computer-assisted program and make economical use of faculty and student time. Although this study had a relatively small sample size (100 students), implementation in a single institution, and a short time between the experiment and the testing for changes, it was an important study because it raised significant research questions that may benefit large numbers of students in terms of efficiency of learning.

Kissinger and Munjas (1981) pointed the way to future research in the area of specific teaching strategies on student achievements. These investigators wanted to determine the relationship among student attributes, teaching methodologies, and ability to apply problem-solving methods to nursing. Impulsiveness, reflectivity, and locus of control were included as variables that influenced performance. This study was the only one in this group for which the investigators used a large sample of baccalaureate nursing students. It is unfortunate that the investigators were unable to select the sample randomly, but the volunteers were drawn from six universities in one region of the United States. The data about teaching method were provided by 77 faculty members from the six schools of nursing. They found that those teaching and testing strategies using clinical problems fostered skill in problem solving. This study may have implications for admission to schools of nursing because it demonstrated that students who scored high on vocabulary tests also scored high in clinical simulations. This study should be replicated because it has the potential of impact on the way problem-solving skills are developed in nursing students.

In four studies investigators approached learning outcomes somewhat differently. Floyd (1975) studied the advantages and disadvantages of team teaching in relation to student outcomes. In surveying one class, baccalaureate nursing students indicated more positive than negative responses to being taught by a group of teachers. Advantages included freedom of choice for the student, greater depth of covered material, and exposure to different values, philosophies, experiences, and sources of information. Highest among the disadvantages were repetition of experiences, lack of student security, and contradictory practices among faculty. This is one of the few recent studies where students' views on both advantages and disadvantages of team teaching were investigated. Chandler and Hunter (1976) provided important information in their descriptive study to determine whether knowing the questions prior to an examination would influence student learning. Their research deserves further study because it raised important questions about the role of anxiety on learning. Brock (1978), in a well-designed experimental study, attempted to determine the impact of a management-oriented course on baccalaureate nursing students' knowledge and leadership skills. Three different teaching strategies were developed, each designed to meet specific course objectives. In an attempt to provide a more refined definition of teaching behavior, Scholdra and Quiring (1973) analyzed the level of questions asked by faculty in a baccalaureate school of nursing. They found that out of a total of 617 questions asked by 16 instructors, only six questions could be considered higher-order questions, although the course objectives specified higher-order cognitive thinking as the desired student outcome. Therefore, the instructors' behavior was not consistent with the course objectives.

Teaching-Learning of Attitudes and Values

A number of variables such as attitudes, values, interests, motivation, appreciation, personal adjustment, self-actualization, and other personality characteristics are considered affective behavior. The term noncognitive is also used to characterize these variables, distinguishing them from the more task-oriented cognitive variables such as achievement and aptitude. Khan and Weiss (1973) pointed out that it is acceptable to include feelings of liking or disliking toward social or psychological objects in the affective domain of teaching-learning research. All of these variables will be considered in reviewing the research on nursing education in this important, but elusive, area of study.

Ten studies included investigation of affective student behaviors. Data were collected by student self-report. Although several investigators used existing measurement scales, in all situations the data were dependent on students' perceptions. Neither observational nor projective techniques were employed. Without question, the general availability and documentation of psychometrically sound attitude scales was far from satisfactory (Khan & Weiss, 1973), and investigators interested in this area of nursing education outcomes should be aware of the limitations of adequate measuring instruments.

One area of continuing interest to faculty is the degree to which their own values and attitudes influence their students. Waltz (1978) found that students' preferences were associated with faculty preferences for the clinical area of nursing practice. A faculty member's reputation among the students and grading practices in clinical courses were also influencing factors. Williams, Bloch, and Blair (1978) confirmed findings of earlier studies (Gordon & Mensh, 1962; Kirchner, 1970) that students' values in graduate programs tended to become more like their faculty's as they progressed in their program. Students showed significant increases in values of support, recognition, and independence. They showed significant decreases in benevolence, conformity, and practical-mindedness. In another study, Gliebe (1977) reported similar findings on student attitudes during their educational process.

Conners (1979) was interested in identifying the student behavior frequently labeled as "professional." She tested the premise that most educators in health professions have definite ideas about the way their profession should be practiced and these attitudes and values are communicated to students in a variety of overt and covert ways. The most important part of this study was the beginning development of an instrument to measure changes in student behaviors.

In two studies (Godejohn, Taylor, Muhlenkamp, & Blaesser, 1975; Mealey & Peterson, 1974), investigators attempted to measure attitude changes in nursing students toward patients with mental illness before and after a course in psychiatric nursing. Godejohn et al. (1975) used simulation gaming as a major teaching strategy and claimed that the sample group of students demonstrated the desired change which provided compelling evidence that simulation gaming is an effective means for changing nursing students' attitudes toward mental illness. Because lifetime personality characteristics are difficult to change as a result of one short experience, this claim should be viewed with caution. The same caution can apply to the study completed by Mealey and Peterson (1974). Their subjects were given the Personal Orientation Inventory (Shostrom, 1964) before and after their psychiatric nursing course. The investigators found changes toward more inner-directedness and slight changes in time-competence.

In two studies, researchers attempted to find if students' attitudes toward human sexuality changed as an outcome of a formal course in human sexuality. Mims, Yeaworth, and Hornstein (1974) administered a pre- and post-test to an interdisciplinary group of students from the health professions and found that the subjects increased their knowledge and changed their attitudes toward sensitive or anxiety reactions related to sexual stimuli. However, students' attitudes about abortion did not change. The investigators confirmed that basic attitudes, particularly those involving value-laden aspects, do not change readiy. In another study, Woods and Mandetta (1975) found that knowledge was increased from a course in human sexuality, but attitudes were not liberalized as a result of the course. Investigators of these two studies urged that replications with larger samples were needed before generalizations could be made.

Burgess (1980) attempted to determine the possible relationship between self-concept of undergraduate nursing students, their performance in clinical situations, and retention in the nursing program. While this study was a noble attempt to determine if selected biographical data were important variables correlating with self-concept, it must be interpreted cautiously because only one self-concept scale was used. Furthermore, the students tested were beginning nursing students, and if attrition factors were being studied it would have been helpful to collect data over a longer period of time.

For a long time investigators have been interested in the affective relationship between student and teacher. Rosendahl (1973) attempted to study the effectiveness of empathy, nonpossessive warmth, and genuineness of self-actualization of nursing students. Although her study involved a small sample she confirmed findings that students felt better and became more self-actualized when personal attributes were present in their teachers. Rosendahl did not depend exclusively on the three written instruments she selected, but included a personal interview for every fifth subject.

A recurring issue for faculty members involved in helping students cope with their educational program through student-centered group meetings is how frequently the teacher must be present. Although there is less emphasis on the group process as a learning tool than in the past, the McLaughlin, Davis, and Reed study (1972) may shed some light on this issue. They found that the leader-resource-person teacher could be on call to the group without loss of student benefit when student sessions were tape-recorded for later analysis and diagnosis.

Teaching Clinical Skills

Seven studies are included in the research on teaching clinical skills. The studies in this group varied widely in their scope. Sweeney, Hedstrom, and O'Malley (1982) asked perhaps the most basic question: What priority do baccalaureate faculty place on the acquisition of psychomotor clinical skills? Using a modified Q-sort and Delphi technique, they randomly selected 15 faculty from one school of nursing. They ambitiously expected 90% agreement from the faculty, and when not realized, this finding led them to conclude that the faculty did not agree on what should be taught. The investigators did not use a panel of judges to determine validity for the skills selected.

In other research, investigators demonstrated specific teaching techniques, but these studies could not be considered truly empirical although the investigators attempted to control variables. For example, Pearson (1974) divided students into an experimental and control group and increased the sensory stimulation for the experimental group to include sound as well as sight. She found no significant differences in the groups but one might wonder why teachers would go out of their way to decrease sensory stimulation. Quiring (1972) found that the autotutorial approach to teaching subcutaneous injections was more effective than the conventional teacher-discussion-demonstration in terms of student learning. Her study confirmed that immediate feedback was most effective in learning manual skills.

Other investigators (Jeffers, 1979; Lehrer, 1980; Sullivan, Grover, Lynaugh, & Levy, 1975) were interested in testing the effectiveness of such teaching methods as video-mediated interaction analyses, using simulation in acquiring clinical observational skills, and using professional patients for helping students learn skills. Although all of these studies indicated some degree of success, it would be difficult to replicate the studies because variables were not clearly stated. Furthermore, the question must be raised whether it is necessary to demonstrate proof for those aspects of the educational process that are quite obvious. For example, in order to learn psychomotor skills one must practice them.

Mitchell and Atwood (1975) provided an interesting contrast. They sought to determine if teaching toward a problem-oriented approach would help students develop critical thinking. The experimental group of students used problem-oriented records and were compared to students taught the more traditional charting. The experimental group consistently identified a greater proportion of nursing-focused problems compared to the control group who identified more technical problems. These investigators developed an interesting method for collecting data in an unobtrusive manner for the student. The student placed carbon paper under the actual charting of observations and care given. These carbon copies were later given to the instructor-investigator for analysis.

Evaluation of Student Performance

Given the amount of time and energy that faculty members spend determining the progress of their students, it was disappointing to find so few studies in this area. Nursing education parallels other educational endeavors in the paucity of studies on student evaluations and grading practices. Four studies widely differing in their scope were identified.

Huckabay (1979) was interested in testing the effect of grading versus nongrading of formative evaluations on cognitive learning and affective behaviors of graduate nursing students. She taught three different student groups, using subsequent classes to test each of her methods. As a result of her findings she suggested that using grades to motivate was not necessary for learning to take place. However, it must be emphasized that these students were graduate students in a course designed to help them become teachers. Therefore, because of its close relationship to their career goals, it can be assumed that they were highly motivated. The issue of investigator bias is prevalent in this type of study and requires the reader to view the conclusions with caution.

Johnson and Wilhite (1973) attempted to determine the validity and reliability of the subjective and objective faculty evaluation of nursing students. They wanted to learn if faculty members' subjective prediction for students' completing the nursing program would correlate with an objective test constructed by three teachers and with NLN achievement tests. Interestingly, the authors acknowledged the fact that objective-type tests were objective only in terms of how they were scored. Considering the low faculty-student ratio (three faculty members teaching 30 students), it is not surprising that the faculty members' ranking of the students correlated with the scores on the tests. Although the investigators are to be commended for the elaborate parametric and nonparametric statistical techniques used, the small number of faculty should not conclude that their evaluations were reliable regardless of the statistical rankings.

In quite a different approach to testing, Dean (1979) questioned whether having a free day prior to mastery testing would be beneficial to students. She found no differences in the students' performances on the mastery testing as a result of having the free day. It is important to note, however, that the students self-selected having the free day or not. This raises the question of whether the students studied or utilized the day for other things.

Acknowledging that observation is a highly subjective technique, Loustau, Lentz, Lee, McKenna, Hirako, Walker, and Goldsmith (1980) were interested in the interrater reliability in clinical evaluations. Results indicated that training sessions for faculty increased the interrater reliability. Because less experienced faculty benefited the most, this study gives direction for inservice education for faculty.

GENERAL CONCERNS

Several conclusions can be drawn from the majority of the studies reviewed on teaching-learning in nursing education. First, most of the studies lack any basis for generalizing to other settings or populations of students. The inadequate controls or sample size, selection of subjects, and research designs make the studies exploratory at best. In many cases the conclusions drawn were beyond the validity of the data. Second, the limited time span used did not allow time for teaching-learning effects to be realized. It is well known that research treatment effects often do not occur until well after the intervention part of the study is completed. A related problem is the one-time measurement of the variables. Since the expected change will occur over a period of time and at differing individual rates, there need to be multiple measurements of the variable(s) of interest, if the effects are to be captured adequately. A third difficulty was the inadequate control of intervening variables. For example, teacher enthusiasm and personal characteristics were not addressed in the studies. Both teachers and students tend to get bored with the same educational routine, and an experimental study brings some excitement into the teaching-learning process. Fourth, there is a lack of systematic and/or direct replication of findings in other settings or populations. Only one investigator extended her work (Huckabay, 1978; Huckabay, et al., 1979).

Another deficiency of these studies was emphasized by Barber (1973). He pointed out that although the investigator and the experimenter can be the same person, their roles are functionally quite different. The investigator decides to conduct a study and then determines how it is to be designed, carried out, analyzed, and interpreted. The experimenter conducts the study, tests the subjects, administers the experimental procedures, and observes and records the subjects' responses. There are powerful influences for each of these roles, and when investigator and experimenter are the same person, the possibility for bias in interpreting results and conclusions is compounded. The investigator's basic assumptions and way of conceptualizing the area of inquiry and related theories determine not only the questions to be asked, what data will be considered relevant, but how the data will be gathered, analyzed, interpreted, and related to the theoretical concepts. Therefore, from the beginning, there is a bias in the questions asked and the hypotheses formulated. The possibility of experimenter bias also exists. Experimenters commonly expect certain results; for example, they expect the experimental group to perform differently than the control group (even when they cautiously state their expectations in terms of a null hypothesis). Perhaps of greatest importance, experimenters commonly desire certain results. They want to see the experimental hypothesis verified.

Barber (1973) concluded his treatise on pitfalls in research with the statement that since experimental research is carried out by fallible individuals, it is open to a wide variety of traps. For experimental research to become a more reliable method for obtaining valid knowledge his suggestions should be heeded. He believed that investigators should make their underlying paradigms and associated theories more explicit and be aware of how paradigms influence every aspect of their research. He suggested that research would be less biased if the investigator who plans the study were not the same person with responsibility for the data analysis. He believed that the person planning the study has a strong commitment to the outcome and should not be the same person serving as experimenter and data collector. He wisely pointed out that, given the many pitfalls in any one experimental study, the results cannot be accepted until they are replicated by a variety of investigators who hold different paradigms or theories.

Problems of reliability in teaching-learning research also exist. Observer reliability is the most common form. Rosenshine and Furst (1973) identified a form of reliability they believed had received too little attention in educational research involving observations of teachers or determining whether a sample of observed behavior is a reliable representative sample of total behavior. Of course, the importance of representativeness depends on the purposes of the study. If the purpose is to relate instructional activities in individual classes to outcomes obtained in these classes, then the problem of representativeness needs further study. It is important to note that observation of teacher-student interactions was used as a measure of teaching outcome in only one study reviewed for this chapter (Scholdra & Quiring, 1973). The heavy reliance on paper-and-pencil testing, existing standardized cognitive and noncognitive tests, and student opinions may be the result of the difficulty in using observation as a means for gathering data in higher education. The sanctity of the classroom is well-respected in higher education. The time involved to observe within classrooms and laboratories is a deterrent. The observer's potential influence on the students and the teacher is an additional problem. Teacher behavior may or may not be similar to what occurs when an observer is not present. Enormous problems of data analysis, from selecting the variables for analysis to statistical procedures, also exist.

It is important to note that these comments on the concerns of teaching-learning research in nursing are consistent with the overall concerns of educational research in general. The investigators who attempted to find answers to the pressing problems of faculty members are to be commended for their efforts.

POSSIBLE REASONS FOR PAUCITY OF RESEARCH

Given the fact that there are approximately 20,000 nurses teaching in schools of nursing (Vaughn & Johnson, 1981), a logical question is: Why are there so few empirical studies in this field? In the past, educational doctorates comprised the major field of study for nurse educators. Review of doctoral dissertation titles from 1971 through 1981 revealed 65 dissertations pertaining to the teaching-learning process in nursing education. Thirty-five of these dissertations were in partial fulfillment of the Doctor of Philosophy degree in education; 29 for the Doctor of Education Degree; and one for the Doctor of Nursing Science degree. Only eighteen of the 65 persons completing the doctoral degree have contributed to nursing literature. Of greater importance is the fact that of the 65 persons completing a doctorate with an emphasis on research on teaching and learning in nursing education, 47 have not published at all.

One can only speculate on the reasons for the lack of continuous research productivity from these nurses. The body of literature in education makes it clear that no one teaching strategy represents the educational panacea. Clifford (1973), in her comprehensive review of the history of the impact of research on teaching, pointed out that one expectation of educational science was that it would stabilize practice, provide technical advice, and legitimize some accepted practices. It is obvious that the body of scientific knowledge about teaching-learning has grown slowly.

There are important social and political influences on nursing faculty and their choice of research they conduct. One could argue that nurse faculty members should be involved in nursing research rather than educational research, and if engaged in nursing research their teaching would improve because they would share with their students new ideas based on their own observations and data. Without doubt, knowing *what* to teach is of greater importance than knowing *how* to teach it. Considering the number of faculty members teaching in nonresearch-oriented institutions without a graduate program in nursing, perhaps one should view the need for teaching-learning research differently. The pendulum has swung away from rewarding research in the teaching-learning process. Dershimer and Iannaccone (1973) pointed out that scientific researchers do not select the problems they study at random. They are influenced by the world around them. In schools of nursing where teaching is the major function of the faculty it follows that faculty will, or should, be interested in learning more about the complex tasks that surround them. Students, as clients or direct purchasers of faculty services, expect that their faculty will be interested in improving those services.

Although there are many articles describing various teaching practices, there are few empirical studies on teaching-learning in the nursing literature. *Nursing Research,* nursing's oldest national journal devoted exclusively to research in nursing, has published the majority of the empirical studies on teaching-learning. It could be debated that although in these studies investigators attempted to answer important questions pertaining to the efficiency and effectiveness of teaching as it relates to outcomes, such studies were not *nursing* research. In other clinical health fields—dentistry, medicine, and pharmacy—journals devoted exclusively to the sharing of research findings and problems of education of future practitioners exist. This journal is the official organ of the association of educators for that health discipline. In reviewing these health profession journals, it was noted that an annual conference is held to share empirical studies and results pertaining to the education of health professionals. The studies, either in abstract or more complete reports, are shared with the members. This helps develop new information about the teaching-learning process and verifies educational improvements. Furthermore, it provides educators with ideas for research replication and extension. Before the first Annual Conference on Nursing Education (sponsored by the University of California, San Francisco, and the *Journal of Nursing Education)* was held in San Francisco, California, in January 1983, nursing educators had no such mechanism to disseminate their studies rapidly. Such conferences offered at periodic intervals should encourage research in nursing education.

FUTURE DIRECTIONS FOR TEACHING-LEARNING RESEARCH

Experimental studies in the nursing educational endeavor have been scarce. Campbell and Stanley (1963) pointed out that the experiment is the means for settling disputes regarding educational practice. It is the only way of verifying educational improvements where new methods can be introduced without the danger of discard of old wisdom in favor of inferior novelties. Of greatest importance in their classic treatise on experimental and quasi-experimental designs for research on teaching was their urging that there be an increase in time-perspective, continuous, and multiple experimentation rather than the once-and-for-all definitive experiments that appear to characterize studies in education. Experiments require replication and cross-validation at other times and under other conditions before they can be interpreted with any degree of confidence. Campbell and Stanley (1963) emphasized that the development of greatly improved statistical procedures and technology developed has aided in handling the complex variables considered in research involving human psychology and learning.

It is clear from recent studies of teaching methods and materials that no clear-cut evidence exists for the superiority of one approach. It is perhaps time that such studies be laid to rest and attention turned to the way strategies are used during the day, the course, or the program to help or promote learning. Studies of the combination and sequences of different instructional strategies may promote understanding of the optimal conditions for learning.

In the review of the studies reported in this chapter, the research questions represent studying traditional educational outcomes such as general problem-solving abilities, achievement of subject-matter knowledge, feelings about the subject or learning in general, development of psychomotor skills, student self-perception, and self-actualization. Given the emphasis on the women's movement and the goal for nurses to function as autonomous professionals and equal partners on the health care team, it is surprising that no studies were found designed to educate teachers on how they could help students become more independent risk-taking decision makers. Much has been written during the past decade on the need to help passive, dependent, and indecisive women develop a sense of self-esteem, power, and personal control (Bush & Kjervik, 1979; Grissum & Spengler, 1976; Muff, 1982). Studies on development and testing of strategies designed to change the behavior of nursing students toward risk-taking and role-breaking behaviors are required. It is necessary to study the effects of specific teaching strategies on the development of inquiry skills. To counteract previous socialization, women entering nursing must have experiences in dealing with power and success, and study of the effects of leadership style on outcomes is needed.

If nursing is to meet its societal mandate of educating skilled practitioners, research on developing clinical decision making in nursing is necessary. Posner and Keele (1973) defined skill as the study of those processes producing expert, rapid, and accurate performance. They pointed out that although use of the term skill is typically confined to motor activity, the study of motor control provides a means for approaching issues of attention and mental operations in general. The performance of clinical skills is exceedingly complex, involving psychomotor skills, judgment, personality factors, and decision-making abilities. Systematic study of the effects of summer clinical experiences, preceptorships, and residencies is needed.

SUMMARY AND CONCLUSIONS

It is clear from reviewing the studies on the teaching-learning process in nursing education that more is unknown than is known. However, this statement holds true for all college and university teaching. Although a number of concerns have been raised about research in this area, it is important to restate the point that investigators attempting to find answers to their problems as instructors are to be commended for their efforts. Some of the probable by-products of their studies have not been published with their results. One could speculate that instructors interested in finding ways to facilitate the learning process are also improving the technology of instruction, even if the studies fail to add to the scientific body of knowledge about teaching-learning. Research in this area is beset with a number of problems. Virtually all of the studies reviewed for this chapter took place within the nursing classroom. As McKeatchie (1974) aptly pointed out, many of the problems in studies within the classroom exist from failure to take into account the important variables in natural educational settings. A reassuring note is in order in summarizing educational research. Cronbach (1975) wrote that although enduring systematic theories are not likely to be achieved, systematic inquiry can hope to make two contributions. One is to assess local events accurately and therefore improve short-run control. The other is to develop explanatory concepts that will help others. Many of the studies reviewed here have achieved one or possibly both of these goals.

REFERENCES

Barber, T. X. Pitfalls in research: Nine investigator and experimenter effects. In R. M. W. Travers (Ed.), *Second handbook of research on teaching*. Chicago: Rand McNally, 1973.

Blatchley, M. E., Herzog, P. M., & Russell, J. D. Effects of self-study on achievement in a medical-surgical nursing course. *Nursing Outlook*, 1978, *26*, 444–447.

Brock, A. M. Impact of a management-oriented course on knowledge and leadership skills exhibited by baccalaureate nursing students. *Nursing Research*, 1978, *27*, 217–221.

Burgess, G. The self-concept of undergraduate nursing students in relation to clinical performance and selected biographical variables. *Journal of Nursing Education*, 1980, *19*(3), 37–44.

Bush, M. A., & Kjervik, D. K. The nurse's self-image. In K. K. Kjervik & I. M. Martinson (Eds.), *Women in stress: A nursing perspective*. New York: Appleton-Century-Crofts, 1979.

Campbell, D. T., & Stanley, J. C. Experimental and quasi-experimental designs for research on teaching. In N. L. Gage (Ed.), *Handbook of research on teaching*. Chicago: Rand McNally, 1963.

Chandler, J. M., & Hunter, M. L. Teaching by testing. *Nursing Outlook*, 1976, *24*, 386–388.

Clifford, G. J. A history of the impact of research on teaching. In R. M. W. Travers (Ed.), *Second handbook of research on teaching*. Chicago: Rand McNally, 1973.

Conners, V. L. Teaching affective behaviors. *Journal of Nursing Education*, 1979, *18*(6), 35–39.

Cronbach, L. J. Beyond the two disciplines of scientific psychology. *American Psychologist*, 1975, *30*, 116–127.

Dean, N. R. Effect of free time the day prior to mastery testing on nursing students' scores. *Nursing Research*, 1979, *28*, 40–42.

Dershimer, R. A., & Iannaccone, L. Social and political influences on educational research. In R. M. W. Travers (Ed.), *Second handbook on research on teaching*. Chicago: Rand McNally, 1973.

Floyd, G. J. Team teaching: Advantages and disadvantages to the student. *Nursing Research*, 1975, *24*, 52–57.

Gliebe, W. A. Faculty consensus as a socializing agent in professional education. *Nursing Research*, 1977, *26*, 428–431.

Godejohn, C. J., Taylor, J., Muhlenkamp, A. F., & Blaesser, W. Effect of simulation gaming on attitudes toward mental illness. *Nursing Research*, 1975, *24*, 367–370.

Gordon, L. V., & Mensh, I. N. Values of medical students at different levels of training. *Journal of Educational Psychology*, 1962, *53*, 48–51.

Grissum, M., & Spengler, C. *Womanpower and health care*. Boston: Little, Brown, 1976.

Huckabay, L. M. Cognitive and affective consequences of formative evaluation in graduate nursing students. *Nursing Research*, 1978, *27*, 190–194.

Huckabay, L. M. D. Cognitive-affective consequences of grading versus nongrading of formative evaluations. *Nursing Research*, 1979, *28*, 173–178.

Huckabay, L. M., Anderson, N., Holm, D., & Lee, J. Cognitive, affective, and transfer of learning consequences of computer-assisted instruction. *Nursing Research*, 1979, *28*, 228–233.

Jeffers, J. M. Using simulation to facilitate the acquisition of clinical observational skills. *Journal of Nursing Education*, 1979, *18*(6), 29–32.

Johnson, D. M., & Wilhite, M. J. Reliability and validity of subjective evaluation of baccalaureate program nursing students. *Nursing Research*, 1973, *22*, 257–262.

Khan, S. F., & Weiss, J. The teaching of affective responses. In R. M. W. Travers (Ed.), *Second handbook of research on teaching*. Chicago: Rand McNally, 1973.

Kirchhoff, K. T., & Holzemer, W. L. Student learning and a computer-assisted instructional program. *Journal of Nursing Education*, 1979, *18*(3), 22–31.

Kirchner, F. P. Values and value changes during and after graduate study in psychology. *Journal of Clinical Psychology*, 1970, *26*, 252–256.

Kissinger, J. F., & Munjas, B. A. Nursing process, student attributes, and teaching methodologies. *Nursing Research*, 1981, *30*, 242–246.

Lehrer, S. S. The professional patient session as a technique for teaching the gynecological examination to nurse practitioner students. *Journal of Nursing Education*, 1980, *19*(5), 38–41.

Loustau, A., Lentz, M., Lee, K., McKenna, M., Hirako, S., Walker, W. F., & Goldsmith, J. W. Evaluating students' clinical performance: Using videotape to estabalish rater reliability. *Journal of Nursing Education*, 1980, *19*(7), 10–17.

Mackie, J. B. Comparison of student satisfaction with educational experiences in two teaching process models. *Nursing Research*, 1973, *22*, 262–266.

McKeatchie, W. J. The decline and fall of the laws of learning. *Educational Researcher*, 1974, *3*(3), 7–11.

McLaughlin, F. E., Davis, M. L., & Reed, J. L. Effects of three types of group leadership structure on the self-perceptions of undergraduate nursing students. *Nursing Research*, 1972, *21*, 244–257.

Mealey, A. R., & Peterson, T. L. Self-actualization of nursing students resulting from a course in psychiatric nursing. *Nursing Research*, 1974, *23*, 138–143.

Mims, F., Yeaworth, R., & Hornstein, S. Effectiveness of an interdisciplinary course in human sexuality. *Nursing Research*, 1974, *23*, 248–253.

Mitchell, P. H., & Atwood, J. Problem-oriented recording as a teaching-learning tool. *Nursing Research*, 1975, *24*, 99–103.

Moser, D. H., & Kondracki, M. R. Comparison of attitudes and cognitive achievement of nursing students in three instructional strategies. *Journal of Nursing Education*, 1977, *16*(1), 14–28.

Muff, J. (Ed.). *Socialization, sexism, and stereotyping*. St. Louis: Mosby, 1982.

Pearson, B. D. Use of the five senses in acquiring professional skills. *Nursing Research*, 1974, *23*, 259–262.

Pensivy, B. A. Traditional versus individualized nursing instruction: Comparison of state board examination scores as a result of these two methods of nursing instruction. *Journal of Nursing Education*, 1977, *16*(2), 14–18.

Posner, M. I., & Keele, S. W. Skill learning. In R. M. W. Travers (Ed.), *Second handbook of research on teaching*. Chicago: Rand McNally, 1973.

Quiring, J. The autotutorial approach. *Nursing Research*, 1972, *21*, 332–337.

Rosendahl, P. L. Effectiveness of empathy, nonpossessive warmth, and genuineness of self-actualization of nursing students. *Nursing Research*, 1973, *22*, 253–257.

Rosenshine, B., & Furst, N. The use of direct observation to study teaching. In R. M. W. Travers (Ed.), *Second handbook on research on teaching*. Chicago: Rand McNally, 1973.

Scholdra, J., & Quiring, J. The level of questions posed by nursing educators. *Journal of Nursing Education*, 1973, *12*(1), 15–20.

Shostrom, E. L. Inventory for the measurement of self-actualization. *Educational Psychology Measurement*, 1964, *24*, 207–218.

Stein, R. F., Steele, L., Fuller, M., & Langhoff, H. F. A multimedia independent approach for improving the teaching-learning process in nursing. *Nursing Research*, 1972, *21*, 436–447.

Sullivan, J. A., Grover, P. L., Lynaugh, J. E., & Levy, A. Video mediated self-cognition and the Amidon-Flanders Interaction Analysis Model in the training of nurse practitioners' history taking skills. *Journal of Nursing Education*, 1975, *14*(3), 42–45.

Sweeney, M. A., Hedstrom, B., & O'Malley, M. Process evaluation: A second look at psychomotor skills. *Journal of Nursing Education*, 1982, *21*(2), 4–16.

Thompson, M. Learning: A comparison of traditional and autotutorial methods. *Nursing Research*, 1972, *21*, 453–457.

Trent, J. W., & Cohen, A. M. Research on teaching in higher education. In R. M. W. Travers (Ed.), *Second handbook of research on teaching*. Chicago: Rand McNally, 1973.

Vaughn, J. C., & Johnson, W. L. *Nursing data book 1981* (Publication No. 19–1882). New York: National League for Nursing, 1981.

Waltz, C. F. Faculty influence on nursing students' preferences for practice. *Nursing Research*, 1978, *27*, 89–97.

White, L. D., & Chavigny, K. H. Direct tape access as an adjunct to learning. *Nursing Research*, 1975, *24*, 295–298.

Williams, M. A., Bloch, D. W., & Blair, E. M. Values and value changes of graduate nursing students: Their relationship to faculty values and to selected educational factors. *Nursing Research*, 1978, *27*, 181–189.

Woods, N. F., & Mandetta, A. Changes in students' knowledge and attitudes following a course in human sexuality. *Nursing Research*, 1975, *24*, 10–15.

CHAPTER 9

Research on Nursing Students

PATRICIA M. SCHWIRIAN
COLLEGE OF NURSING
THE OHIO STATE UNIVERSITY

CONTENTS

The research related to nursing students has been very diverse. It was conducted by investigators with a wide range of interests; most of the investigators conducted one or two studies, then carried the work no further. The resulting literature is largely fragmented, noncumulative, and characterized by a lack of clear direction and unifying themes. A second characteristic of the research is that it was problem-driven rather than theory-driven. That is, the study questions were prompted by processes and problems of concern to nurse educators, rather than intended to guide the development, explication, or testing of nursing-related or learning-related theory.

The critical review presented in this chapter pertains to research on nursing students reported between 1965 and 1982. With few exceptions, the material was published in refereed journals. In general, four broad questions were addressed by investigators in this area. The first two questions were: Who chooses nursing as a profession and why? and What characterizes students who persist in nursing school, as opposed to those who drop out? The other two general questions were: What factors are associated with various academic and attitudinal outcomes in nursing school? and What factors are associated with performance on the state board nursing registration examinations? The content of this chapter is organized accordingly.

The major portion of the chapter is devoted to a review and summary of the content and methods of research on nursing students. Within each group of studies that addressed the above general questions are embedded subcategories of studies organized according to the nursing student attributes of interest to the investigators, such as demographics, cognitive attributes, and noncognitive, psychosocial characteristics. Following the summary, there is a discussion of general methodological issues and problems that tended to characterize this research literature. Finally, some observations regarding trends and future directions for research on nursing students are presented.

RESEARCH RELATED TO ADMISSION, ATTRITION, AND RETENTION

The recruitment, selection, and admission of students to schools of nursing are processes that require a considerable expenditure of resources. Thus, it is important that the students selected for admission are those who will continue their studies to the completion of the program. The two general questions to which this body of research pertained were: Who chooses nursing as a profession and why? and What characterizes students who persist in nursing school as opposed to those who drop out?

Prospective Nursing Students

During the 1960s and into the 1970s a series of studies were reported that described the characteristics of students who had expressed the intent to pursue their education in nursing (American Council on Education Policy Analysis Service—USPHS, 1974; Bailey, 1968; Pavalko, 1969; Richek & Nichols, 1973; Roraback, 1968/1969). A potpourri of variables was examined. These included socioeconomic status, father's occupation, personality factors, values, size of community of origin, work values, and high school course preferences. As noted in an earlier examination (Schwirian, 1977a) of that literature, the methods, measures, and objectives of the studies varied so widely that no profile of the typical aspirant to the nursing profession emerged. Interest in this area appears to have waned, since reports of similar studies have not been published in major nursing journals in recent years.

Admitted Nursing Students

Like prospective students, newly admitted students received considerable attention from investigators in the 1960s and into the middle 1970s. Few reports of the same descriptive nature were published since that time. The data that described and compared the students typically were gathered during the students' first year of nursing school. Schwirian (1977b) found that many schools of nursing used extensive batteries of cognitive and noncognitive measures to evaluate prospective and newly admitted students. These were the data sources for many of the studies reported in the 1960s and early 1970s.

Demographic characteristics of nursing students were described by a number of investigators (Johnson, 1974; Knopf, 1972; Levine, 1968/1969; Miller, 1972; Montag, 1972; Nash, 1975; Wren, 1971). The general pattern that emerged from these studies was that: (a) nursing students tended to come from middle-middle to lower-middle class homes, (b) the vast majority of students were women and white, and (c) the majority were entering the study of nursing directly from high school.

The studies in which students in different types of programs were compared (Bullough & Sparks, 1975; Knopf, 1972; Nash, 1975; Schwirian, 1979a; Wren, 1971) revealed that associate degree (AD) programs had more students who were married, were men, were black, lived closer to the nursing school, and came from lower socioeconomic backgrounds than students in diploma and baccalaureate programs. In the early years of AD programs, students in those programs usually were older than baccalaureate and diploma students. This is changing to more of a bimodal distribution for both associate and baccalaureate groups, as more nontraditional students are seeking baccalaureate degrees in nursing. Factors related to economics, such as shorter length of program, lower tuition, and less travel time required were cited consistently as reasons for choosing the AD program in nursing.

Cognitive and academic attributes also were examined. Comparisons of students who entered nursing and those in other areas (Johnson & Leonard, 1970; Pavalko, 1969) indicated that nursing students had attained higher scores on selected measures of intelligence than their nonnursing counterparts. When cognitive attributes of students in three different types of nursing programs—baccalaureate, diploma, and AD—were compared (Katzell, 1968; Litherland, 1966; Schwirian, 1979a; Wren, 1971), students in baccalaureate programs had obtained high Scholastic Aptitude Test (SAT) scores and achieved higher grades in high school than students in the other programs. AD students usually had the lowest average scores on indicators of prior academic achievement.

A number of investigators in the 1960s attempted to characterize the personality and attitudinal components of nursing students. The picture that emerged from most of those studies (Adams & Klein, 1970; Aldag & Christensen, 1967; Bailey, 1969; Baker, 1965; Bernstein, Turrell, & Dana, 1965; Casella, 1968; Garvin, 1976; Gunter, 1969a; Johnson & Leonard, 1970; Levine, 1968/1969; Mayes, Schultz, & Pierce, 1968; Smith, 1968) was the nursing student as a traditional female with low needs for autonomy and high needs for nurturance; generous, dependent, passive; and who adhered to values toward work and women's roles that also were traditional.

More recent studies suggested that this picture may have changed. For example, Kahn (1980) found that nursing students did not display the low autonomy needs that characterized students in earlier studies. Meleis and Dagenais (1981) reported that, contrary to much of the earlier work (e.g., Aldag, 1970; Aldag & Christensen, 1967; O'Neill, 1973), nursing students did not have a more feminine sex-role identity than that of college students not enrolled in nursing.

In terms of decisions related to their choice of nursing and motives for entering that profession, nursing students tended to cite altruistic, caring, and security-related motives rather than economic ones. Nursing students also typically reported having made their decision to enter the profession at an earlier age than women studying for other professions. The most-often cited influence to enter nursing was the presence of a significant other who was a nurse (Davis, 1973; Miller, 1972; Montag, 1972; Morris & Grassi-Russo, 1979; Schwirian, 1979a; Taylor, 1970).

Beginning nursing students also were described in terms of their perceptions of the nursing profession. In general, investigators found that students had perceptions of the traditional, technical image of the nursing role (Collins & Joel, 1971; Gunter, 1969b; Skipper, 1965).

Retention and Attrition in Diploma Schools of Nursing

The investigators who examined cognitive and academic predictors of persistence in diploma schools (Gerstein, 1965; Katzell, 1968; Klahn, 1969; Plapp, Psathas, & Caputo, 1965; Thurston, Brunclik, & Feldhusen, 1968) generally found that prenursing measures such as high school achievement, SAT scores, and intelligence (IQ) test scores were useful as predictors of attrition in the first year of nursing, but their utility did not persist over time for students in diploma schools of nursing.

The focus of investigators studying noncognitive predictors varied widely. The investigators examined: vocational interest (Gerstein, 1965; Klahn, 1969); personality as measured by the Sixteen Personality Factor Questionnaire (16-PF), Edwards Personal Preference Schedule (EPPS), and the Minnesota Multiphasic Personality Inventory (MMPI) (Smith, 1965; Thurston, et al., 1968); self-concept (Klahn, 1969); attitudes (Thurston, Brunclik, & Feldhusen, 1969); and satisfaction and stresses (Katzell, 1968). These investigators identified no definitive noncognitive predictors of persistence or attrition in diploma programs of nursing.

Retention and Attrition in Associate Degree Nursing Programs

The study of attrition in AD and baccalaureate programs increased in the early 1970s at the same time the studies of diploma programs were declining in number. Most investigators who examined cognitive predictors focused on measures of achievement such as the National League for

Nursing (NLN) Pre-Nursing and Guidance Examination, high school grade point average (GPA), GPA earned in prenursing college courses, and verbal ability (Donsky & Judge, 1981; Katzell, 1968; Lamoureux & Johannsen, 1977; Stankovich, 1977). Backman and Steindler (1971a) used IQ as measured by the Wechsler Adult Intelligence Scale (WAIS) as a cognitive predictor. Results from these studies showed that higher scores on preexisting cognitive and achievement measures were associated positively with student persistence in AD nursing programs.

Fewer studies of noncognitive predictors of persistence were conducted in AD programs than had been reported in diploma programs (Baker, 1975; Jones, 1975; Lamoureux & Johannsen, 1977; Miller, 1974). These investigators also were unable to identify any personality or values characteristics predictive of persistence or attrition. However, Baker (1975) and Donsky and Judge (1981) reported that the more mature, married female students admitted to AD programs were the most likely to continue to graduation.

Retention and Attrition in Baccalaureate Nursing Programs

Measures of prior achievement and academic aptitude were used as predictors of attrition in many baccalaureate programs. It is common that colleges and universities require SAT or American College Tests (ACT) testing for all applicants, and many schools of nursing do not admit students as majors until they have attained sophomore or junior status in the university. Thus, a broader base of academic aptitude data is available to baccalaureate educators than to either diploma or AD educators. Investigators who studied the predictive utility of prenursing measures of academic aptitude and achievement consistently reported a positive association between those measures and the likelihood that students would complete the baccalaureate program (Allchnie & Bellucci, 1981; Katzell, 1968; Knopke, 1979; Kovacs, 1970; Levitt, Lubin, & Dewitt, 1971; Raderman & Allen, 1974; Wittemeyer, Camiscioni, & Purdy, 1971).

Once again, the utility of noncognitive predictors of persistence or attrition was largely unconvincing. Even measures that were used in several studies, such as the EPPS, the 16–PF, and the MMPI, provided no consistent pattern of findings from study to study. Factors that may have been associated with attrition in one study showed no relationship at all in other studies (e.g., Anderson, 1968; Hegarty, 1976; Knopke, 1979; Levitt et al., 1971; Liddle, Heywood, & Morman, 1971; May, 1967; Miller, 1974; Wittemeyer et al., 1971).

RESEARCH RELATED TO OUTCOMES OF NURSING PROGRAMS

This large group of studies was divided into two major subsets—the studies of students while they were still enrolled in schools of nursing, and those related to their postgraduation performance on State Board Testing Pool Examinations (SBTPE). The in-school research was classified as studies (a) dealing with the prediction of academic achievement in nursing school; (b) describing attitudinal outcomes; (c) describing changes in student characteristics over time in school; and (d) comparing attributes of students who obtained their nursing education in AD, diploma, and baccalaureate schools of nursing.

Prediction of Academic Achievement

This group constitutes the single largest category of studies reviewed for this chapter. Investigators studied the predictive validity of cognitive and noncognitive variables. The findings from the studies of cognitive predictors were highly consistent; those from studies of noncognitive predictors showed no such consistency.

Cognitive predictors. The cognitive predictor used most frequently was academic achievement as measured by grade point average (GPA) or class standing. Prior academic achievement was highly predictive of subsequent academic achievement in nursing for students in AD programs (Backman & Steindler, 1971a; Munday & Hoyt, 1965; Owen, Feldhusen, & Thurston, 1970) and diploma programs (Litherland, 1966; Michael, Haney, & Jones, 1966; Michael, Haney, Lee, & Michael, 1971; Munday & Hoyt, 1965; Plapp et al., 1965). GPA also was highly predictive of grades earned in baccalaureate programs of nursing (Allchnie & Bellucci, 1981; Anderson, 1968; Burgess & Duffey, 1969; Chissom & Lanier, 1975; Lewis & Welch, 1975; Litherland, 1966; Munday & Hoyt, 1965; Reekie, 1971; Rezler & Moore, 1978; Stankovich, 1977; Tillinghast & Norris, 1968;

Trussell & Pappas, 1974). Many of these investigators examined multiple predictors in their studies, and GPA often was identified as the best predictor of subsequent academic achievement.

Plapp et al. (1965) and Finegan (1967) studied the relationship of SAT scores to achievement of diploma students. Owen et al. (1970) and Backman and Steindler (1971a) studied AD students. Both groups found that SAT scores were significant predictors of achievement in nursing school. Investigators who focused on baccalaureate students (Allchnie & Bellucci, 1981; Chissom & Lanier, 1975; Tillinghast & Norris, 1968) reported that while SAT scores were associated positively with achievement, prior GPAs showed an even stronger association. Findings from studies of ACT scores were very similar (Ledbetter, 1968/1969; Lewis & Welch, 1975; Munday & Hoyt, 1965; Trussell & Pappas, 1974).

A variety of other standardized measures of cognitive ability and functioning also were associated positively with academic achievement in nursing school. These included the California Achievement Test (Michael et al., 1966; Michael et al., 1971); the Iowa Test of Educational Development (Litherland, 1966); SCAT (Anderson, 1968; Burgess & Duffey, 1969); the Wechsler Adult Intelligence Scale (WAIS) (Backman & Steindler, 1971a; Burgess & Duffey, 1969); and the College Qualification Test (CQT) (Johnson & Leonard, 1970).

Noncognitive predictors. The large number of studies cited in the preceding section shows that program outcomes in terms of student grades were of interest to many investigators during the past two decades. However, as Taylor, Nahm, Quinn, Harms, Mulaik, and Mulaik (1965) pointed out, while measures of academic achievement and cognitive ability were highly predictive of behaviors such as achievement in content and theory courses, their utility was limited because they predicted only a narrow spectrum of achievement. This concern prompted a number of studies of noncognitive predictors of achievement in nursing programs. The 16–PF was examined by Bittman (1973/1974), Johnson and Leonard (1970), Michael et al., (1966); and Michael et al., (1971). Scores on the MMPI were studied by Anderson (1968), Burgess and Duffey (1969), and Burgess, Duffey, and Temple (1972). The EPPS was studied by Michael et al., (1966). These studies failed to reveal any predictive validity for these measures of personality.

Other investigators examined a variety of noncognitive predictors of achievement such as: vocational interest (Anderson, 1968; Elton & Rose, 1970; Johnson & Leonard, 1970, Mowbray & Taylor, 1967); values (Allchnie & Bellucci, 1981; Finegan, 1967; Trussell & Pappas, 1974);

self-concept (Burgess, 1980; Burgess et al., 1972; Burgess & Duffey, 1969; Komorita, 1972); biographical factors (Burgess & Duffey, 1969; Reekie, 1971); and attitudes (Burgess et al., 1972; Morman, Liddle, & Haywood, 1965; Owen et al., 1970). In a series of studies conducted by investigators working out of Purdue University (e.g., Owen et al., 1970; Owen & Feldhusen, 1970; Reed, Feldhusen, & VanMonfrans, 1973), it was shown that adding noncognitive measures to a battery of cognitive measures in a regression equation added to the predictive value of the whole battery. By themselves, however, the noncognitive measures bore little relationship to academic achievement in nursing school.

Attitudinal Outcomes

While many investigators were concerned with the cognitive performance of students in schools of nursing, a much smaller group examined non-cognitive outcomes such as attitudes.

Studies of nursing students' attitudes toward the elderly were conducted by three investigators. Robb (1979) developed instruments to measure beliefs and behavioral intentions toward the elderly. She found that experience in a course of gerontologic nursing was associated with slightly more favorable attitudes toward the elderly and that these attitudes persisted up to two years after the course. Damrosch (1982) found that senior baccalaureate nursing students expressed more favorable attitudes toward sexually active elders than toward old people who were not described as sexually active. Sedhom (1982) reported that students' attitudes toward old people were associated positively with self-concept and related significantly to the quality of the students' past experiences with the elderly.

Nursing student attitudes toward rape victims was the subject of another study by Damrosch (1981). Students were less able to like and identify with a hypothetical rape victim who was perceived as careless, and to whom they attributed more responsibility for the rape than to another hypothetical victim who was perceived as being more careful.

Worsley (1980) used factor analysis to study Australian student nurses' stereotypes of patients and factors associated with those stereotypes. Three primary dimensions emerged from the analysis: cooperation, patient's state, and demandingness. Felton, Reed, and Perla (1981) also used factor analysis in their study of students' attitudes toward cancer, persons with cancer, and cancer nursing. They found that the attitudes of nursing students and nurses were similar, and both were different from those of a sample of physicians, particularly in attitudes toward aggressive treatment of cancer.

Changes in Student Attributes during Nursing School

One approach to the investigation of student outcomes associated with the nursing experience was to study the differences in attributes of students at different stages in their study of nursing. While longitudinal designs would be the most useful in carrying out such studies, limitations of time and resources usually prompted one-time comparisons of different student cohorts. These studies were grouped into four categories: (a) studies related to professional image and professional socialization; (b) studies of elements of personality and values; (c) studies of nursing students' self-concepts; and (d) a small group with miscellaneous foci.

Professional image. Since the purposes, measures, and methods of these studies varied widely, a pattern of findings was not apparent. Coe (1965) found that diploma students identified with nursing more strongly at the end of their first year than they had at the beginning of the year. Schoeberle and Craddick (1968) found more identification with the profession among diploma seniors than among freshmen, but the association was weak. The studies of both Bittman (1973/1974) and Psathas (1968) suggested that students in diploma programs became increasingly technique-oriented during their time in school.

Findings from several studies of baccalaureate nursing students indicated that students' images of nursing became more professional over time as did their identification with the profession (Ichilov & Dotan, 1980; Sharp & Anderson, 1972; Stein, 1969a, 1969b). Gunden (1980) concluded that seniors' views of the ideal nurse were much more congruent with faculty views than those of sophomore students. However, the studies reported by Brown, Swift, and Oberman (1974), Pallone and Hosinski (1967), and Siegel (1968) showed no professional socialization differences in seniors and younger nursing students.

Personality and value. Studies of changes in personality and value structures produced mixed results. Three studies in which investigators used the EPPS (Psathas & Plapp, 1968; Schultz, 1965; Stein, 1969a, 1969b) demonstrated no consistent pattern of differences over time. Values were examined by May and Ilardi (1970) using the Allport Vernon Lindzey Study of Values (AVL), and Blomquist, Cruise, and Cruise (1980) used the

Rokeach Values Survey in a study of over 1,000 freshman and senior students in secular and religious baccalaureate schools of nursing. The first study showed lower senior scores of theoretical and religious values and higher scores on aesthetic and political values. The Blomquist et al. study showed that seniors had significantly different rankings than freshmen for 17 of the 36 possible values, including higher values accorded to independence, imagination, honesty, freedom, and self-respect. Seniors also placed a lower value on helpfulness than freshmen students.

Self-concept. The self-concept of nursing students was the subject of a handful of change studies. Studies by Pallone and Hosinski (1967), Klahn (1969), Dietz (1973/1974), and Ellis (1980) showed inconclusive results regarding changes in self-concept during nursing school.

Miscellaneous. The last category of change studies covers miscellaneous topics. It includes the study by Lenburg, Burnside, and Davitz (1970), who showed that second-year associate degree students inferred more psychological stress to patients in illness situations, while first-year students inferred more physical pain. Bailey, McDonald, and Claus (1970) found that students farther along in an experimental nursing curriculum displayed more verbal creativity, and McIntyre, McDonald, Bailey, and Claus (1972) observed increased skills in communication, data collection, and decision making among senior students in a baccalaureate program. However, Thomas (1979) found that the creativity of senior students was actually lower than that demonstrated by younger students.

Comparison of Students in Three Types of Nursing Programs

The student characteristics typically associated with professional socialization were the subject of between-school-type comparisons in several studies. Richards (1972) found that baccalaureate students held a more professional image of nursing than did associate or diploma students, and Lynn (1981) determined that AD students had a more traditional orientation toward nursing than baccalaureate students. Bullough and Sparks (1975) characterized AD students as having more of a cure orientation, while baccalaureate students held a strong care orientation.

Meleis and Dagenais (1981) determined that AD and baccalaureate nursing students perceived their own degree of professionalism higher than did diploma students. Murray and Morris (1982) observed that students in baccalaureate programs were much stronger advocates of nursing autonomy and patients' rights than students in either AD or diploma schools. No differences were found by Connelly (1970) in the motivation and career selection patterns, nor by Meleis and Farrell (1974) when comparing students' responses on the Leadership Opinion Questionnaire. Snyder (1981) also reported no program difference in students' attitudes toward the professional concept of the health care team.

In terms of personality traits, no differences in AD, diploma, and baccalaureate students were found by Bailey (1969) using the EPPS, by Richards (1972) using the Gordon Personal Profile, nor by Meleis and Dagenais (1981) in terms of sex-role identity. However, two other studies did show personality differences. Meleis and Farrell (1974) concluded that AD students were higher on structure and diploma students were lower on autonomy. Goldstein (1980) found that baccalaureate students scored slightly higher on self-actualization as measured by the Personality Orientation Inventory (POI) than a comparable group of AD students.

Prediction of State Board Test Pool Examination Performance

Educators have had considerable interest in students' postgraduation performance on the State Board Test Pool Examination (SBTPE). The volume of research on this topic was almost as large as that focused on prediction of academic achievement in nursing schools. It showed a similar pattern and consistency in findings. The most commonly used predictor variable in the SBTPE prediction studies was academic achievement as measured by GPA or class standing. The cumulative high school GPA was used often (Backman & Steindler, 1971b; Kovacs, 1970; Litherland, 1966; Miller, Feldhusen, & Asher, 1968; Mueller & Lyman, 1969; Reed & Feldhusen, 1972; Tillinghast & Norris, 1968). All of these investigators, except Tillinghast and Norris, reported that high school GPA had a significant positive association with SBTPE scores. Other investigators used GPA at various points in the nursing program as predictors of SBTPE performance (Baldwin, Mowbray, & Taylor, 1968; Behm & Warnock, 1978; Brandt, Hastie, & Schumann, 1966; Dubs, 1976; Ledbetter, 1968/1969; Miller et al., 1968; Muhlenkamp, 1971; Perez, 1977; Reed & Feldhusen, 1972; Reekie, 1971; Stankovich, 1977; Ussery & Little, 1979). Except for Baldwin et al., these investigators reported that nursing GPA was highly predictive of SBTPE scores.

The most commonly used college entrance tests, the SAT and ACT, also were investigated as predictors of SBTPE performance. Positive associations were reported by Backman and Steindler (1971b), Tillinghast and Norris (1968), Miller et al., (1968), Muhlenkamp (1971), and Reed and

Feldhusen (1972). Kovacs, Backman and Steindler, and Reed and Felhusen stated that among the variables they examined, including high school rank and IQ, SATs were the best predictors. Muhlenkamp concluded that the SAT was predictive, but that performance on NLN Achievement Tests was an even better predictor of SBTPE scores. The ACT examination scores were studied by Ledbetter (1968/1969) and they also had a significant positive association with SBTPE scores.

Students in many schools of nursing take NLN Achievement Tests when they are near the end of their nursing studies. A number of investigators found these scores were highly predictive of SBTPE performance (Baldwin et al., 1968; Bell & Martindill, 1976; Brandt et al., 1966; Deardorff, Denner, & Miller, 1976; Ledbetter, 1968/1969; Mueller & Lyman, 1969; Muhlenkamp, 1971; National League for Nursing, 1970; Papcum, 1971). Kovacs (1970) and Backman and Steindler (1971b) reported that measures of IQ also were associated positively with achievement on the state board examinations.

A few investigators examined the predictive validity of some noncognitive predictors of SBTPE performance. Miller et al. (1968) included anxiety and memory traits; Mueller and Lyman (1969) administered the 16–PF; and Reekie (1971) included other personality measures in their studies. None of these measures had significant value as predictors of SBTPE performance. The only noncognitive variables shown to be associated with higher board scores were higher socioeconomic status and age (Miller et al., 1968; Reed & Feldhusen, 1972).

METHODOLOGICAL ISSUES

Sampling

Nursing students have been the subjects of a considerable amount of research. Four major factors contributed to this situation. First, the education of nurses is one of the largest single activities within the profession: thus the attention was warranted. Second, the individuals with an inclination toward conducting research were located in colleges and universities. Third, the relative novelty of nursing research often made it difficult for nurses to gain entré to patient care facilities for the conduct of clinical research. Finally, nursing students constitute a large, easily available body of potential subjects. However, the easy availability created a design weakness that characterized most of the studies. Investigators usually used nonrandom convenience samples consisting of all the members of one or more classes or cohorts of students. This strategy tended to limit severely the generalizability of the findings.

A second factor limiting the generalizability of many of the studies (with the exception of school comparison studies) was that they commonly used single-site samples. There were notable exceptions to both of those sampling patterns, such as Katzell's (1968) study of students'stress, expectations, and attrition; Knopf's (1972) career pattern study; and Schwirian's (1977a, 1977b, 1978, and 1979a, 1979b) performance prediction studies in the middle 1970s. While sampling strategy was a common limitation, sample sizes usually were quite adequate in the studies of nursing students, since whole classes participated as subjects. In summary, investigators must attend to sampling strategies, as well as sample size, to enhance the reliability of their findings.

Academic Setting

A common deficiency of the studies was that there were virtually no descriptions of the students' academic environments beyond the fact that they were located in an AD, diploma, or baccalaureate program. It has been common in the studies of both nursing students and nurses for investigators to focus solely on the performer to the total exclusion of the performance environment. Students do not perform in a vacuum. Each school, like each work setting, has its own particular ambience which is bound to affect behaviors of all kinds. More attention should be paid to the student-learning environment interaction when nursing student studies are conducted and reported.

Measurement

A problem shared by most investigators in the area of nursing performance has been the lack of sound measures of important variables. The area of research on nursing students has been no exception. Measures of academic ability and achievement have been the most reliable, and it was shown consistently that the best predictor of academic achievement is prior academic achievement. However, practice in a caring profession requires affective attributes that cannot be measured by grade point averages. Valid, reliable measures of these attributes have remained elusive.

Nurse investigators have been cautious about developing noncognitive measures specific to their own needs, opting instead for more standardized measures developed within such other disciplines as psychology and sociology. The development and testing of good measurement tools is acknowledged to be a complex, time-consuming process. However, it is the only way investigators will be able to quantify and subsequently study the attributes of particular relevance to nurses and nurse educators. As these groups become more clear and more definitive as to the behavioral, attitudinal, and value-related outcomes associated with quality patient care, they will be able to structure learning opportunities and environments that are more supportive of the development of those desired behaviors, attitudes, and values.

Analysis

Analytical techniques based on correlation formed the core of the studies designed to identify predictors of attrition and retention, academic achievement, and SBTPE performance. The most productive strategies were those using multiple correlation techniques. The same observation was made by Taylor, Nahm, Loy, Harms, Berthold, and Wolfer (1966) in their review of prediction studies that were conducted up to the summer of 1965. As Schwirian (1981) pointed out, the studies that henceforth will provide the most useful information for descriptive or predictive purposes will employ fairly sophisticated multivariate techniques. Techniques such as path analysis, factor mapping, canonical correlation, and discriminant analysis are now widely available to investigators. Moreover, they generally are part of well-documented statistical packages supported by most university computer systems. Thus, the days of using only zero-order Pearson r's and simple t tests are long past.

The need for the development of valid, reliable measures of student behavior variables was cited above. This vital research effort also must be supported by the use of powerful statistical tools such as factor analysis, multidimensional scaling, and latent structure analysis.

Models

It was noted at the beginning of this chapter that the problem-driven nature of research on nursing students has produced a literature that is fragmented and largely noncumulative. Without some integrating mechanism or strategy, future research in the area likely will be the same; this would be neither useful nor cost effective. Desirable and necessary behavioral outcomes for nursing students must be defined; then models must be developed and tested to determine the best sets of personal, situational, and educational variables that can produce the desired outcomes. The information sources for investigators who would use modeling strategies are abundant. These include concepts and theories from nursing and related disciplines, as well as the findings from earlier investigators such as those mentioned in this chapter. There are many approaches to devising explanatory models: Schwirian (1981) described one approach—a variable-blocking technique (Namboodiri, Carter, & Blalock, 1975). Many other causal modeling strategies have been presented (e.g., Blalock, 1971; Goldberger & Duncan, 1973; Maki & Thompson, 1973); some will prove to be useful, and others will not. Only systematic application and testing in the nursing and nursing education settings will establish the model-based knowledge foundations the nursing profession requires. In short, it is time for the research on nursing students to move from being problem-driven to being model-driven.

TRENDS AND FUTURE RESEARCH DIRECTIONS

In the nearly twenty years covered by this review, the quality of the published research on nursing students have improved considerably, especially in the past five years. There have been marked advances in the sophistication of both design and analysis. However, as the quality has improved, the quantity has diminished sharply and more research is reported focusing on clinical problems and theory building. As the quality of nursing research expands in all areas it is important to maintain publication opportunities for investigators in this substantive area.

On the basis of the trends and issues associated with nursing education for the remainder of this century, four areas were identified that deserve careful research attention. The first area is the health of nursing students. This is consistent with the women's health movement and the growing recognition that the role of the caretaker is very demanding, very stressful, and claims many casualties. Many health attitudes and practices are developed while young people are in college. A few investigators have explored nursing students and health. Schwirian and Kisker (1977) examined baccalaureate students' perception of the concept of health, and

Camooso, Greene, Hoffman, Leuner, Mattis, Ptaszynski, Reiley, Silver, Winfrey, and Winland (1980) studied changes in students' preventive health practices. Murray, Swan, and Mattar (1981) explored smoking practices among new student nurses. Student concerns and stress were studied by Carter (1980), Gunter (1969c), and Packard, Schwebel, and Ganey (1979). Sheehan, O'Donnell, Fitzgerald, Hervig, and Ward (1981–1982) reported a study designed to devise a prediction model for accident/error rates among students using preexisting stressors as predictors. In general, the area of nursing student health is open for a substantial amount of significant research.

A second area that offers opportunities for needed research is that of the "second-step" programs that provide opportunities for diploma and AD nurses to obtain baccalaureate degrees in nursing. The learners in these programs are often nontraditional compared to most generic students. They tend to be older, to have greater personal and family responsibilities, to have had experience in the real world, and they have different developmental tasks to achieve. Finally, their reasons for being in school and, thus, their learning needs are very different from those of their generic counterparts. It is likely that the program outcomes for these students also will be different. Much has been written describing what educators *do* and what they *should do* with and for these students, but to date little empirical evidence in the area exists.

A few investigators studied registered nurse (RN) students enrolled in baccalaureate programs. Their results may provide useful ideas and background data for new investigations. Gortner's (1968) study provided baseline data regarding comparisons of generic and RN students on many variables, but little was written about them during the 1970s. Recently, several investigators reported studies based on the second-step project at Sonoma State University (e.g., Church, Brian, & Searight, 1980; Jako, 1980; Little & Brian, 1982; Wilson & Levy, 1978). Little and Brian (1982) identified "challengers," "interactors," and "mainstreamers" among RN students, thus suggesting a typology that other investigators might use and test in their own studies of this special group of nursing students. In two other studies, Rezler and Moore (1978) developed a multiple regression model for predicting final GPAs of RN students, and Belock (1980) compared academic achievement of RNs from AD and diploma programs and found no differences in their academic performance as baccalaureate students.

A third area in which a large number of studies doubtless will be conducted in the next few years is prediction of performance on the new state board examinations—the National Council Licensure Examination (NCLEX). While performance on such tests is not performance in nursing practice, it is agreed that knowledge of the content included in the examinations must be assured before one should be admitted to the practice of nursing. Data from sound, multivariate, model-driven studies of examination achievement could be used productively by those who plan and implement nursing school curricula.

An important area of investigation related to the NCLEX is the examination of the quality of the test itself. It is imperative that the experts in test development and evaluation ensure this quality control and share the information with the nursing education and practice communities.

Finally, an area in need of much careful attention from investigators is that focused on the students enrolled in graduate programs in nursing. To date, few investigators (Ainslie, Anderson, Colby, Hoffman, Meserve, O'Connor, & Quimet, 1976; Brogan, 1982; Miller, 1980; Stein & Green, 1970; Tripp & Duffey, 1981) have studied nursing graduate students. However, as graduate programs increase and mature—particularly doctoral programs—good empirical data and models are needed to evaluate program outcomes and to serve as a foundation for further improvement.

REFERENCES

Adams, A., & Klein, L. R. Students in nursing school: Considerations in assessing characteristics. *Nursing Research,* 1970, *19,* 362–366.

Ainslie, B. S., Anderson, L. E., Colby, B. K., Hoffman, M. A., Meserve, K. P., O'Connor, C., & Quimet, K. M. Predictive value of selected admission criteria for graduate nursing education. *Nursing Research,* 1976, *25,* 296–299.

Aldag, J. C. Occupational and non-occupational interest characteristics of men nurses. *Nursing Research,* 1970, *19,* 529–534.

Aldag, J. C., & Christensen, C. Personality correlates of male nurses. *Nursing Research,* 1967, *16,* 375–376.

Allchnie, M. C., & Bellucci, J. T. Prediction of freshman students' success in a baccalaureate nursing program. *Nursing Research,* 1981, *30,* 49–53.

American Council on Education Policy Analysis Service—USPHS. *Trends and career changes of college students in the health field* (Department of Health, Education and Welfare Publication No. HRA 76–54). Washington, D.C.: U.S. Government Printing Office, 1974.

Anderson, W. Predicting graduation from a school of nursing. *Vocational Guidance Quarterly,* 1968, *16,* 295–300.

Backman, M., & Steindler, F. Let's examine—Cognitive abilities related to attrition in a collegiate nursing program. *Nursing Outlook,* 1971, *19,* 807–808. (a)

Backman, M., & Steindler, F. Let's examine—Prediction of achievement in a collegiate nursing program and performance on state board examinations. *Nursing Outlook*, 1971, *19*, 487. (b)

Bailey, J. Comparative analysis of the personality structure of nursing students. *Nursing Research*, 1969, *18*, 320–326.

Bailey, J., McDonald, F. J., & Claus, K. E. Evaluation of the development of creative behavior in an experimental nursing program. *Nursing Research*, 1970, *19*, 100–107.

Bailey, P. Some comparisons of occupational therapy biographical facts with implications for recruiting. *American Journal of Occupational Therapy*, 1968, *22*, 259–263.

Baker, E. J. Associate degree nursing students: Non-intellective differences between dropouts and graduates. *Nursing Research*, 1975, *24*, 42–44.

Baker, S. R. The relationships of social attitudes to manifest needs. *Nursing Research*, 1965, *14*, 345–346.

Baldwin, J. P., Mowbray, J. K., & Taylor, R. G. Factors influencing performance on state board test pool examinations. *Nursing Research*, 1968, *17*, 170–172.

Behm, R. J., & Warnock, F. N. State board examinations and associate degree program effectiveness. *Nursing Research*, 1978, *27*, 54–56.

Bell, J. A., & Martindill, C. F. A cross-validation study for predictors of scores on state board examinations. *Nursing Research*, 1976, *25*, 54–57.

Belock, S. *Comparison of the grade point averages of registered nurses from diploma programs with registered nurses from associate degree programs*. Castelton, Vt.: Castelton State College, 1980. (ERIC Document Reproduction Service No. ED 188 728).

Berstein, L., Turrell, E. S., & Dana, R. H. Motivation for nursing. *Nursing Research*, 1965, *14*, 222–226.

Bittman, S. A. Prediction of patient-technique orientation of student nurses after one year of nursing school (Doctoral dissertation, Texas Technological University, 1973). *Dissertation Abstracts International*, 1974, *34*, 4622B–4623B. (University Microfilms No. 74–5795)

Blalock, H. M. (Ed.). *Causal models in the social sciences*. Chicago: Aldine-Atherton, 1971.

Blomquist, B. L., Cruise, P. D., & Cruise, R. J. Values of baccalaureate nursing students in secular and religious schools. *Nursing Research*, 1980, *19*, 379–383.

Brandt, E. M., Hastie, B., & Schumann, D. Predicting success on state board examinations: Relationships between course grades, selected test scores, and state board examinations. *Nursing Research*, 1966, *15*, 62–69.

Brogan, D. R. Professional socialization to a research role: Interest in research among graduate students in nursing. *Research in Nursing and Health*, 1982, *5*, 113–122.

Brown, J., Swift, Y. B., & Oberman, M. L. Baccalaureate students' image of nursing: A replication. *Nursing Research*, 1974, *23*, 53–59.

Bullough, B., & Sparks, C. Baccalaureate vs. associate degree nurses: The care-cure dichotomy. *Nursing Outlook*, 1975, *23*, 688–692.

Burgess, G. The self-concepts of undergraduate nursing students in relation to clinical performance and selected biographical variables. *Journal of Nursing Education*, 1980, *19*(3), 37–44.

Burgess, M. M., & Duffey, M. The prediction of success in a collegiate program of nursing. *Nursing Research*, 1969, *18*, 68–72.

Burgess, M. M., Duffey, M., & Temple, F. G. Two studies of prediction of success in a collegiate program of nursing. *Nursing Research*, 1972, *21*, 357–366.

Camooso, C., Greene, M., Hoffman, J., Leuner, J., Mattis, C., Ptaszynski, E., Reiley, P., Silver, S., Winfrey, M. E., & Winland, J. Preventive health practices of generic baccalaureate nursing students. *Nursing Research*, 1980, *29*, 256–257.

Carter, E. W. Stress in nursing students: Dispelling some of the myth. *Nursing Outlook*, 1980, *30*, 248–251.

Casella, C. Need hierarchies among nursing and non-nursing college students. *Nursing Research*, 1968, *17*, 273–275.

Chissom, B. S., & Lanier, D. Prediction of first quarter freshman GPA using SAT scores and high school grades. *Educational and Psychological Measurement*, 1975, *35*, 461–463.

Church, E. F., Brian, S., & Searight, M. W. Describing a new baccalaureate nursing population: The second step. *Western Journal of Nursing Research*, 1980, *2*, 575–587.

Coe, R. M. Self-conception and professional training. *Nursing Research*, 1965, *14*, 49–52.

Collins, D. L., & Joel, L. A. The image of nursing is not changing. *Nursing Outlook*, 1971, *19*, 456–459.

Connelly, T. Nursing career commitment. *Hospitals*, 1970, *44*, 142–143; 146; 148; 150.

Damrosch, S. P. How nursing students' reactions to rape victims are affected by a perceived act of carelessness. *Nursing Research*, 1981, *30*, 168–170.

Damrosch, S. P. Nursing students' attitudes towards sexually active older persons. *Nursing Research*, 1982, *31*, 252–255.

Davis, A. J. Self-concepts, occupational role expectations, and occupational choice in nursing and social work. In A. Heiss, J. Mixer, & J. Paltridge (Eds.), *Participants and patterns in higher education: Research and reflections*. Berkeley: University of California, The Program in Higher Education, 1973.

Deardorff, M., Denner, P., & Miller, C. Selected National League for Nursing Achievement Test scores as predictors of state board examination scores. *Nursing Research*, 1976, *25*, 35–38.

Dietz, M. R. A study of self-concept of diploma nursing school students (Doctoral dissertation, University of Pittsburgh, 1973). *Dissertation Abstracts International*, 1974, *34*, 3878B (University Microfilms No. 74–2083)

Donsky, A. P., & Judge, A. J. *Academic and nonacademic characteristics as predictors of persistence in an associate degree nursing program*. Minneapolis, Minn.: Annual Forum of the Association for Institutional Research, 1981. (ERIC Document Reproduction Service No. ED 205 076)

Dubs, R. Comparison of student achievement with performance rating of graduates and state board examination scores. *Nursing Research*, 1975, *24*, 59–63.

Ellis, L. S. An investigation of nursing student self-concept levels: A pilot survey. *Nursing Research*, 1980, *29*, 389–390.

Elton, C. F., & Rose, H. Aspirations: Fulfilled or forgotten? *Nursing Research,* 1970, *19,* 72–75.

Felton, G., Reed, P., & Perla, S. Measurement of nursing students' attitudes toward cancer. *Western Journal of Nursing Research,* 1981, *3,* 62–74.

Finegan, A. The predictive value of measured motivational factors in evaluating nurse candidates. *Psychiatric Quarterly Supplement,* 1967, *41,* 77–85.

Garvin, B. J. Values of male nursing students. *Nursing Research,* 1976, *25,* 352–357.

Gerstein, A. Development of a selection program for nursing candidates. *Nursing Research,* 1965, *14,* 254–257.

Goldberger, A. S., & Duncan, O. S. *Structural equation models in the social sciences.* New York: Seminar Press, 1973.

Goldstein, J. O. Comparison of graduating AD and baccalaureate nursing students' characteristics. *Nursing Research,* 1980, *29,* 46–49.

Gortner, S. R. Nursing majors in twelve western universities: A comparison of registered nurse students and basic senior students. *Nursing Research,* 1968, *17,* 121–129.

Gunden, E. A. *A comparative study of perceptions of sophomore nursing students, senior nursing students, nursing faculty, and clients as to the importance of empathy as an attribute of the "ideal" nurse.* Indianapolis: Indiana University School of Nursing, 1980. (ERIC Document Reproduction Service No. ED 189 999)

Gunter, L. M. The developing nursing student: Part I. A study of self-actualizing values. *Nursing Research,* 1969, *18,* 60–64. (a)

Gunter, L. M. The developing nursing student: Part II. Attitudes toward nursing as a career. *Nursing Research,* 1969, *18,* 131–136. (b)

Gunter, L. M. The developing nursing student: Part III. A study of self-appraisals and concerns reported during the sophomore year. *Nursing Research,* 1969, *18,* 237–242. (c)

Hegarty, W. H. Organizational and sociological factors affecting attrition in collegiate schools of nursing. *International Journal of Nursing Studies,* 1976, *12,* 217–222.

Ichilov, O., & Dotan, M. Formation of professional images among Israeli student nurses. *International Journal of Nursing Studies,* 1980, *17,* 247–259.

Jako, K. L. Defining and measuring student success: A three-dimensional approach. *Western Journal of Nursing Research,* 1980, *2,* 462–477.

Johnson, R. W., & Leonard, L. C. Psychological test characteristics and performance of nursing students. *Nursing Research,* 1970, *19,* 147–150.

Johnson, W. L. Admissions of men and ethnic minorities to schools of nursing, 1971–1972. *Nursing Outlook,* 1974, *22,* 45–49.

Jones, C. W. Why associate degree nursing students persist. *Nursing Research,* 1975, *24,* 57–59.

Kahn, A. M. Modifications in nursing student attitudes as measured by the EPPS: A significant reversal from the past. *Nursing Research,* 1980, *29,* 61–63.

Katzell, M. E. Expectations and dropouts in schools of nursing. *Journal of Applied Psychology,* 1968, *52,* 154–157.

Klahn, J. E. Self-concept and change-seeking need of first-year student nurses. *Journal of Nursing Education,* 1969, *8,* 11–16.

232   RESEARCH ON NURSING EDUCATION

Knopf, L. *From student to R.N.: A report of the nurse career pattern study* (Department of Health, Education and Welfare Publication No. NIH 72–130). Washington, D.C.: U.S. Government Printing Office, 1972.

Knopke, H. J. Predicting student attrition in a baccalaureate curriculum. *Nursing Research*, 1979, *28*, 224–227.

Komorita, N. I. Self concept measures as related to achievement in nursing education (Doctoral dissertation, Wayne State University, 1972). *Dissertation Abstracts International*, 1972, *32*, 6809A. (University Microfilms No. 72–14584)

Kovacs, A. R. Uniform minimum admission standards. *Nursing Outlook*, 1970, *18*, 54–56.

Lamoureux, M. E., & Johannsen, C. *Multiple criteria development for the selection of community college nursing program students*. Edmonton, Alberta, Canada: Association of Canadian Community Colleges, 1977. (ERIC Document Reproduction Service No. ED (163 032)

Ledbetter, P. J. An analysis of the performance of a selected baccalaureate program in nursing with regard to selected standard examinations (Doctoral dissertation, University of Alabama, 1968). *Dissertation Abstracts International*, 1969, *29*, 3381A. (University Microfilms No. 69–6549)

Lenburg, C. G., Burnside, H., & Davitz, L. J. Inferences of physical pain and psychological distress. III: In relation to length of time in the nursing education program. *Nursing Research*, 1970, *19*, 399–401.

Levine, A. G. Marital and occupational plans of women in professional schools: Law, medicine, nursing, teaching (Doctoral dissertation, Yale University, 1968). *Dissertation Abstracts International*, 1969, *30*, 829A. (University Microfilms No. 69–13, 353)

Levitt, E., Lubin, B., Dewitt, K. N. An attempt to develop an objective test battery for the selection of nursing students. *Nursing Research*, 1971, *20*, 255–258.

Lewis, J., & Welch, M. Predicting achievement in an upper-division bachelor's degree nursing major. *Educational and Psychological Measurement*, 1975, *35*, 467–469.

Liddle, R. L., Heywood, H. L., & Morman, R. R. Predicting baccalaureate degree attainment for nursing students: A theoretical study using the TAV system. *Nursing Research*, 1971, *20*, 258–261.

Litherland, R. L. Iowa tests of educational development as a predictor of success in Iowa schools of professional nursing (Doctoral dissertation, The University of Iowa, 1966). *Dissertation Abstracts International*, 1966, *27*, 1240A. (University Microfilms No. 66–11673)

Little, M., & Brian, S. The challengers, interactors and mainstreamers: Second step education and nursing roles. *Nursing Research*, 1982, *31*, 239–245.

Lynn, M. R. *The professional socialization of nursing students: A comparison based on type of educational program*. Los Angeles, Calif.: American Education Association, 1981. (ERIC Document Reproduction Service No. ED 201 268)

Maki, D. P., & Thompson, M. *Mathematical models and applications*. Englewood Cliffs, N.J.: Prentice-Hall, 1973.

May, T. W. Differences between nursing student dropouts and remainers on the Study of Values. *Psychological Reports 19, Part 1*, 1967, *41*, 491.

May, T. W., & Ilardi, R. L. Change and stability of values in collegiate nursing students. *Nursing Research*, 1970, *19*, 359–362.

Mayes, N., Schultz, M., & Pierce, C. M. Commitment to nursing—How is it achieved? *Nursing Outlook*, 1968, *16*, 29–31.

McIntyre, H. M., McDonald, F. J., Bailey, J. T., & Claus, K. K. A simulated clinical nursing research test. *Nursing Research*, 1972, *21*, 229–235.

Meleis, A. I., & Dagenais, F. Sex-role identity and perception of professional self. *Nursing Research*, 1981, *30*, 162–167.

Meleis, A. I., & Farrell, K. Operation concern: A study of senior nursing students in three nursing programs. *Nursing Research*, 1974, *23*, 461–468.

Michael, W. B., Haney, R., & Jones, R. A. The predictive validities of selected aptitude and achievement measures and of three personality inventories in relation to nursing training criteria. *Educational and Psychological Measurement*, 1966, *26*, 1035–1040.

Michael, W. B., Haney, R., Lee, Y. B., & Michael, J. J. The criterion-related validities of cognitive and noncogitive predictors for nursing candidates. *Educational and Psychological Measurement*, 1971, *31*, 983–987.

Miller, C. L. Factors in graduate nursing student performance. *International Journal of Nursing Studies*, 1980, *17*, 39–45.

Miller, C. L., Felhusen, J. F., & Asher, W. J. The prediction of state board examination scores of graduates of an associate degree program. *Nursing Research*, 1968, *17*, 555–558.

Miller, M. H. On blacks entering nursing. *Nursing Forum*, 1972, *2*, 248–263.

Miller, M. H. A follow-up of first-year nursing student dropouts. *Nursing Forum*, 1974, *13*, 32–47.

Montag, M. L. *Evaluation of graduates of associate degree nursing programs*. New York: Teachers College, Columbia University, 1972.

Morman, R. R., Liddle, R. L., & Haywood, H. L. Prediction of academic achievement of nursing students. *Nursing Research*, 1965, *14*, 227–230.

Morris, P. B., & Grassi-Russo, N. Motives of beginning students for choosing nursing school. *Journal of Nursing Education*, 1979, *18*(5), 34–40.

Mowbray, J. K., & Taylor, R. G. Validity of interest inventories for the prediction of success in a school of nursing. *Nursing Research*, 1967, *16*, 78–81.

Mueller, E. J., & Lyman, J. B. The prediction of scores on state board test pool examinations. *Nursing Research*, 1969, *18*, 263–267.

Muhlenkamp, A. F. Let's examine—Prediction of state board scores in baccalaureate programs. *Nursing Outlook*, 1971, *19*, 57.

Munday, L., & Hoyt, D. P. Predicting academic success for nursing students. *Nursing Research*, 1965, *14*, 341–344.

Murray, L. M., & Morris, D. R. Professional autonomy among senior nursing students in diploma, associate degree, and baccalaureate nursing programs. *Nursing Research*, 1982, *31*, 311–313.

Murray, M., Swan, A. V., Mattar, N. Smoking among new student nurses. *Journal of Advanced Nursing*, 1981, *6*, 255–260.

Namboodiri, N. K., Carter, L. F., & Blalock, H. M. *Applied multivariate analysis and experimental designs*. New York: McGraw-Hill, 1975.

Nash, P. M. *Evaluation of employment opportunities for newly licensed nurses*

(Department of Health, Education and Welfare Publication No. HRA 75–12). Washington, D.C.: U.S. Government Printing Office, 1975.

The National League for Nursing. *A validation study of the NLN pre-nursing and guidance examination and related studies emerging from data gathered from the validation study.* New York: Author, 1970.

O'Neill, M. F. A study of baccalaureate nursing student values. *Nursing Research,* 1973, *22,* 437–442.

Owen, S. V., & Feldhusen, J. F. Effectiveness of three models of multivariate prediction of academic success in nursing education. *Nursing Research,* 1970, *19,* 517–525.

Owen, S. V., Feldhusen, J. F., & Thurston, J. R. Achievement prediction in nursing education with cognitive, attitudinal and divergent thinking variables. *Psychological Reports,* 1970, *26,* 867–870.

Packard, K. L., Schwebel, A. I., & Ganey, J. S. Concerns of final semester baccalaureate nursing students. *Nursing Research,* 1979, *28,* 302–304.

Pallone, N. J., & Hosinski, M. Reality testing a vocational choice: Congruence between self, ideal, and occupational percepts among student nurses. *Personnel and Guidance Journal,* 1967, *45,* 666–670.

Papcum, I. Let's examine—Results of achievement tests and state board tests in an associate degree program. *Nursing Outlook,* 1971, *19,* 341.

Pavalko, R. M. Recruitment to nursing: Some research findings. *Nursing Research,* 1969, *18,* 72–76.

Perez, T. L. Investigation of academic moderator variables to predict success of state board of nursing examinations in a baccalaureate nursing program. *Journal of Nursing Education,* 1977, *16*(8), 16–23.

Plapp, J. M., Psathas, G., & Caputo, D. V. Intellective predictors of success in nursing school. *Educational and Psychological Measurement,* 1965, *25,* 565–577.

Psathas, G. The fate of idealism in nursing school. *Journal of Health and Social Behavior,* 1968, *9,* 52–64.

Psathas, G., & Plapp, J. M. Assessing the effects of a nursing program: A problem in design. *Nursing Research,* 1968, *17,* 336–342.

Raderman, R., & Allen, D. Registered nurse students in a baccalaureate program: Factors associated with completion. *Nursing Research,* 1974, *23,* 71–73.

Reed, C. L., & Feldhusen, J. F. State board examination score prediction for associate degree nursing program students. *Nursing Research,* 1972, *21,* 149–153.

Reed, C. L., Feldhusen, J. F., & Van Monfrans, A. P. Prediction of grade point averages using cognitive and noncognitive predictor variables. *Psychological Reports,* 1973, *32,* 143–148.

Reekie, E. Personality factors and biographical charcateristics associated with criterion behaviors of success in professional nursing (Doctoral dissertation, University of Washington, 1971). *Dissertation Abstracts International,* 1971, *31,* 5212A. (University Microfilms No. 71–8534)

Rezler, A. G., & Moore, J. S. Correlates of success in the baccalaureate education of registered nurses. *Research in Nursing and Health,* 1978, *1,* 159–164.

Richards, M. A. B. A study of differences in psychological characteristics of students graduating from three types of basic nursing programs. *Nursing Research*, 1972, *21*, 258–261.

Richek, H. G., & Nichols, T. Personality and cognitive characteristics of prenursing majors. *Nursing Research*, 1973, *22*, 443–448.

Robb, S. S. Attitudes and intentions of baccalaureate nursing students toward the elderly. *Nursing Research*, 1979, *28*, 43–50.

Roraback, C. The college bound high school senior girls and nursing as a major field of study (Doctoral dissertation, Columbia University, 1968). *Dissertation Abstracts International*, 1969, *29*, 3802B. (University Microfilms No. 69–6038)

Schoeberle, E. A., & Craddick, R. A. Human figure drawings by freshmen and senior student nurses. *Perceptual and Motor Skills*, 1968, *27*, 11–14.

Schultz, E. D. Personality traits of nursing students and faculty concepts of desirable traits: A longitudinal comparative study. *Nursing Research*, 1965, *14*, 261–264.

Schwirian, P. M. *Prediction of successful nursing performance, Part 1: A review of research related to the prediction of successful nursing performance 1965–1975* (Department of Health, Education, and Welfare Publication No. HRA 77–27). Washington, D.C.: U.S. Government Printing Office, 1977. (a)

Schwirian, P. M. *Prediction of successful nursing performance, Part 2: Admission practices, evaluation strategies, and performance prediction among schools of nursing* (Department of Health, Education, and Welfare Publication No. HRA 77–27). Washington, D.C.: U.S. Government Printing Office, 1977 (b)

Schwirian, P. M. Evaluating the performance of nurses: A multidimensional approach. *Nursing Research*, 1978, *27*, 347–351.

Schwirian, P. M. *Prediction of successful nursing performance, Part 3: Evaluation and prediction of the performance of recent nurse graduates* (Department of Health, Education, and Welfare Publication No. HRA 79–15). Washington, D.C.: U.S. Government Printing Office, 1979. (a)

Schwirian, P. M. *Prediction of successful nursing performance, Part 4: Nurse graduate performance: An in-depth analysis of selected pertinent factors* (Department of Health, Education, and Welfare Publication No. HRA 719–15). Washington, D.C.: U.S. Government Printing Office, 1979. (b)

Schwirian, P. M. Toward an explanatory model of nursing performance. *Nursing Research*, 1981, *30*, 247–253.

Schwirian, P. M., & Kisker, K. L. Perceptions of health among baccalaureate nursing students. *Journal of Nursing Education*, 1977, *16*(60), 2–9.

Sedhom, L. N. Attitudes toward the elderly among female college students. *Image*, 1982, *14*, 81–85.

Seither, F. F. Prediction of achievement in baccalaureate nursing education. *Journal of Nursing Education*, 1980, *19*(3), 28–36.

Sharp, W. H., & Anderson, J. C. Changes in nursing students' descriptions of the personality traits of the ideal nurse. *Measurement and Evaluation in Guidance*, 1972, *5*, 339–344.

Sheehan, D. V., O'Donnell, J., Fitzgerald, A., Hervig, L., & Ward, H. Psychosocial predictors of accident/error rates in nursing students: A prospective study. *International Journal of Psychiatry in Medicine*, 1981–1982, *11*, 125–136.

Siegel, H. Professional socialization in two baccalaureate programs. *Nursing Research*, 1968, *17*, 403–407.

Skipper, J. K. The role of the hospital nurse: Is it instrumental or expressive? In J. K. Skipper & R. C. Leonard (Eds.), *Social Interaction and Patient Care*. Philadelphia: Lippincott, 1965.

Smith, G. M. The role of personality in nursing education. *Nursing Research*, 1965, *14*, 54–57.

Smith, J. E. Personality structure in beginning nursing students: A factor analytic study. *Nursing Research*, 1968, *17*, 140–145.

Snyder, M. Preparation of nursing students for health care teams. *International Journal of Nursing Studies*, 1981, *18*, 115–122.

Stankovich, M. J. *The statistical probability of the academic performance of registered nursing students at Macomb*. Project No. 0141-77. Warren, Mich.: Macomb County Community College, 1977. (ERIC Document Reproduction Service No. ED 161 501)

Stein, R. F. The student nurse—A study of need, roles, and conflicts, Part 1. *Nursing Research*, 1969, *18*, 308–315. (a)

Stein, R. F. The student nurse—A study of needs, roles, and conflicts, Part 2. *Nursing Research*, 1969, *18*, 440–443. (b)

Stein, R. F., & Green, E. J. The graduate record examination as a predictive potential in the nursing major. *Nursing Research*, 1970, *19*, 44–47.

Taylor, C. W., Nahm, H., Loy, L., Harms, M., Berthold, J., & Wolfer, J. A. *Selection and recruitment of nurses and nursing students: A review of research studies and practices*. Salt Lake City: University of Utah Press, 1966.

Taylor, C. W., Nahm, H., Quinn, M., Harms, M., Mulaik, J., & Mulaik, S. A. *Report of measurement and prediction of nursing performance, Part 1. Factor analysis of nursing students' application data, entrance test scores, achievement test scores, and grades in nursing school*. Salt Lake City: University of Utah Press, 1965.

Taylor, J. K. Recruiting: Nurse power is the answer. *RN*, 1970, *33*, 61–63.

Thomas, B. Promoting creativity in nursing education. *Nursing Research*, 1979, *28*, 115–119.

Thurston, J. R., Brunclik, H. L., & Feldhusen, J. F. The relationship of personality to achievement in nursing education, Phase 2. *Nursing Research*, 1968, *17*, 265–268.

Thurston, J. R., Brunclik, H. L., & Feldhusen, J. F. Personality and the prediction of success in nursing education. *Nursing Research*, 1969, *18*, 252–262.

Tillinghast, B. S., & Norris, B. Let's examine—The relation of selected admission variables to student achievement. *Nursing Outlook*, 1968, *16*, 58.

Tripp, A., & Duffey, M. Discriminant analysis to predict graduation-nongraduation in a master's degree program in nursing. *Research in Nursing and Health*, 1981, *4*, 345–353.

Trussell, R. P., & Pappas, J. P. *Some variables for student nurse selection* (Rocky Mountain Psychological Association Report No. 47). Salt Lake City: University of Utah Press, 1974.

Ussery, R. M., & Little, B. E. *A study of nursing curriculum factors and achievement on the North Carolina state board test pool nursing examination*.

Summary report. Greenville, N.C.: East Carolina University, 1979. (ERIC Document Reproduction Service No. ED 176 654)

Wilson, H. S., & Levy, J. Why RN students drop out. *Nursing Outlook*, 1978, *26*, 437–441.

Wittemeyer, A. L., Camiscioni, J. S., & Purdy, P. A. A longitudinal study of attrition and academic performance in a collegiate nursing program. *Nursing Research*, 1971, *20*, 339–347.

Worsley, A. Exploration of student nurses' stereotypes of patients. *International Journal of Nursing Studies*, 1980, *17*, 163–174.

Wren, G. Some characteristics of freshman students in baccalaureate, diploma, and associate degree nursing programs. *Nursing Research*, 1971, *20*, 167–172.

CHAPTER 10

Curricular Research in Nursing

Marilyn L. Stember
School of Nursing
University of Colorado Health Sciences Center

CONTENTS

An awareness has emerged in nursing about the need to articulate and build a scientific body of knowledge about nursing practice, education, and administration (de Tornyay, 1977; Gortner, 1980). The purpose of this review is to summarize and assess the accumulated state of knowledge regarding curricula in nursing. Studies that could contribute to the scientific basis were analyzed with respect to substantive areas emphasized, as well as methodological quality. Considering both these elements and the consistency of findings across the more rigorous research, the cumulative development of knowledge was assessed. Important issues to address in future research also are suggested.

SELECTION OF STUDIES FOR REVIEW

As the focal topic for this review, curriculum was defined broadly as the structure and content of all courses collectively offered to produce a total effect (Wu, 1979). A minimum requirement for inclusion of a study was

239

that a scientific approach was taken to assess systematically one or more types of curricula or at least one element of the curriculum design or process. This included studies in which investigators examined such areas as conceptual frameworks, content, or course placements. Studies were also included if investigators related antecedent or concurrent variables to curriculum variables or if they focused on the relationship of various curricular models and their outcomes. A delimiter on this general perspective was the knowledge that other specific reviews in this series were planned to address the following areas: research on teaching strategies; research on student selection, retention, and outcomes; and research on educational administration. Studies of practical nursing curricula were excluded, as well as studies related to continuing education curricula.

A further decision was made to focus on relatively recent research that could contribute to the current base of nursing curricular knowledge. Thus, the analysis of studies in this review was concentrated on research published in the past 15 years. Readers who are interested in earlier studies are referred to several articles on research in nursing education (Abdellah, 1970; Clarke, 1977; Gortner & Nahm, 1977; Hill, Gortner, & Scott, 1980). Particularly comprehensive is Gortner and Nahm's historical account. Another valuable article is Abdellah's description of educational studies sponsored by the United States Department of Health and Human Services' Division of Nursing between 1955 and 1968.

A search was made to identify the studies that could be evaluated for their contribution to the current knowledge base. A computerized search was done, using the MEDLARS and ERIC data bases and specifying key words that included curriculum, educational research, and nursing programs. These terms were linked with research terms such as surveys, follow-up studies, evaluation studies, and questionnaires. The resulting citations were screened for their appropriateness for inclusion. Nonempirically based articles describing the design or implementation of curricula were excluded. Books, monographs, and reports were other sources for curricular research. However, no categorized, comprehensive list of these publications was available.

A large number of studies regarding nursing curricula have been conducted as part of the educational requirements of the researcher. Master's and doctoral theses were other sources considered. However, no centralized listing of Master's theses has been compiled. One hundred eighty-one abstracts of research relating to nursing curricula were found in *Dissertation Abstracts International* volumes published since 1970. These abstracts were read and analyzed briefly. Although some general statements are made about these studies, they were excluded from the central analysis because many of the full studies were not readily available to be evaluated methodologically, and the more important research was likely to have been published.

Finally, manual searches were done in several ways. Some tracking of citations from one study to another was done. Earlier cited research was examined for its inclusion in the review. In addition, *Nursing Research* and the *Journal of Nursing Education*, the two journals thought most likely to publish nursing curricula research, were reviewed issue by issue for the most recent 15 years.

Forty-seven published studies met the above inclusionary criteria. Although the selection of studies for this review was systematic and quite comprehensive, some studies inadvertently may have been omitted. Furthermore, if all potentially relevant research had been included, some earlier studies should have been reviewed and a wider range of sources (i.e., general education literature, medical education studies) would have been necessary. The listing is not complete and is probably biased toward more successful curricula studies, since unsuccessful projects are less likely to be submitted or accepted for publication. Although the 47 studies identified are not an exhaustive collection of all research on nursing curricula, they provided the domain from which an analysis could be made.

CATEGORIZING THE STUDIES FOR AN OVERVIEW

Studies that met the criteria were categorized according to the main purpose of the study, type of research design, and various conceptual and methodological issues. A summary of the 47 studies presented in Table 10–1 shows the clustering of studies into five major areas. From this collation, it is evident that studies about specific content in the curriculum (28%) and evaluative studies of various curriculum models (23%) were investigated most frequently. Nine studies (19%) comprised a third category; these were designed to compare differences in the graduates of different types and lengths of nursing curricula that prepare registered nurses. Seven other studies (15%) were about curricula for nontraditional baccalaureate students. The remaining 7 studies (15%) were descriptions of conceptual frameworks or structural approaches used in nursing curricula.

Among the studies reviewed, the most frequently employed designs were cross-sectional surveys (45%) and quasi-experimental designs (53%). Stevens (1971) used an historical research design. While many of the

Table 10–1. Categories of Research about Nursing Curricula with Topics and Citations

Categories, Topics, Researchers, Dates

Organizational Patterns in Nursing Curricula
Conceptual frameworks in BS programs—Part 1 (DeBack, 1981)
Theorists in use in conceptual frameworks (Hall, 1979)
Blocked and integrated curriculums in use—Part 1 (Pardue, 1979)
Models used to organize curricula (Quiring & Gray, 1982)
Conceptual frameworks in BS and MS programs (Santora, 1980)
Structural approaches used in nursing curricula (Stevens, 1971)
Conceptual frameworks in BS curricula (Torres & Yura, 1974)

Evaluation of Curricular Organization
Comparison of problem solving with control (Bailey, McDonald, & Claus (1971)
Evaluation of one curriculum (Brandt, Hastie, & Schumann (1967)
Comparison of diagnostic ability in curricula types—Part 2 (DeBack, 1981)
Comparison of old and new curricula (Koehler, 1982)
Evaluation of one curriculum (LaBelle & Egan, 1975)
Evaluation of one curriculum (Marriner, Langford, & Goodwin, 1980)
Evaluation of one integrated curriculum (Melcolm, Venn, & Bausell, 1981)
Comparison of blocked and integrated curricula—Part 2 (Pardue, 1979)
Comparison of blocked and integrated curricula (Richards, 1977)
Comparison of body systems and concepts curricula (Schoen, 1975)
Comparison of old and new curricula (Stone & Green, 1975)

Examination of Specific Content
Master's core content (Beare, Daniel, Gover, Gray, Lancaster, & Sloan, 1980)
Alcohol and drug abuse content (Burkhalter, 1975)
Group dynamics course (Garner & Lowe, 1965)
Gerontological content (Gunter, 1971)
Alcoholism content (Gurel, 1974)
Effect of alcoholism course (Harlow & Goby, 1980)
Public health content in curricula (Holt, 1970)
Effect of aging content (Kayser & Minnigerode, 1975)
Core content in master's program (McLane, 1978)
Student attitude about evening courses (Robbins, 1973)
Influence of geriatric content (Tollett & Thornby, 1982)
Experimental community health course (Warner & Walsh, 1968)
Human sexuality course (Woods & Mandetta, 1975)

Comparison of Types of RN Curricula
Educational level and performance (Dyer, Cope, Monson, & Van Drimmelen, 1972)
AD versus BS on self-actualization (Goldstein, 1980)
AD versus BS on professional practice (Gray, Murray, Roy, & Sawyer, 1977)
AD, diploma, and BS on employer's ratings (Howell, 1978)
AD, diploma, and BS on autonomy (Murray & Morris, 1982)

AD, diploma, and BS on competencies (Nelson, 1978)
AD, diploma, and BS on psychological measures (Richards, 1972)
Diploma and BS self-rated performance (Smoyak, 1972)
AD versus BS on clinical practice (Waters, Chater, Vivier, Urrea & Wilson, 1972)
Baccalaureate Curricula for Nontraditional Students
Characteristics of Second Step programs (Church, Brian & Searight, 1980)
Characteristics of open curricula (Lenburg & Johnson, 1974)
Professional changes in Second Step curricula (Little & Brian, 1982)
Open curriculum study (Notter & Robey, 1979)
Comparison of articulated and nonarticulated (Schoenmaker, 1975)
Comparison of accelerated and generic (Tierney, 1979)
Evaluation of one Second Step curriculum (Wilson, Vaughan & Gaff, 1977)

---

studies had a longitudinal element, none of the investigators used a time series or repeated measures design. Neither phenomenological nor ethnographic studies were found, although qualitative methods were used by some investigators.

The investigators who implemented a quasi-experimental design selected comparison or control groups. Researchers in eight studies used previous cohorts of students as control groups. This was particularly common in research designed to test the effectiveness of a new curriculum or course. A few investigators (Garner & Lowe, 1965; Harlow & Goby, 1980; Stone & Green, 1975) identified a simultaneous nonequivalent control group to use as a comparison. In many of the quasi-experimental studies, preexisting differences between groups and uncontrolled external events raised concern about internal validity and precluded drawing conclusions about the treatment variable. Although experimental designs were implemented successfully in many nonlaboratory settings, none of the studies included random assignment of subjects to experimental and control groups.

In 12 other studies, the nature of the research question influenced the researcher to compare two or more intact groups. For example, students in a baccalaureate (BS) program were compared with students in an associate degree (AD) program, or graduating generic baccalaureate students were compared with graduating registered nurse (RN) baccalaureate students. Although the demographic characteristics often were examined in both groups, these variables rarely were included as covariates in statistical testing between groups. Unfortunately, if differences were found, they were attributed to the experimental condition (i.e., type of curriculum) rather than to unknown selection differences.

Few studies were designed to test a theory. The linking of brief theoretical ideas and previous research in the area created the general frameworks for the studies. The research was marked by a lack of commonality in theoretical models. Concept identification and definitions were inconsistent. It was not obvious that these studies were built upon other studies, either in conceptual or methodological dimensions.

The samples used for these studies were predominantly convenience samples. Of more concern was the observation that in over half of the studies, only one school or hospital was used. Twenty studies were conducted in only one institution while investigators of three more studies used two or three schools but only one institution of each type required. Clearly these studies must be criticized for their lack of external validity. In five studies (Little & Brian, 1982; Richards, 1972; Smoyak, 1972; Tollett & Thornby, 1982; Waters, Chater, Vivier, Urrea, & Wilson, 1972), investigators used a slightly broader convenience sample employing from 6 to 13 schools or institutions. A regional or statewide target population was intended in four studies (Goldstein, 1980; Holt, 1970; Howell, 1978; Nelson, 1978). The universe of subjects was the target of eight surveys. The target population for most of these surveys was all BS and/or master's (MS) programs accredited by the National League for Nursing (NLN) during a specified time period.

Another interesting observation was that random selection was rarely used in the sampling procedure. An exception was DeBack (1981), who randomly selected five schools from each of four categories of curriculum types and then used random selection to identify 10 students from each of the 20 schools. Similarly, Pardue (1979) randomly selected four blocked and four integrated curricula after determining the kind of framework used in all NLN-accredited baccalaureate programs. Quiring and Gray (1982) used a 50% random selection for their survey. However, in most of the studies, no attempt was made to define the target population and to select a sample consonant with that population. In some studies the criteria for selection were not explicit.

The sampling loss was reported in the majority of studies. When the research was a part of the academic program requirements, investigators were able to achieve a nearly perfect sample retention, regardless of the method of data collection. For 11 of the surveys, investigators reported response rates greater than 70%, while 7 reported a 50 to 69% return rate. A high sampling loss was reported by some investigators. Goldstein (1980) reported participation rates of 14% and 25% at 2 schools in her study. A wide range of sampling loss (40% to 98%) was found in Tollett and Thornby's (1982) survey in 12 schools. The sampling loss was not reported in seven studies.

The sample sizes planned and obtained were generally adequate for the design specified and the number of variables identified. The Woods and Mandetta study (1975) of 11 women and 12 men who took one course is an exception. This pre- posttest, no-control group design with a small sample clearly had major limitations. Many studies had extraordinarily large sample sizes. For example, one of the open curriculum studies (Lenburg & Johnson, 1974) involved 2,282 programs. Some of the quasi-experimental studies had several hundred students in each of the treatment and control conditions.

Strategies for measurement and methods for data collection were varied. Some researchers carefully defined variables and specified operational definitions. In these studies, instruments tended to be described with information about their previously established reliability and validity; none reported the psychometric properties attained in their samples. However, the majority of studies used self-made questionnaires, interview guides, or tests. These investigators frequently did not identify the specific variables they were trying to measure and the instruments had not undergone psychometric testing. If any work was done in measurement, face and content validity was established through jury and literature justification. The instruments used with greatest frequency in these studies were State Board Examination scores and NLN Achievement Test scores. However, none of the users reported reliability or validity data on these tools.

The most common form of data production was the questionnaire; this method of data collection was used in 27 of the studies. Written tests or paper and pencil instruments were used in 18 of the studies. Interviews were used in 6 investigations (Marriner, Langford, & Goodwin, 1980; Robbins, 1973; Stone & Green, 1975; Tollett & Thornby, 1982; Waters et al., 1972; Wilson, Vaughan, & Gaff, 1977). Waters et al. (1972) and Marriner et al. (1980) also used observation as one data collection strategy. Secondary data were used in many of the studies; some investigators relied extensively on the content analysis of documents (Church, Brian, & Searight, 1980; DeBack, 1981; Santora, 1980; Torres & Yura, 1974). Other investigators located test scores and demographic information in student and alumni files.

The necessity to control for investigator bias was not acknowledged by most of the researchers. Whether this resulted from ignorance, lack of rigor, or practicality could not be discerned. Many studies were carried out by curriculum coordinators or evaluators who obviously were aware of the group membership. Raters were sometimes faculty members who were not using blind review principles.

ASSESSMENT OF SUBSTANTIVE AREAS

As identified in the previous section, five substantive areas were investigated to some extent in nursing curricula. In this section, the studies in each group are evaluated and examined together for their contribution to a knowledge base.

Organizational Patterns in Nursing Curricula

The explosion of knowledge in recent decades encouraged the identification and use of structural patterns to assist organization of the curricula. Subsequent to the NLN accreditation requirement that schools of nursing have a conceptual framework, several investigators examined the organizing frameworks for curricula in nursing programs.

Two content analyses of NLN accreditation documents were done. Torres and Yura (1974) examined the frameworks reported in the 50 BS programs that submitted documentation for accreditation from 1972 to 1973. They found considerable confusion about frameworks, but found that the major concepts were man, society, health, and nursing. Similarly, Santora (1980) analyzed NLN reports submitted by the 61 schools that offered both master's and baccalaureate programs and applied for accreditation between 1972 and 1978. Santora found that the leading concepts were health, man, nursing, nursing process, and environment. She found that one-third had no framework or an ambiguous framework. The majority of others were cast as adaptation frameworks. Systems and developmental frameworks were found in combination with other orientations.

Information about conceptual frameworks in use was obtained by two investigators in their phase one studies. Pardue (1979) was identifying the sampling frame for selecting blocked-content and integrated-content schools. Using a definition of blocked-content as organization according to the medical model, and integrated-content as curricular organization around concepts so that medical specialties were not distinguishable, 204 NLN-accredited schools were surveyed. Sixty-three percent were described as integrated-content, 27% as partially integrated, and 10% as blocked-content programs. Using a different classifying scheme and precise definitions derived from the literature, DeBack (1981) identified four curricular models: developmental, systems, interaction, and medical. From her first phase survey of 270 NLN-accredited programs, 50% were classified as systems models, 19% were developmental models, 6% were interaction models, and none were medical models. The remaining 24% were classified as mixed models. Both investigators found their classification schemes were not exhaustive nor mutually exclusive.

Hall (1979) was interested in whether nursing programs were basing their curricula on leading nursing theorists and whether the same framework was used in both baccalaureate and master's programs. In a descriptive study using a national sample, Hall (1979) surveyed 76 schools with higher education programs in nursing to determine if their conceptual frameworks were based on one or more of six identified nursing theorists: Orem, Rogers, Levine, King, Roy, and Johnson. Hale found that faculty used established theorists in undergraduate programs to a greater extent than in graduate programs. Of the BS programs, 41% of the respondents indicated their curriculum was based on one or more identified theorists. Most graduate programs were based on unique conceptual frameworks. Santora (1980) noted differences in frameworks between programs within schools. She found that BS and MS programs shared the framework in only 32 of the 61 schools studied.

Using an historical method, Stevens (1971) analyzed nursing curricula with the framework of four major structural approaches used in building curricula: logistic, dialectical, operational, and problematic. Stevens concluded that prior to the 1950s, a disease-centered, body systems approach in the logistic tradition was the common structure in nursing education. Since that time, various curricula forms that were derived from other structural approaches have been implemented. Stevens suggested that the problematic method was then in vogue and had the potential for expansion, but she predicted a return to the logistic method accompanied by computerized technology.

To determine the methods and models employed to organize curricula, Quiring and Gray (1982) randomly sampled one-half of the NLN-accredited four-year programs. Respondents were given eight categories including concepts, threads, nursing principles, organizing themes, disease orientation, nursing process, body systems orientation, and other. These terms were not defined for the respondent. These researchers found an overwhelming majority of schools attempted to integrate curricular components through the use of some combination of concepts, threads, and nursing process orientation. However, the authors acknowledged that these terms may not be differentiated, since respondents tended to use the terms interchangeably in open-ended responses.

Some investigators were interested in whether the selection and use of a particular framework was related to other variables. DeBack (1981) found that developmental and interaction models were more common in schools where the enrollment was less than 300. However, Santora (1980) found neither enrollment size nor presence of a university hospital were related to the type of framework. Some regional differences were noted in the use of nursing theorists as a basis for the curriculum (Hall, 1979).

In summary, in the surveys conducted on the topic of organizational patterns in nursing curricula, investigators used national target populations and samples achieved through respectable return rates; the findings would be expected to have some generalizability. However, there was evidence that the terms used in this area of research were open to ambiguity on the part of both investigators and respondents. Since the classification schemes differed across studies, the findings were not directly comparable. In general, the research about conceptual frameworks used in nursing curricula suggested that while prominent in the past, the use of the medical or disease model as an organizing schema was very limited in the last decade. In use were curricular models based on nursing concepts, threads, and processes; the curricula were organized around man as a total person with presenting or potential problems. The discrepancies about the frequency of usage of each type of conceptual framework could result from the different classification schemes, definitions used by the investigators, or from actual trends in usage. Little evidence has been amassed to link the choice of conceptual framework with other school, faculty, or professional variables.

Evaluation of Curricular Organization

Investigators in the second group of research attempted to evaluate the outcome of one or more types of curricular organization. The general form of these studies was a quasi-experimental design to compare two or more types of curricular structure. A number of variables served as measures or indicators of the success of these curricula. With the exception of DeBack (1981) and Pardue (1979), convenience samples were used and a comparison group selected from previous classes. Analysis of variance was used to test for significant differences.

In more than half of the studies a knowledge indicator was used. State Board Examination scores were used in five studies (Koehler, 1982; Pardue, 1979; Richards, 1977; Schoen, 1975; Stone & Green, 1975), with consistency in the findings. State Board Examination scores were significantly higher in more traditional, blocked curricula than in integrated, concept-oriented curricula. In three studies, NLN Achievement Test scores also were compared. Two investigators (Schoen, 1975; Stone & Green, 1975) found that students in the blocked curriculum did better, but Richards (1977) found mixed results. Even though these two tests were standardized, widely used, and presumably reliable, their use raised a validity question. These measures, organized in the medical model tradition, may be inadequate for determining the effectiveness of both curricular approaches.

Differences in students' ability were examined across types of curricula. Integrative curricula were hypothesized to increase critical thinking. Pardue (1979) found no difference as measured by the Cornell Critical Thinking Test, Level Z (Ellis & Milliman, Note 1). Using the Watson-Glaser (1964) Critical Thinking Appraisal, Richards (1977) found less critical thinking ability in students in the new integrated curriculum. DeBack (1981) found that among four types of curriculum models (systems, developmental, interaction, and mixed), there were no differences in the students' ability to formulate nursing diagnoses. Bailey, McDonald, and Claus (1971) found no difference in problem-solving abilities as a result of implementing a problem-solving framework. In a comparative study (Richards, 1977) at one school, students in the integrated curriculum possessed a higher degree of leadership and empathetic ability than students in the previous blocked curriculum.

Faculty satisfaction was compared in schools with integrated versus blocked curricula. Pardue (1979) found no differences on the Purdue Teacher Opinionnaire (Bentley & Rempel, Note 2), a 100-item instrument designed to measure 10 satisfaction factors.

Several single case curricular evaluation studies were reported in the literature. Although they have little generalizability, they may elucidate some methodological or conceptual clarification. Two research teams (LaBelle & Egan, 1975; Marriner et al., 1980) advocated the use of the countenance framework for describing and judging educational programs and demonstrated the approach in single case studies. In another study, Brandt, Hastie, and Schumann (1967) examined the fit of specific program objectives with performance of the graduates in the work setting. Melcolm, Venn, and Bausell (1981) studied the relationships between NLN Achievement Test scores, grades, and State Board Examination scores in an integrated curriculum in a single school. They found essentially the same correlational magnitude as reported in the literature for other curricular patterns of organization.

One difficulty with all of the studies in this area was the incomplete and imprecise description of the curricula under study. Some researchers included only a brief description of the organizational structure, while others made little attempt at description. The lack of specification of the independent variables in these studies makes replication impossible and interpretation of the results across studies difficult.

One consistent finding was that students in traditional, blocked curricula scored better on standardized knowledge tests than students in integrated, concept-oriented curricula. However, these tests may not be valid and appropriate measures of professional nursing knowledge. Insufficient research has been done on other outcomes of curricular patterns to evaluate whether curricular pattern has any important consequences.

Examination of Specific Content

Another group of nursing investigations about curricula includes studies concerned with certain content areas. Some studies were designed to describe content that either was or should be included in nursing curricula. Other studies were evaluations of a certain course or component.

Some studies were designed to identify current content emphasis and placement. Motivated by the trend for increased delivery of health services in the community, Holt (1970) asked faculty of 13 BS programs in six New England states about the extent and placement of community content in the curriculum. However, she found that public health concepts were not initiated early in the curriculum and only one program integrated community concepts at every level. Most programs projected future curricular change; about three-fourths expected to have integrated public health content at some unspecified future date.

Two studies were designed to determine the need for curricular content regarding alcoholism and drug abuse. Burkhalter (1975), in a survey of RNs (53% responded) in one hospital, found nurses reported they were better prepared in alcoholism than drug use. From a questionnaire completed by faculty at one school, Gurel (1974) determined the amount of hours of instruction devoted to alcoholism and faculty's support for more content or courses on the subject. These studies have limited value for the scientific basis about curricula.

The identification of core content for master's curricula was the purpose of two studies. Researchers for both efforts (Beare, Daniel, Grover, Gray, Lancaster, & Sloan, 1980; McLane, 1978) sent questionnaires to large national samples. Beare et al. used a content inventory to determine real and ideal core content in NLN-accredited master's programs. McLane asked graduate program directors, deans, directors of nursing, and graduate students about core competencies. In both studies, a core was identified that included research, leadership, interpersonal skills, and knowledge of the discipline.

The increasing percentage of elderly people and the nursing manpower shortage in this specialty prompted some schools to add gerontological content and experiences in the curriculum, with the hope of influencing student attitudes about the elderly and increasing students' likelihood of working with this population. Using the Tuckman-Lorge Attitude (TLA) questionnaire (Tuckman & Lorge, 1953), both Gunter (1971) and Kayser and Minnigerode (1975) examined pre- and posttest scores relative to a particular set of experiences. They found that while stereotypical attitudes were reduced, the gerontological content either made no difference in their willingness to work in these settings, or it decreased an already low preference for this area. In a study of 570 students in 12 BS programs, Tollett and Thornby (1982) found no correlation between amount of gerontology in the curriculum and student attitudes about aging as measured on the TLA.

Harlow and Goby (1980) used a quasi-experimental design to determine if an experience that included working with alcoholics would yield positive changes in knowledge and attitudes among the students. Expected differences were found on all scales. When an experimental course in community health was compared with the traditional course, Warner and Walsh (1968) found no differences in NLN Achievement tests, teacher-made tests, or clinical performance.

Other studies in this area had major methodological weaknesses. Although Garner and Lowe (1965) found differences in students who took a group dynamics course, the instruments were developed and used without psychometric testing and the experimental and control groups were confounded by also having different clinical majors. The differences that occurred were erroneously ascribed to one course. The Woods and Mandetta (1975) pre- and posttest no-control group study of 23 students in one human sexuality course also had limitations. Robbin's (1973) investigation of a group of her own students about their attitude toward evening clinical experience may have been subject to bias; the brief interviews were conducted by the instructor just prior to clinical evaluation conferences.

In summary, the detailed descriptive findings about ideal core curricular content for master's programs provides a beginning empirical basis for graduate nursing educators. The studies of gerontological content are informative in that they challenge a common assumption that more knowledge and exposure will contribute to a greater willingness to work with special populations. Other findings are suggestive of societal and professional trends that may influence curricular offerings, but the process may take a period of time. Many of the studies about specific content contribute little to the knowledge base because they lack internal and external validity.

Comparison of Types of RN Curricula

Registered nurses receive basic education in associate degree, diploma, or baccalaureate degree programs. Considerable debate has occurred about whether there are sufficient differences in the curricula (other than length of program) or outcomes that can be distinguished. As the profession discussed a change to a two-level educational and professional structure, several studies were done to document similarities and differences. These studies are described in the next section.

In the majority of studies, investigators used supervisory ratings to measure nursing performance among graduates from these curricular types. In a study of directors of nursing in Oregon (only 58% responded), Howell (1978) found significant differences in new graduates of different programs. BS graduates were rated highest on thinking skills. Diploma graduates were rated highest on bedside skills, but BS rated higher than AD graduates. Howell also found a rater bias among the 50 directors in the study; diploma-prepared directors rated diploma graduates highest, while baccalaureate- and master's-prepared administrators rated BS graduates superior. All directors rated AD graduates inferior to other graduates. In a study conducted in 31 Veterans Administration hospitals, Dyer, Cope, Monson, and Van Drimmelen (1972) obtained positive relationships between level of education and some professional performance characteristics.

Waters et al. (1972) asked immediate supervisors and directors of nursing to rate practice levels of 24 AD and 24 BS nurses. Although some discrepancies in the data obtained in different ways were noted, AD graduates were seen to be hospital-oriented, mechanical, and routine. BS nurses were viewed as more independent, comprehensive, and supportive. Nelson (1978) also used supervisory ratings to evaluate 329 new graduates from nine schools of nursing in North Dakota. Using a 35-item inventory developed by the investigator, supervisors rated the technical, communicative, and administrative skills of baccalaureate graduates significantly higher than associate or diploma nurses.

Self-reports of performance also were used. Nelson (1978) paralleled her supervisory reports with ratings by the graduates. In overall competence, the diploma graduates rated themselves significantly higher than the other two groups, but baccalaurate graduates rated themselves higher than AD graduates. When each skill group was compared, diploma nurses scored higher in technical and administrative skills and BS nurses scored higher in communication skills. Nurses from the three types of curricula and their respective supervisors differed significantly in perceptions of the graduate's overall competence. Smoyak (1972) also used a self-reported performance method to compare BS and diploma graduates from 13 schools selected to represent various areas of the country. Using an investigator-developed tool, few differences were found in the two groups.

Members of the research team evaluated nursing performance in other comparative investigations. Gray, Murray, Roy, and Sawyer (1977) constructed a paper-and-pencil clinical situation to compare AD and BS students at one school. The rationale for selecting extremes for the sample was unclear. Clear differences were noted between the AD and BS graduates that were consistent with the curricular expectations.

Other investigators compared personal and professional characteristics. Murray and Morris (1982) found in a study of senior students in a diploma, an AD, and a BS program that the BS students scored significantly higher on professional autonomy. Self-actualization as measured by the Personal Orientation Inventory (Shostrom, 1966) was compared by another researcher (Goldstein, 1980). In a study in 10 schools, Goldstein noted that BS students scored significantly higher than AD students on one of the two major scales. However, caution is necessary in interpreting findings from this study, since the response rates in some schools were as low as 14% and 25%. Furthermore, in neither of these studies was it known if the groups differed on these variables prior to entering the programs. In another study, Richards (1972) administered the Cottell and Cottell (1962) intelligence test called the IPAT (Institute for Personality and Ability Testing), a personality inventory, Gordon Personal Profile (1963), and a professionalism scale, to graduates of 13 schools in three western states. No statistical differences among the three types of students were found in intelligence or personality, but BS students had significantly higher scores on some professionalism dimensions.

In studies where investigators compared the professional performance of students or graduates of the three major types of curricula for preparing registered nurses, findings were similar. It is more difficult to distinguish between the baccalaureate and diploma prepared nurses, but they are both clearly superior to the AD nurse. The research evidence concerning possible differences in personal characteristics is too weak to draw any conclusions.

Baccalaureate Curricula for Nontraditional Students

Historically, the various kinds of nursing educational programs (practical, AD, diploma, and BS) developed as independent options without considering an educational career ladder within the nursing occupation. Furthermore, no provisions were made for other nontraditional students to gain lateral access to nursing education. In the last two decades, a movement was launched to facilitate upward mobility among nurses and to recruit nontraditional nursing students. These developments stimulated a number of research questions. Research on baccalaureate curricula for nontraditional students forms the last group of studies in this review.

The NLN Open Curriculum Study Project (Lenburg & Johnson, 1974; Notter & Robey, 1979) deserves special recognition. Spanning the decade of the 1970s, the project personnel conducted a number of studies, national in scope and detailed in nature. Only a few of the findings are presented here. In a 1975 survey, faculty of 1,765 programs reported some type of open curriculum practice (Notter & Robey, 1979). From their analysis of data from a 1972 survey, Lenburg and Johnson (1974) identified four distinctive patterns of open curricula: programs accepting only licensed personnel; advanced placement programs; multiple exit option programs; and external degree programs for which degrees were awarded on the basis of credit by examination without required attendance in the program. The reports contained description of curricula, faculty, students, and policies and practices implemented.

In another descriptive study, Church et al. (1980) attempted to survey all baccalaureate programs especially designed for RNs. A Second Step program was identified in 75 responding schools. All programs were less than 10 years old; 86% had less than five years of experience with students. However, more than 5,000 students had graduated. Only 16% of the programs were accredited by the NLN. The typical curricula in these programs as judged by a document review included courses in community health, leadership, research, problem solving, health care system, professional attitudes, and independent study. Themes and concepts frequently seen by researchers included biopsychosocial, holistic, nursing process, change agents, client advocacy, and health-illness continuum.

In two studies, investigators examined the professional aspect of the preparation of technically oriented registered nurses in open curricular BS programs. Little and Brian (1982) used a pre- and posttest design with no control group to assess the impact of the curriculum on professional orientation. Using a subset of the Second Step data ($n = 236$) from the six accredited programs, they found that students made statistically significant gains on eight of the twelve measures of the Omnibus Personality Inventory (Heist & Yonge, 1968), with the greatest changes in intellectual characteristics. Students also gained significantly in self-assessments of professional interests, competency, and commitment.

A different methodology was used in another study concerning professionalism. In a qualitative and quantitative study of 197 students from one Second Step program, Wilson et al. (1977) used a scheduled battery of questionnaires, standardized tests, and interviews to study changes in attitudes, values, opinions, and personality orientations as they related to nursing and to life in general. Students qualitatively described how the curriculum expanded both their professional and personal lives.

Access to BS nursing education has also been enhanced by implementing articulation plans. This often included a pattern of two years of transfer curriculum at another university and an upper division nursing major. Schoenmaker (1975) addressed the question of whether the articulated students did as well in the upper division nursing components as the regularly matriculated students. No differences in attrition or grade point average were found.

Another nontraditional BS curriculum is the accelerated model which is designed for individuals who hold a bachelor's or higher degree in a major other than nursing. In a comparative study of 77 accelerated graduates and randomly selected basic graduates, Tierney (1979) showed that accelerated students scored higher on all five State Board Examination scores and all but one NLN Achievement Test. On self and supervisory ratings of work performance, no significant differences were noted. The accelerated students also had a different personality profile, suggesting that accelerated students who choose nursing as a second career may be different from those who select nursing at the time of high school graduation.

In summary, research in this area suggests that nursing curricula designed for registered nurses, college graduates, and other nontraditional students were implemented only recently and grew rapidly. Surveys of schools offering these curricula have assisted in elucidating the procedures, policies, and themes. Although the studies were limited in number, some evidence suggested that RN students believed they had a different professional perspective after the baccalaureate program. The comparative studies also were few, but it appeared that graduates who studied in BS curricula designed for nontraditional students were as effective as graduates who were prepared in a generic baccalaureate curricula.

DISCUSSION AND SUGGESTIONS FOR FUTURE RESEARCH

The knowledge generated by curricular research has not been impressive. While it would be wrong to conclude that no substantive gains in knowledge building have been made, the research efforts have been fragmented, imprecise, and often nongeneralizable. This reviewer concurs with Reres (1979) who stated in an editorial:

> Here we are at the end of the 20th century with very little reliable data to indicate the ideal way that nursing education might be brought to the learner. We have little real knowledge of even such pragmatic factors as the safe ratio of clinical instructors to students, let alone evaluation of all the complex variables. (p. 162)

The major impediment to the formulation of a scientific basis about nursing curricula is conceptual. First, the concepts employed appear to be inadequate for describing the structure and processes of the curriculum as well as for describing antecedent factors or expected outcomes. Some empirical descriptive work has been done to elucidate these concepts and their categories; much more work is needed. Systematic mapping of the entire range of independent, dependent, and mediating variables is essential for the cumulation of research findings in a form suitable for theory building. Many of the inconclusive and sometimes contradictory results of past research derived from a lack of concept identification, definition, and operational indicators.

More importantly, there is an absence of an adequate nursing curricular paradigm that facilitates the study of curricula in the context of how it is influenced by or may influence other phenomena. In the studies reviewed, most investigators had no theoretical frame of reference. Others presented a limited theoretical rationale for the relationship between several variables. Only a small minority of investigators appeared concerned with the development of science; most conducted studies to answer specific pragmatic questions.

In an attempt to facilitate some organization for research about nursing curricula, a model was developed. As seen in Figure 10–1, curricula are shaped by the broad historical and social context. These global factors influence the professional status of nursing, current or potential practice roles, available technology, and the scientific basis of the discipline, which in turn influence curricular characteristics. For example, the women's movement and changes in the health care delivery system influence the

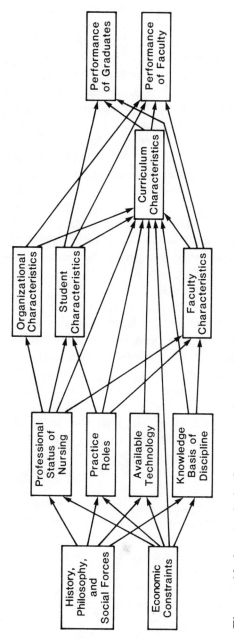

Figure 10–1. Analytic framework for organizing nursing curricular knowledge

257

professional status of nursing and practice roles. Developments in the physical and social sciences potentially influence the scientific basis of the discipline of nursing. Likewise, legislation, computer technology, health needs, population characteristics, and consumer demands are likely to influence directly or indirectly nursing curricula.

Through the model, it is suggested that background factors affect institutional, student, and faculty characteristics. As the professional status of nursing changes, for example, different types of faculty or students might be attracted. Organizational, student, and faculty characteristics are postulated to influence directly the curricula characteristics. Finally as shown in the model, some curriculum characteristics are related to certain graduate and faculty outcomes. The outcomes used to date have been somewhat limited to knowledge, attitude, and performance measures. To the extent other outcomes are important, such as manpower distribution, serving underserved populations could be examined. Moreover, all of the postcurricular outcomes can be affected by a number of variables other than the curricula; for example personal and setting variables must be built into the design as control variables.

This model is presented as a beginning analytic framework for planning and designing curricular research. It makes apparent how few of the possible relationships have been explored. Few influences of philosophical, social, political, or economic forces were documented. Except for Hall (1979), the relationship of the scientific basis of the discipline to the curricula has been neglected by investigators. Few researchers examined how current or potential practice roles might influence the curricula. The relationship of organizational characteristics to the curricula was largely unexplored. A number of investigators examined the relationship between student characteristics and the type of curricula, but the majority of the nondescriptive studies related content or curricula characteristics to various student outcomes.

The research needed will require greater diversity, sophistication, and rigor in research design. More qualitative studies are needed to elucidate concepts and categories. Psychometric testing and validity issues are prerequisite for future research. In order to test relationships, it will be necessary to look at designs other than single case studies, surveys, and comparative designs. Since the curriculum and the system in which it is embedded are complex, multivariate strategies such as structural equation modeling may be useful, as well as data reduction strategies such as factor or cluster analysis. More variables must be controlled statistically in quasi-experimental studies.

A cadre of scholars committed to developing a scientific knowledge base is needed. Based on the large numbers of dissertations written about nursing curricula in the past decade, there are substantial numbers of potential scholars. Exchanges such as those established at the first Research in Nursing Education Conference in 1982 will be invaluable. Another fact of concern is that much of the dissertation work is unpublished. Perhaps the quality was inadequate; maybe editors of major journals lack interest in curricular research, or possibly, in their research training, investigators were not socialized as to the need to publish articles from their dissertation. As scholars begin the endeavor of building a scientific knowledge base, perhaps other publication outlets will develop.

A number of investigators have made an effort to examine empirically the design and effects of nursing curricula. The research completed has suffered from methodological weaknesses and has lacked guidance by substantive theoretical perspectives. Thus, the existing data are highly descriptive, often particular to only one or several schools, and they lack coherence for contributing to a theoretical research paradigm that sharpens important issues and future research needs. A beginning conceptual model and directions for future research were suggested.

REFERENCE NOTES

1. Ennis, R., & Millman, J. *Manual for Cornell Critical Thinking Test*. Urbana, Ill.: University of Illinois, 1971.
2. Bentley, R. R., & Rempel, A. M. *Manual for Purdue Teacher Opinionnaire*. West Lafayette, Ind.: Purdue University Bookstore, 1970.

REFERENCES

Abdellah, F. G. Overview of nursing research, 1955–1968, Part III. *Nursing Research*, 1970, *19*, 239–252.

Bailey, J. T., McDonald, F. J., & Claus, K. E. *Experimental curriculum evaluation project*. Belmont, N.Y.: Wadsworth Publishing, 1971.

Beare, P. G., Daniel, E. D., Gover, V. F., Gray, C. J., Lancaster, J., & Sloan, P. E. The real vs. ideal content in master's curricula in nursing. *Nursing Outlook*, 1980, *28*, 691–694.

Brandt, E. M., Hastie, B., & Schumann, D. Comparison of on-the-job perfor-

260   RESEARCH ON NURSING EDUCATION

mance of graduates with school of nursing objectives. *Nursing Research*, 1967, *16*, 50–57.

Burkhalter, P. Alcoholism, drug abuse and drug addiction: A study of nursing education. *Journal of Nursing Education*, 1975, *14*(2), 30–36.

Cattell, R. B. & Cattell, A. K. S. *IPAT Test of "g" test manual*. Champaign, Ill.: Institute for Personality and Ability Testing, 1962.

Church, E. F., Brian, S., & Searight, M. W. Describing a new baccalaureate nursing population: The second step. *Western Journal of Nursing Research*, 1980, *2*, 574–592.

Clarke, M. Research in nurse education. *Nursing Times*, 1977, *73*, 25–28.

DeBack, V. The relationship between senior nursing students' ability to formulate nursing diagnoses and the curriculum model. *Advances in Nursing Science*, 1981, *33*, 51–66.

de Tornyay, R. Nursing research: The road ahead. *Nursing Research*, 1977, *26*, 404–407.

Dyer, E. D., Cope, M. J., Monson, M. A., & Van Drimmelen, J. B. Can job performance be predicted from biographical personality, and administrative climate inventories? *Nursing Research*, 1972, *21*, 294–304.

Garner, G. S., & Lowe, A. Group dynamics in graduate education of nurses. *Nursing Research*, 1965, *14*, 146–150.

Goldstein, J. O. Comparison of graduating AD and baccalaureate nursing students' characteristics. *Nursing Research*, 1980, *29*, 46–49.

Gordon, L. V. *Gordon Personal Profile Test manual*. New York: Harcourt, Brace & World, 1963.

Gortner, S. R. Nursing science in transition. *Nursing Research*, 1980, *29*, 180–183.

Gortner, S. R., & Nahm, H. An overview of nursing research in the United States. *Nursing Research*, 1977, *26*, 10–33.

Gray, J. E., Murray, B. L. S., Roy, J. F., & Sawyer, J. R. Do graduates of technical and professional nursing programs differ in practice? *Nursing Research*, 1977, *26*, 368–373.

Gunter, L. M. Students' attitudes toward geriatric nursing. *Nursing Outlook*, 1971, *19*, 466–469.

Gurel, M. Should courses for nurses that deal solely with alcoholism be taught at universities? A preliminary report. *Nursing Research*, 1974, *23*, 166–169.

Hall, K. V. Current trends in the use of conceptual frameworks in nursing education. *Journal of Nursing Education*, 1979, *18*(4), 26–29.

Harlow, P. E., & Goby, M. J. Changing nursing students' attitudes toward alcoholic patients: Examining effects of a clinical practicum. *Nursing Research*, 1980, *29*, 59–60.

Heist, P., & Yonge, G. *The manual for the Omnibus Personality Inventory*. New York: Psychological Corporation, 1968.

Hill, M. S., Gortner, S. R., & Scott, J. M. Educational research in nursing: An overview. *International Nursing Review*, 1980, *27*, 10–17.

Holt, F. A. Public health nursing concepts in the basic curriculum. *Journal of Nursing Education*, 1970, *9*(1), 15–21.

Howell, F. J. Employers' evaluations of new graduates. *Nursing Outlook*, 1978, *26*, 448–451.

Kayser, J. S., & Minnigerode, F. A. Increasing nursing students' interest in working with aged patients. *Nursing Research*, 1975, *24*, 23–26.

Koehler, M. L. Evaluating a curriculum. *Journal of Nursing Education*, 1982, *21*(1), 32–39.

LaBelle, B. M., & Egan, E. C. Follow-up studies in nursing: A case for determining whether program objectives are achieved. *Journal of Nursing Education*, 1975, *14*(3), 7–13.

Lenburg, C., & Johnson, W. Career mobility through nursing education: A report on NLN's open curriculum. *Nursing Outlook*, 1974, *22*, 265–269.

Little, M., & Brian, S. The challengers, interactors and mainstreamers: Second step education and nursing goals. *Nursing Research*, 1982, *31*, 239–245.

Marriner, A., Langford, T., & Goodwin, L. D. Curriculum evaluation: Wordfact, ritual, or reality. *Nursing Outlook*, 1980, *28*, 228–232.

McLane, A. M. Core competencies of masters-prepared nurses. *Nursing Research*, 1978, *27*, 48–53.

Melcolm, N., Venn, R., & Bausell, R. B. The prediction of state board test pool examinations scores within an integrated curriculum. *Journal of Nursing Education*, 1981, *20*(5), 24–28.

Murray, L. M., & Morris, D. R. Professional autonomy among senior nursing students in diploma, associate degree and baccalaureate nursing programs. *Nursing Research*, 1982, *31*, 311–313.

Nelson, L. F. Competence of nursing graduates—technical, communicative, and administrative skills. *Nursing Research*, 1978, *27*, 121–125.

Notter, L. E., & Robey, M. *The open curriculum in nursing education: Final report of the NLN open curriculum study*. (NLN Publication No. 19–1799). New York: National League for Nursing, 1979.

Pardue, S. F. Blocked- and integrated-content baccalaureate nursing programs: A comparative study. *Nursing Research*, 1979, *28*, 305–311.

Quiring, J., & Gray, G. Organizing approaches used in curriculum design. *Journal of Nursing Education*, 1982, *21*(2), 38–44.

Reres, M. E. Educational research, but never on the curriculum. *Western Journal of Nursing Research*, 1979, *1*, 161–162.

Richards, M. A. A study of differences in psychological characteristics of students graduating from three types of nursing programs. *Nursing Research*, 1972, *21*, 258–261.

Richards, M. A. One integrated curriculum: An empirical evaluation. *Nursing Research*, 1977, *26*, 90–95.

Robbins, J. Students' attitudes toward evening experience. *Nursing Outlook*, 1973, *21*, 169–170.

Santora, D. *Conceptual frameworks used in baccalaureate and master's degree curricula* (NLN Publication No. 15–1828). New York: National League for Nursing, 1980.

Schoen, D. C. Comparing the body-systems and conceptual approaches to nursing education. *Nursing Research*, 1975, *24*, 383–387.

Schoenmaker, A. An articulated nursing program: Five years later. *Nursing Outlook*, 1975, *23*, 110–113.

Shostrom, E. L. *Personal Orientation Inventory*. San Diego: Education and Industrial Testing Service, 1966.

Smoyak, S. A. A panel study comparing self reports of baccalaureate and diploma nurses before graduation and after their first work experience in hospitals. In E. Jacobi, & L. E. Notter. *American Nurses' Association Eighth Nursing Research Conference.* Washington, D.C.: United States Department of Health Education and Welfare, 1972.

Stevens, B. J. Analysis of structural forms used in nursing curricula. *Nursing Research,* 1971, *20,* 388–397.

Stone, J. C., & Green J. L. The impact of a professional baccalaureate degree program. *Nursing Research,* 1975, *24,* 287–292.

Tierney, C. C. An accelerated baccalaureate curriculum in nursing. In *Innovative approaches to baccalaureate programs in nursing.* (NLN Publication No. 15–1804). New York: National League for Nursing, 1979.

Tollett, S. M., & Thornby, J. I. Geriatric and gerontology nursing curricular trends. *Journal of Nursing Education,* 1982, *21*(6), 16–23.

Torres, G., & Yura, H. *Today's conceptual framework: Its relationship to the curriculum development process* (NLN Publication No. 15–1529). New York: National League for Nursing, 1974.

Tuckman, J., & Lorge, I. Attitudes toward old people. *Journal of Social Psychology,* 1953, *37,* 249–260.

Warner, B. A., & Walsh, J. E. A comparative study of two undergraduate courses in community nursing. *Nursing Research,* 1968, *17,* 71–74.

Waters, V. H., Chater, S. S., Vivier, M. L., Urrea, J. H., & Wilson, H. S. Technical and professional nursing: An exploratory study. *Nursing Research,* 1972, *21,* 124–131.

Watson, G., & Glaser, E. *Watson-Glaser Critical Thinking Manual.* New York: Harcourt, Brace, Jovanovich, 1964.

Wilson, H. S., Vaughan, H. C., & Gaff, J. G. The second step model of baccalaureate education for registered nurses: The student's perspective. *Journal of Nursing Education,* 1977, *16*(6), 27–35.

Woods, N. F., & Mandetta, A. Changes in students' knowledge and attitudes following a course in human sexuality. *Nursing Research,* 1975, *24,* 10–15.

Wu, R. R. Designing a curriculum model. *Journal of Nursing Education,* 1979, *18*(3), 13–21.

PART IV

Research on the Profession of Nursing

CHAPTER 11

Information Processing in Nursing Practice

MARGARET R. GRIER
COLLEGE OF NURSING
UNIVERSITY OF ILLINOIS AT CHICAGO

CONTENTS

In information science, the concern is knowledge about the collection, classification, storage, retrieval, and dissemination of data for deriving information. Inquiry in this area thus is focused on the measurement of data in terms of information content, distinguishing characteristics, alternative choices, and efficiency of processing, particularly between human beings and machines. The purpose of this review was to synthesize knowledge about the processing of information to make patient care decisions. The research findings from 1900 to 1982 accumulated about this topic were organized and summarized, generalizations were derived, and hypotheses or questions for future research formulated. The following definitions were used as a framework for the study:

1. Collection of nursing data—Identifying and acquiring the patient information needed for nursing practice.
2. Organization of nursing data—Structuring and classifying nursing data for use and/or storage.
3. Use of nursing data—Evaluating information for making patient care decisions.
4. Storage of nursing data—Recording information cognitively, manually, or by machine, for use in nursing practice.

265

The population for study was the research reports and theoretical papers on nursing information published through 1982. The works were identified by colleagues, by tracking citations from one study to another, by searching literature indexes and computer listings, and by systematically reviewing nursing journals. The most productive keywords for the computerized searches were *nursing informatics* on the Health Planning and Administration File and *nursing process* on Medline of Medlars II. Other keywords used were *information systems, automated data processing, computers,* and *nurses* on Medical Subject Headings. In addition, the following journal volumes were searched systematically: *Advances in Nursing Science,* Volumes 1 to 4, *Image,* Volumes 1 to 15, *Journal of Advanced Nursing,* Volumes 1 to 7, *Journal of Nursing Education,* Volumes 1 to 21, *Nursing Outlook,* Volumes 1 to 30, *Nursing Research,* Volumes 1 to 31, *Public Health Nursing,* Volumes 1 to 42, *Research in Nursing and Health,* Volumes 1 to 6, and *Western Journal of Nursing Research,* Volumes 1 to 4. From this population, about 250 papers and 6 books were selected for review according to the definitions presented. Topics excluded were information used by patients and for administrative or educational purposes. Although part of the science of nursing information, work on nursing diagnoses also was not included in this review, since that topic is planned for Volume 3 of the *Annual Review of Nursing Research.*

The main interest was reports of descriptive, quasi-experimental, and experimental research, as well as theoretical papers in which hypotheses were presented and/or discussed. To make this selection, the papers reviewed were classified as to theory, research, empirical study, summary of research, documented article, general information, and opinion or editorial (Basson, 1967). The analysis consisted of assessing the selection, number, and description of the subjects for study; describing the measures, their reliability, and analysis; judging the controls for potential threats to the validity of the results; and listing the findings and conclusions.

RESULTS FROM THE SEARCHES

Research findings on the collection, organization, use, and storage of nursing data are summarized in this section. Although these artificial divisions are made for this report, in practice, the steps are interrelated; many findings reported under one area are relevant to another. After the summary of findings, the knowledge gained and methodologies used are discussed, possible generalizations presented, and future research suggested. Unless otherwise noted, the findings presented were judged reasonably valid within the limitations of the reported study.

Collection of Nursing Data

Research on the collection of nursing data can be organized under three headings: (a) identifying patient characteristics about which information is needed, (b) organizing the collection of data, and (c) acquiring the data by observation and measurement. The research reports on the first and third topics, identifying and acquiring data, are summarized below; works related to organizing data are presented in the next part since that process also applies to using and storing data. It should be noted, however, that organization of data is a necessary part of identifying and acquiring data.

Identifying data. Hammond, Kelly, Schneider, and Vancini (1966a) found that textbooks did not agree on patient cues of secondary shock nor describe patient cues for pain, but noted that an exception to this finding was a textbook published by Beland (1965). Grier and Grier (1978) also reported that textbooks lacked information for making decisions about pain medications, and went on to describe the resulting adverse consequences.

When the necessary data for their study were not found in textbooks, Hammond and his colleagues (1966a) surveyed nurses across the United States about cognitive tasks of patients with abdominal pain after abdominal surgery. Within the 212 cognitive tasks reported, 165 cues of patient pain and 17 types of nursing actions for the pain were identified. But the cues conveyed only minimal information (Hammond, Kelly, Castellan, Schneider, & Vancini, 1966) and were not associated with four groupings of the nursing actions (Hammond et al., 1966a); a list of the 165 pain cues was not published. Broderick and Ammentorp (1979) described 12 categories of 59 data items about unspecified patient pain (available from the author), but found that additional data also were requested by nurses in choosing an action for the pain. In their report, Hammond et al. (1966a) concluded that the cognitive tasks in nursing are complex in regard to the number and dependability of patient cues, a conclusion supported by others. Bailey, McDonald, and Claus (1973) thought nursing students used too much data. Cianfrani (1982) described adverse effects from increasing amounts of irrelevant data. Gordon (1973, 1980) found greater diagnostic accuracy and tolerance of risk with restricted amounts of data. Abdellah (1957), Broderick and Ammentorp (1979), and Wilcox (1961) spoke to the need to identify relationships between items of patient data. Broderick and Ammentorp (1979) thought that the way nurses emphasized and sampled certain data items showed that relationships between the elements were being sought.

One way of identifying the data to collect is by using preinformation about a patient (i.e., admission note) to predict possible diagnoses, and then selecting data to test those hypotheses (Hammond, 1966). Gordon (1980) found that 60 nurses requested less contextual information (i.e., time and type of surgery) to predict a diagnosis with amounts of data restricted than with amounts of data unrestricted. Accurate nurses ceased testing contextual data in the first half of the diagnostic process, while inaccurate nurses continued to use the strategy in the second half of the task. Gordon concluded that contextual data may help limit the hypotheses for specific and direct testing late in the diagnostic process. Kraus (1976) reported preinformation about patient-directed nurse observations of a filmed patient, but gave no evidence to support this finding. In fact, the lack of interaction between the preinformation conditions and the importance assigned to data found in the study could indicate the opposite. Lagina (1971) also gave no evidence to support her statement that nurses relied on knowledge of the diagnosis in determining anxiety. These studies indicate that preinformation or contextual information may help confirm patient observations (or vice versa), but the extent to which these types of data are useful for forming hypotheses and/or guiding data collection remains an intriguing question. Cianfrani's (1982) findings indicated that if the correct nursing diagnosis was among those hypothesized, the correct final diagnosis was highly likely. Methods to help nurses hypothesize patient problems could be more beneficial than approaches for arriving at a final diagnosis. This is particularly true given the potential for computerized aids to make the final diagnosis, a technology that will increase the importance of hypothesizing diagnoses.

Gordon (1973) and Hammond et al. (1966a) investigated nurses' strategies in selecting patient data to accept or reject hypotheses about patient states. Gordon (1973) found the simultaneous testing of multiple hypotheses by 60 nurses decreased across the diagnostic process while sequential testing of single hypotheses increased. Counter to theoretic expectations, this same mixed strategy was used when information was restricted for one health problem and unrestricted for another health problem. In the first half of the process the nurses seemed to want as much information as possible while eliminating hypotheses as rapidly as possible. Of five nurses studied, Hammond et al. (1966a) found that three tended to use sequential scanning of data and two simultaneous scanning, but the majority of strategies were undefined. Of particular note for future re-searchers was the variance of 0 to 1.00 among the five nurses in using strategies to select data. Thus, the strategies nurses use to select patient data appear complex and variable.

Acquiring data. Acquiring patient data is the hallmark of a profession-al nurse (Abdellah, 1957; Nightingale, 1894/1907; Verhonick, 1961). Supporting this, Wolfe (1965) concluded that two nurses were more skilled observers of patient care than two nonnurse observers. Of the 236 blind judgments of the recordings rendered by a 19-member panel, 179 were that the nurses' recordings contained *more* information. From a national study of 1,965 nurses, Verhonick, Nichols, Glor, and McCarthy (1968) reported that skills in observing patient data increased with educational level; rel-evant observations increased and supportive nursing actions were more related to the observations. Takacs and Valenti (1982) determined that measuring temperature with a glass thermometer was a function of other activities, but this was not found with electronic thermometers. Other studies, however, revealed that nurses were imprecise in measuring and estimating patient characteristics (Choi, Boxerman, & Steinburg, 1978; Gunn, Sullivan, & Glor, 1966; Higgins, 1982; Wilcox, 1961).

Wilcox (1961) found that 10% to 20% of 349 nurses measured blood pressures incorrectly. Variances in the measures were random and related to the diastolic and hypertensive pressures; differences between the nurses who made and did not make the erroneous measures could not be identified. Findings of Choi et al. (1978) supported those of Wilcox; they found that in recording systolic and diastolic pressures, respectively, nursing students had more of the terminal digits as 0 (28% and 33%), and fewer as 6 (16% and 13%) than the 20% expected ($SD = 6.0$ to 9.9). The percentage of the 0 to 9 terminal digits for weights also differed from the 10% expected. About 40 of the 120 nursing students did not differ from the expected in their recordings; 50% of the terminal digits were recorded as 0 by only 5% of the students. The investigators stated that rounding error was even greater for three cardiologists than for the student nurses, but these data were not reported. Gunn et al. (1966) found that differences in blood pressure readings were due to the measurement procedures used, rather than the two nurse observers. These latter investigators noted that no information is preferable to wrong information, and questioned the clinical costs relative to the benefits of standardized and controlled procedures for measuring blood pressure.

Higgins (1982) measured nurses' accuracy in estimating amounts of blood on peripads. Although the estimates were consistent, 71% were overestimations and 25% underestimations. As could be predicted, the greatest variance was in estimating very large and small amounts. While finding problems with the extremes of measurement scales is not surprising, they are of concern since theoretically the extreme values are more critical in patient care. However, no studies of the clinical significance of these findings in terms of quality or cost of health care were found.

Despite evidence of the complexity and difficulties of data collection in nursing practice, and the assumption that improved data collection would improve care, investigations of methods to aid in acquiring nursing data were few. Bonney and Rothberg (1963) evaluated a quantitative tool for obtaining patient data and making nursing diagnoses; Fedder (1956) developed a method to base care plans on scientific principles; McCain (1965a, 1965b) proposed a tool for systematic assessment of patient functioning; Simon (1961) and Simon and Chastain (1960) presented scales for rating patient welfare; and Taylor and Johnson (1974) developed computer forms for collecting nursing data. Verhonick (1961) reported efforts to develop objective measures of decubitus ulcers.

In most instances, evaluation of methods to acquire patient data were limited, and few of the tools were widely used. In addition to the complexity of nursing data, the lack of scientific knowledge about nursing information and of conceptual frameworks for nursing practice are major factors in not developing ways to aid in identifying, organizing, and acquiring patient data. Systematic methods for identifying and acquiring data help structure the data collected. Efforts to organize data for collection, use, and storage are presented below.

Organization of Nursing Data

As noted earlier, organization is necessary if data are to be collected, used, and stored efficiently and effectively. The review revealed conceptual frameworks specifically for nursing information, but little evidence about how exhaustive, exclusive, and independent the schemes are. These theoretical works are included in this review because of their importance in developing a science of nursing information and their potential for helping with information processing in nursing.

Over time much attention has been given to methods for organizing the collection, use, and storage of nursing data (e.g., Bonney & Rothberg, 1963; Committee on Records, 1925, 1933; Fedder, 1956; Harmer & Henderson, 1939, 1955; McCain, 1965a, 1965b; National League for Nursing, 1974; Orlando, 1961; Taylor & Johnson, 1974; Wald & Leonard, 1964; Werley & Grier, 1981; Yura & Walsh, 1973). The best known and most widely used scheme is the nursing process. According to Henderson (1982), this analytical procedure evolved (Harmer & Henderson, 1939, 1955) from a unit on planning patient care included within the curriculum proposed by the National League of Nursing Education (1937). From a comparison of two types of patient records, Sullivan (1981) found that the process components of assessment, problem, and action were described more frequently than those of goal, evaluation, and data reprocessing. Grier (1981) questioned the analytical properties of the nursing process and expanded it to include cognitive steps for clinical decision making. She and others reported research using such a framework (Bailey, McDonald, & Claus, 1973; Broderick, & Ammentorp, 1979; Cianfrani, 1982; Corcoran, 1983; Grier, 1976; Grier & Grier, 1978; Grier, Howard, & Cohen, 1979; Grier & Schnitzler, 1979). Related frameworks are those of Finch (1969), Kelly (1964, 1966), Hammond (1964, 1966), and Hansen and Thomas (1968).

Howland and McDowell (1964) presented a framework that included concepts of decision making, as well as concepts of cybernetics and homeostasis. In their schema the nurse-patient-physician triad regulated patient homeostasis by monitoring, comparing, and regulating information; data about desired and actual patient states were most important, and members of the triad had to be prepared as information processors. Chow (1969) based her study of nursing actions on this framework. Fox (1964) proposed a method by which the transmission of information between the monitor, comparator, and regulator could be studied. He said the important measures were: rationale for selecting data, information content of data, agreement between senders and receivers, and efficacy of processing information.

The characteristics of unitary man were set forth as a theoretical framework for nursing diagnoses (Kim & Moritz, 1981). Included were awareness (waking, feeling, knowing), interaction (exchanging, communicating, relating); and acting (valuing, choosing, moving). Another framework proposed for nursing diagnoses (Kim & Moritz, 1981) was that of Orem (1971). Orem's theory was used to organize nursing data on outcomes of care (Horn & Swain, 1977), and study of the quality of care using decision making and outcome criteria (Padilla & Grant, 1982).

Efforts to computerize nursing data have led to the development of other frameworks. Neal (1981) described a system for retrieving nursing information organized around the concepts of motion, sensation, cognition, affiliation, and patient expressions and indicators of these concepts and nursing actions. Simmons (1980) described an information system for community nursing that included four domains: environmental, psychosocial, physiological, and health behaviors; nursing diagnoses and desired outcomes were included within each domain. Cook and Mayers (1981) and Romano, McCormick, and McNeely (1982) described computerized information systems within clinical settings.

Frameworks that conceptualize nursing practice are necessary for efficient and effective processing of information. Conceptualization is necessary for efficient data collection in complex settings, and for efficient processing of related data sets. Conceptualization also is necessary for structuring meaningful, and thus useful, systems for gathering and storing data. While frameworks for nursing information have been proposed, only the nursing process has been tested or widely used.

Use of Nursing Data

The use of nursing data requires the evaluation of obtained information for use in making choices among alternatives. In nursing practice the major decisions are judgment about a patient problem (a diagnosis) and selection of a nursing action (a decision) for the selected diagnosis. Thus, the research on using patient data is organized under the diagnostic process, the decision process, and the influences on these two processes.

Diagnostic process. The rationale for Abdellah's (1957) study of overt and covert nursing problems was that correctly diagnosing patient problems influences subsequent decisions about nursing actions. Abdellah found that nurses and physicians identified a similar number of problems, but nurses determined more emotional problems and physicians more physical problems. McLaughlin, Cesa, Johnson, Lemons, Anderson, Larson, and Gibson (1979) found that nurse practitioners used a psychosocial model to manage care more so than family practice physicians, but the two groups were similar in the use of a pathophysiological model. Others (Hefferin & Hunter, 1975; Suhayda & Kim, in press) found that nurses documented and acted on more physiological problems. Kraus (1976) found that nurses placed more importance on, and were less certain about, disease data than emotional or neutral data. Cianfrani (1982) found differences between diagnosing three patient problems, but the differences were greater between the psychosocial problem of pain and the two physiological problems. Lagina (1971) found that nurses referred more frequently to subjective than objective data in diagnosing anxiety. Rausch and Rund (1981) found that nurses relied more on subjective data in judging urgency of illnesses, and more on objective data in judging urgency of injuries.

In testing a diagnostic aid, Aspinall (1979) found that a decision tree helped nurses with less education and experience, as well as those with more than 10 years of clinical experience. The controversial nature of the decisions Aspinall studied should not detract from the finding that the decision aid helped in making those choices.

Hammond, Kelly, Schneider, and Vancini (1967) compared revisions of nursing judgments with those of a normative model (Bayes theorem) when new information was presented. Taking into account the nurses' restricted use of the probability range, the investigators found that the nurses revised their probabilities consistently and logically, but only one-third as much as proposed in the model. In the study, the nurses did not use the entire range of possible probability estimates; their certainty as to the presence and absence of a patient state rarely exceeded 85% and 15%, respectively. These findings were further evidence of nurses' uncertainty about data. Nurses were rarely either 75% certain or 25% uncertain about the meaning of data on a patient characteristic; their probabilities were about 50% (i.e., a diagnosis may or may not be present).

Contained in this report (Hammond et al., 1967) was an excellent description of Bayes theorem and the application of this model to nursing problems. The investigators discussed the either-or type of judgment used in their study, the atypical presentation and use of nursing data, and the fit of the model to cognitive nursing tasks. The model worked best with clearly defined alternative judgments and assumption of independence of data items. In contrast, nursing diagnoses usually involved many diffuse alternatives based on highly related patient cues.

The cognitive task of arriving at a nursing diagnosis frequently has been viewed as one of concept attainment, requiring skills in critical thinking (e.g., Gordon, 1973; Hammond, 1966). For small samples of undergraduate and graduate nursing students, Matthews and Gaul (1979) reported correlations showing that concept mastery was related to perception of patient cues for undergraduate students, but not graduate students; no relationship between critical thinking and the diagnosing of a nursing problem was found. Grier and Schnitzler (1979) found that nurses with master's degrees won appreciably more money than associate degree nurses collecting data for number judgments ($.40 versus $.18), but not for nursing judgments ($.34 versus $.31). Perhaps education leads to cognitive skills that help the nurse reduce uncertainty, but does not help reduce the uncertainty associated with nursing data per se.

Decision process. Nurses favored physiological nursing actions as opposed to those of a psychosocial nature (Suhayda & Kim, in press). From 100 randomly selected abdominal surgery cases described by field nurses, Bailey (1967) identified five discrete and valid domains of action taken by nurses for reducing patients' pain. The clearest pattern of action was to comfort and evaluate the patient, and give medication. The single nursing action not included among the domains was psychological support which correlated negatively ($r = -.32$) only with the domain of notifying the physician and avoiding inquiry about the patient. This indicated that nurses supported the patient psychologically when not involving the physician. It is interesting given the other findings that nurses are skilled in psychosocial care, but place greater emphasis on physiological data and actions.

From a review of public health records, Walker and Deuble (1968) found that about 33% of 1,525 home visits involved accident prevention. Subsequent record analysis revealed that nurses helped patients identify dangerous consequences and carry out activities to avoid them; the main goal was maintaining the patient's safety. This goal required adherence to a safe margin without widening that margin by fear. The nurses had to estimate the risk of an accident and act to reduce that risk to attain the goal. Based on these findings, the investigators recommended studies of the criteria nurses use to estimate risk. Avoidance of risk to patients appeared to be a major nursing goal (Grier & Grier, 1978), but attention has not been given to the accompanying risk assessment and trade-offs. "Potential problem" was the judgment leading to this goal, and triage and monitoring activities were initiated to protect the patient from risk (Moreland & Grier, in press).

In their continuing study, Hammond, Kelly, Schneider, & Vancini (1966b) found that nurses differed widely in choosing 16 actions; one nurse chose one of the actions for only one case, while another nurse chose that same action for 33 cases. The hypothesis of a high degree of confidence in decisions for cases where there was a large number of useful patient cues was not confirmed, $r = .01$ to $.20$. The six nurses tended to indicate all cues as very useful, and varied little in their moderate certainty about choices of nursing action. In other words, the nurses did not discriminate among the data presented and lacked confidence in their decisions. Even given the limitations of the study (N of 100 for a 16 by 2 contingency table), the investigators concluded that if the information necessary for decision making existed, these nurses did not know it, did not agree to it, or did not use it consistently. As noted by Broderick and Ammentorp (1979), discrimination between patient states so as to choose appropriate nursing actions depends on identifying relationships between data elements.

Corcoran (1983) described how nurses evaluated alternative nursing actions as they occurred and failed to evaluate all the options generated. In other words, they did not identify a set of options for evaluation, comparison, and choice. Nurses who developed consistent and appropriate plans used an opportunistic approach (jumped from one problem to another) in more complex cases, but were more systematic in less complex cases. The successful nurses may have been trying to use simultaneous evaluation of multiple actions to reduce cognitive strain in the complex situations and sequential hypotheses testing for the less complex cases (Gordon, 1973; Hammond, 1966). Overall these findings indicated that nurses did not use efficient and systematic strategies for choosing actions, that inappropriate choices of action could result, and that even the strategies used by skilled nurse decision makers broke down in complex situations.

Grier (1976), Grier and Grier (1978), and Grier et al. (1979) studied a decision aid in choosing nursing actions. They found that the aid led to choices of action more in keeping with goals of the nurses studied, that nurses performed well in estimating occurrences of events, and that the aid was useful for identifying, describing, and analyzing the critical parameters of a decision. Where the aid probably was most beneficial was in structuring and systematizing the decision-making process.

Influences. Hansen and Thomas (1968) defined five sets of interacting variables for their study of decisions by public health nurses (see also Grier, 1976). Those variable sets were situational, contextual, decision maker, associated strategies, and decisions. A number of studies demonstrated these influences on nursing decisions. In studies of decision maker variables, Crisham (1981) and Ketefian (1981a, 1981b) found that the higher the level of education and critical thinking, the more advanced was moral reasoning; no relationship between clinical experience and moral judgments was found. Grier et al. (1979) and Mickey (1958) reported differences between hospital nurses in choosing analgesic medication and public health nurses in choosing family visits, respectively, that could have been due to different beliefs and value systems.

Grier and Schnitzler (1979) found greater willingness to accept risk, and better risk-taking strategies with increasing levels of education— diploma, associate (AD), baccalaureate (BS), and master's (MS) degrees. Differences between the groups were shown most clearly in the nursing skills game. The MS and BS degree nurses bet an average of $.48 on their resuscitation skills and AD and Diploma nurses $.24; MS and BS nurses predicted they would achieve the desired pressure 62% of the time, and AD and Diploma nurses prediced success 47% of the time; MS and BS nurses sought winnings of $2.50, while AD and Diploma nurses sought winnings of $.86. The above differences occurred despite the fact that the groups reported similar experience with resuscitation and achieved the desired level of pressure at almost the same rate (68%). Thus, with increasing levels of education the nurses took greater risk on their skill, sought higher gains, and were more accurate in predicting the outcome of their action.

Broderick and Ammentorp (1979) found that experienced nurses and nursing students categorized pain data in a similar fashion, and used those data in a similar order, but the experienced nurses requested more data and a wider range of data than the student nurses. In her comparison of expert and novice nurses, Corcoran (1983) found that experts recognized more patient problems, had more knowledge of alternative actions, developed more consistent plans of care, failed to address all the problems identified, and did not combine information. Novices, on the other hand, did not recognize as many problems, were slightly more consistent in addressing the identified problems, lacked the necessary knowledge, oversimplified the planning problem, and failed to combine information. These findings seemed to support those of others that the processing of nursing information improves with education (Crisham, 1981; Ketefian, 1981a, 1981b; Verhonick et al., 1968). The findings of Sparks (1979) provided insight as to why differences between nurses according to educational level may not always be revealed. She found no difference between 188 bacculaureate and 128 associate degree students on a simulated patient management problem, but did find differences between the two groups on an inventory of care planning. When process was examined, as opposed to decisions, differences were revealed (Corcoran, 1983). For the simulated patient management problems, investigators frequently used proficiency and efficiency scores that masked how information was obtained and used for making decisions (Dincher & Stidger, 1976).

Cianfrani (1982) studied the situational variables of amounts and relevance of data. While there were differences across the three nursing problems studied, increasing amounts of irrelevant data influenced adversely the diagnostic process, irrelevance more so than amounts. Cianfrani concluded that the identification of the critical data for making nursing judgments would aid the diagnostic process in two ways, specify relevant data and reduce the amounts of data that had to be processed.

Bailey (1967) studied the context for making decisions by comparing the actions chosen by nurses in clinical practice with those chosen by nurses in the experimental situation. The similarity in choices between three experimental nurses was considerably higher than that for the 100 field nurses. This indicated that the paper and pencil method of choosing actions elicited responses unlike those of a nurse in clinical practice. Thomas and Hansen (1969) studied the decisions of public health nurses, while Gordon (1973, 1980) and Hammond and colleagues (1966a, 1966b) studied strategies nurses use to make decisions.

Storage of Nursing Data

There are many articles of opinion and "how to" on record keeping, but few research reports. Other than the mind of a nurse, there are two major ways for storing nursing data, in a written record or in a computer. In this section, studies on the use of the written record and computer are presented; material on cognitive processes is presented in the parts of this chapter on collecting and using data.

Written record. From an audit of 500 patient records, Phaneuf (1968) found that the overall documentation was excellent in 24%, good in 36%, incomplete in 27%, and poor in 13%. In these records, documentation on executing physician orders was excellent (92%), on managing care was moderately good (64% to 67%), and on implementing nursing procedures and promoting health was poor (33% to 58%).

Records of nursing care were found lacking in several studies (Chow, 1969; Cline, 1959; Damrosch & Soeken, 1983; Derryberry, 1939a, 1939b; Suhayda & Kim, in press; Sullivan, 1981). Damrosch & Soeken reported variation and inconsistency in the verbal expressions of nurses. For example the *SD* for the term "certain" = 8.47, for "always" = 14.64, for "normally" = 29.38, and for "never" = 28.17. As noted by the authors, numbers did not resolve uncertainty, but clearly expressed uncertainty. Roose (1963) found different interpretations of the physician order for bedrest among nurses and between nurses and physicians. Cline (1959) identified a mean of 3.76 spelling errors in 24-hour reports; 45% of these spelling errors were lay terms and 55% professional terms. There is no reason to believe that spelling in recording clinical data has improved since 1959.

Sullivan (1981) compared 100 source-oriented (traditional, narrative type) and 100 problem-oriented records on the presence and absence of components of the nursing process. The source-oriented records contained 40% of the possible components and the problem-oriented records 32%; the proportion of completed chains was greater in the source-oriented record (7.1%) than in the problem-oriented record (1.5%). The components of assessment, patient problems, and nursing actions were described more than goals, evaluation, and reprocessing data, regardless of record type. Chow (1969) found that nurses did not record all their observations. One nurse measured blood pressure 41 times and recorded it 23 times; three nurses measured and regulated intravenous flow 43 times, but only recorded this activity periodically. On the other hand, more written recordings of respirations were made than the nurses were discerned measuring on the videotape. Suhayda and Kim (in press) also found unsystematic and inconsistent documentation in their study of critical care records, and suggested a different format than narrative for recording the basis for nursing judgments and decisions.

Walker and Selmanoff (1964) studied nurses' notes as a ritualistic activity. They found that the average time spent writing nurses' notes on the day shift was 18 and 32 minutes at a university and private hospital respectively, or 28 and 40 seconds per patient. The nursing staff and physicians in both settings reported infrequent use of nursing notes, and this was confirmed by observations (nurses averaged .63 and .52 referrals per patient day and physicians averaged .06 and .30 referrals per patient day). Nursing personnel made more referrals on the medical units than on the surgical units. Further study revealed an omission rate of 62 items of patient care data for every 100 items charted; 12% of the items charted were inaccurate. The investigators concluded that charting had changed from a ritualistic to a meaningless activity.

But use of nurses' notes was reported by a majority of physicians and nurses in a study by Healy and McGurk (1966), and very few thought the notes were not helpful. Only 19% of the nurses said they recorded immediately after an activity, 68% recorded notes when time was available. There was both agreement and disagreement between nurses and physicians on items to include in the nurses' notes. The greatest discrepancy was on patient teaching; 74% of the nurses and 6% of the physicians said this item should be charted. The area of patient teaching was not among the authors' recommendations of items to include in a patient record.

Steckel (1976) found that the amount of charting increased with positive reinforcement. The major increases were in number of charts on which the nurses wrote, and in the amount charted under various components of the nursing process. The findings showed that feedback alone was not a sufficient reinforcer for increased charting; gains were achieved only when charting goals were identified and their attainment rewarded. Breu and Gawlinski (1981) found that when the documentation of cardiac arrhythmias was increased from once every eight hours to every two hours the number of arrhythmias detected increased from 39% to 63%, and the number of complete documentations about the arrhythmias increased from .33 to 2.4 per patient.

Computer. Lagine (1971) developed a computer program for diagnosing anxiety. Data were obtained from 50 patients by interview and fed into a computer programmed to diagnose mild, moderate, or severe anxiety. The computerized diagnoses were compared to nurse ratings of patient anxiety, a standard anxiety scale score, and patient galvanic skin reactivity scores. Agreement was low, but a cluster analysis revealed an intercorrelation of .64 between 7 of the 18 anxiety symptoms measured. Goodwin and Edwards (1975) reported on the development of a computer program to aid in diagnosing skin functions. While the program demonstrated a technique for recording and analyzing data, and reinforced the acquisition of appropriate data, it required over an hour to run.

Rosenberg, Glueck, Strachel, Reznikoff, and Ericson (1969) described a computerized form for recording observations of psychiatric patient behavior. While taking about the same time as written notes, the automated form was more efficient and complete because of automated editing, and structured, standardized data gathering. A study by Ravensborg (1970) supported the Rosenberg et al. findings that automated nursing notes improved the observation, recording, and transmitting of patient information. Stein (1969) compared an automated form for collecting data with narrative notes and found that the automated forms provided more information at first, but this difference was not apparent one year later. The reduction in completed automated forms could have resulted from repeated use (redundancy fatigue) as discussed by Stein, but it also could have come from learning the computerized system of data collection. Stein also noted the lack of agreement among nurses on the content of nurses' notes, and that the automated note did not allow for unusual occurrences for which special reports may be needed.

In discussing the necessity of nurse involvement in decision making about computer applications, Farlee and Goldstein (1971) reported findings from their study of a computer system that is no longer in operation. They hypothesized that computerized hospital units in use the longest would be evaluated most positively. The sequential order of implementing the system was: admissions, medications, laboratory, x-ray, and nursing orders. The percentages of nurses satisfied were laboratory (74%), medications (71%), x-ray (69%), admissions (56%), and nursing orders (41%). Only 50% of the nurses thought computerized nursing notes improved care and only 40% thought they aided efficiency. Overall, only about 40% of the nurses were satisfied with the system. A major difficulty in evaluating computerized information systems is the failure to collect baseline data on the manual system for comparison. Given the findings on nursing notes, the nurses Farlee and Goldstein studied probably were not satisfied with the manual notes either.

Several studies of the attitudes of nurses and other health care workers toward computers were conducted. Rosenberg, Reznikoff, Stroebel, and

Ericson (1967) found that the attitudes of nursing students exposed to clinical use of a computer improved, while the attitudes of students not exposed did not. Startsman and Robinson (1972) found that medical students, medical record librarians, medical house staff, and medical faculty favored computer use slightly more than nurses, nursing students, and ancillary personnel. Thies (1975) found that those most likely to have negative attitudes toward computers were in rural areas, female, less experienced, and had no prior contact with computers. Negative perceptions of computer training significantly influenced attitudes.

Certainly there is abundant evidence that written records of patient care are invalid. If adequate data are to be obtained for patient care and for reimbursement of services, the nursing role in information processing must be recognized, rewarded, and new approaches explored. Automated storing, processing, and transmitting of data could help data collection and use, but reports on this technology are few. Goodwin and Edwards (1975) and Lagina (1971) showed that much can be learned about patient data by development of this technology, and identification of data could be a major benefit from computerizing nursing information. Computerized systems of nursing information must be based on studies of information needs and processing and on conceptual frameworks appropriate to nursing practice, if the systems are to be meaningful and thus useful.

DISCUSSION AND FUTURE RESEARCH DIRECTIONS

There is beginning support for a science of nursing based on information processing. While limited, a body of knowledge about nursing information was identified in this chapter. Conceptual frameworks for the collection, organization, use, and storage of information exist, and relationships between variables of decision makers, decision situations and contexts, and decisions and strategies have been described. Although the existing knowledge about nursing information is confined to research settings, rapid movement toward interactive study from laboratory description to clinical tests of explanations and predictions can be anticipated. Knowledge about nursing information is summarized below.

Despite the importance of information processing in nursing practice, nursing data are not clearly identified as shown by the amounts of uninformative data collected and used. To reduce the resulting uncertainty, nurses collect too much data and use strategies that are complex and probably inefficient for making decisions. Nursing decisions probably are more appropriate when data are relevant and restricted in amount. Nurses are imprecise in collecting and recording both qualitative and quantitative data, particularly the more critical extreme values. Education leads to differences in the process of making decisions, and these differences appear positive. However, education does not increase certainty about nursing data, nor lead to more effective strategies for making complex nursing decisions. Structured and systematic procedures for collecting, using, and storing data are beneficial. Decision making varies greatly among nurses, among situations, and among contexts.

The biggest impediment to expanding this body of knowledge is the unclear definition of nursing data. If existing computerized systems of information could be exploited for nursing research, or if such systems could be developed specifically for research, there probably would be an explosion of knowledge about information processing and decision making in nursing. Only with computers can the vast and complex arrays of nursing data be processed so that limited amounts of the most sensitive data can be identified. Additionally, the relationships among the data elements and the reliabilities of these data can be assessed. There are indications that increased knowledge about nursing information would lead to better and more cost-effective patient care.

In addition to data identification, the focus of future research should be in two other areas: description of skills in processing nursing information and testing of improved strategies, aids, and systems for processing information. Emphasis should be on identifying skilled nurse decision makers and describing their information processing strategies, rather than on identifying deficiencies in processing information. In-depth study of skilled strategies could be most productive for improving decision-making skills and for developing new methods for information processing.

Laboratory-type studies are appropriate, given the current knowledge about nursing information. Random selection of real patient descriptions would strengthen such studies, however, and the goal should be laboratory description followed by clinical testing of derived explanations and predictions. Studies conducted within real-life settings should be defined as narrowly as possible, and confined to restricted (but large) populations of decision situations and/or decision makers. Variables of the choice situation, the decision makers, and the context of the study must be controlled. Hanchett (1981) noted the limitations of record review and time-sampling from her study of a computer implementation. She found that the relationship between one patient problem and one nursing action could be ascertained, but confounded patient problems and nursing actions, as well as changing patient needs, were problematic.

A number of methods for studying nursing information have been described. A major purpose of the articles by Kelly, Hammond, and others was to describe approaches nurses could use to study information processing. Included in these reports were methods for data analysis (Thomas & Hansen, 1969). In addition, nurse researchers should examine methods from signal detection theory (Swets & Pickett, 1982) and artificial intelligence. The latter may be particularly appropriate for data identification and development of computer systems.

Projective techniques to trace information processing appear useful for describing cognitive strategies of skilled nurse decision makers. Since only a few subjects can be studied, their selection is critical. Several investigators used video recordings of actual or simulated patient situations, that more appropriately might be translated to computer technology. Computer simulations provide for collection of large amounts of data; comparison with a standard, accurate recording of rapid and confounded problems and actions; and selectivity and decreasing vigilance in observing.

Two methods, while useful, should be employed only with full appreciation of their considerable limitations—vignettes and simulations of patient situations (Farrand, Holzemer, & Schleutermann, 1982; Holzemer, Schleutermann, Farrand, & Miller, 1981). The results will be influenced by the content, by how the choice is framed, and will not generalize to other contexts. These methods are useful for analyzing specific decision variables, examining consistency in choices and comparisons across decision makers, and identifying influences of variables within the choice situation or context.

Throughout the history of modern nursing the collection, organization, use, and storage of nursing information received considerable attention. There have been efforts to base patient data on scientific facts, improve the process of data collection, systematically organize and store data, and describe data use. A body of knowledge about nursing is being built based on information processing. The further development of this body of knowledge should be a national priority because nursing information is the foundation of clinical science. As Nightingale (1894/1907) said: "Observation tells us the fact, reflection the meaning of the fact. . . . Observation tells how the patient is, reflection tells what is to be done. . . . The trained power of attending to one's own impressions made by one's own senses, so that these should tell the nurse how the patient is, is the *sine qua non* of being a nurse at all" (pp. 254–255).

REFERENCES

Abdellah, F. G. Methods of identifying covert aspects of nursing problems. *Nursing Research,* 1957, *6,* 4–23.

Aspinall, M. J. Use of a decision tree to improve accuracy of diagnosis. *Nursing Research,* 1979, *28,* 182–185.

Bailey, D. E. Clinical inference in nursing: Analysis of nursing action patterns. *Nursing Research,* 1967, *16,* 154–160.

Bailey, J. T., McDonald, F. J., & Claus, K. E. An experimental curriculum. In F. G. Abdellah, I. L. Beland, A. Martin, & R. V. Matheney (Eds.), *New directions in patient centered nursing.* New York: Macmillan, 1973.

Basson, P. H. The gerontological nursing literature. *Nursing Research,* 1967, *16,* 267–271.

Beland, I. L. *Clinical nursing: Pathophysiological and psychosocial approaches.* New York: Macmillan, 1965.

Bonney, V., & Rothberg, J. The League exchange: Nursing diagnosis and therapy. New York: National League for Nursing, 1963.

Breu, C. S., & Gawlinski, A. A comparative study of the effects of documentation on arrhythmia detection efficiency. *Heart & Lung,* 1981, *10,* 1058–1062.

Broderick, M. E., & Ammentorp, W. Information structures: An analysis of nursing performance. *Nursing Research,* 1979, *28,* 106–110.

Choi, S. C., Boxerman, S. B., & Steinburg, L. Nurses' preference of terminal digits in data reading. *Journal of Nursing Education,* 1978, *17*(9), 38–41.

Chow, R. Postoperative cardiac nursing research: A method for identifying and categorizing nursing action. *Nursing Research,* 1969, *18,* 4–13.

Cianfrani, K. L. The influence of amounts and relevance of data on identifying health problems (Doctoral dissertation, University of Illinois, 1982). *Dissertation Abstracts International,* 1982, *43,* 34B–35B. (University Microfilms No. 83–05276)

Cline, D. S. An analysis of spelling errors made by professional nurses. *Nursing Outlook,* 1959, *6,* 400–402.

Committee on Records. Activities of the national organization for public health nursing. *The Public Health Nurse,* 1925, *17,* 389–390.

Committee on Records. The why of nursing records. *Public Health Nursing,* 1933, *25,* 642–647.

Cook, M., & Mayers, M. Computer-assisted data base for nursing research. In H. H. Werley & M. R. Grier (Eds.), *Nursing information systems.* New York: Springer, 1981.

Corcoran, S. A. Nursing care planning by hospice nurses (Doctoral dissertation, University of Minnesota, 1983). *Dissertation Abstracts International,* 1983, *44*(9B).

Crisham, P. Measuring moral judgment in nursing dilemmas. *Nursing Research,* 1981, *30,* 104–110.

Damrosch, S. P., & Soeken, K. Communicating probability in clinical reports: A preliminary study of nurses' numerical associations to verbal expressions. *Research in Nursing and Health,* 1983, *6,* 85–87.

Derryberry, M. Do case records guide the nursing service? *Public Health Reports,* 1939, *54,* 66–76. (a)

Derryberry, M. Nursing accomplishments as revealed by case records. *Public Health Reports*, 1939, *54*, 2035–2043. (b)

Dincher, J. R., & Stidger, S. L. Evaluation of a written simulation format for clinical nursing judgment. *Nursing Research*, 1976, *25*, 280–285.

Farlee, C., & Goldstein, B. A role for nurses in implementing computerized hospital information systems. *Nursing Forum*, 1971, *10*, 339–357.

Farrand, L. L., Holzemer, W. L., & Schleutermann, J. A. A study of construct validity: Simulations as a measure of nurse practitioners' problem-solving skills. *Nursing Research*, 1982, *31*, 37–42.

Fedder, H. J. Basic science concepts essential in planning nursing care. *Nursing Research*, 1956, *4*, 100–124.

Finch, J. Systems analysis: A logical approach to professional nursing care. *Nursing Forum*, 1969, *8*, 176–189.

Fox, D. J. A proposed model for identifying research areas in nursing. *Nursing Research*, 1964, *13*, 29–36.

Goodwin, J. O., & Edwards, B. S. Developing a computer program to assist the nursing process: Phase 1. From systems analysis to an expandable program. *Nursing Research*, 1975, *24*, 299–305.

Gordon, M. Information processing strategies in nursing diagnosis. In the *Ninth Nursing Research Conference, San Antonio*. Kansas City, Mo.: American Nurses' Association, 1973.

Gordon, M. Predictive strategies in diagnostic tasks. *Nursing Research*, 1980, *29*, 39–45.

Grier, M. R. Decision making about patient care. *Nursing Research*, 1976, *25*, 105–110.

Grier, M. R. The need for data in making nursing decisions. In H. H. Werley & M. R. Grier (Eds.), *Nursing information systems*. New York: Springer, 1981.

Grier, M. R., & Grier, J. B. The system for delivering pain medication: The patient's pain, the doctor's order, the nurse's choice. In B. T. Williams (Ed.), *Fourth Illinois Conference on Medical Information Systems*. Urbana: Regional Health Resource Center, 1978.

Grier, M. R., Howard, M., & Cohen, F. Beliefs and values associated with administering narcotic analgesics to terminally ill patients. In *Clinical and scientific sessions*. Kansas City, Mo.: American Nurses' Association, 1979.

Grier, M. R., & Schnitzler, C. P. Nurses' propensity to risk. *Nursing Research*, 1979, *28*, 186–191.

Gunn, I. P., Sullivan, E. F., & Glor, G. A. K. Blood pressure measurement as a quantitative research criterion. *Nursing Research*, 1966, *15*, 4–11.

Hammond, K. R. An approach to the study of clinical inference in nursing. Part 2. Clinical inference in nursing: A methodological approach. *Nursing Research*, 1964, *13*, 314–320.

Hammond, K. R. Clinical inference in nursing: 2. A psychologist's viewpoint. *Nursing Research*, 1966, *15*, 27–38.

Hammond, K. R., Kelly, K. J., Castellan, Jr., N. J., Schneider, R. J., & Vancini, M. Clinical inference in nursing: Use of information-seeking strategies by nurses. *Nursing Research*, 1966, *15*, 330–336.

Hammond, K. R., Kelly, K. J., Schneider, R. J., & Vancini, M. Clinical inference in nursing: Analyzing cognitive tasks representative of nursing problems. *Nursing Research*, 1966, *15*, 134–138. (a)

Hammond, K. R., Kelly, K. J., Schneider, R. J., & Vancini, M. Clinical inference in nursing: Information units used. *Nursing Research*, 1966, *15*, 236–243. (b)

Hammond, K. R., Kelly, K. J., Schneider, R. J., & Vancini, M. Clinical inference in nursing: Revising judgments. *Nursing Research*, 1967, *16*, 38–45.

Hanchett, E. S. Appropriateness of nursing care. In H. H. Werley & M. R. Grier (Eds.), *Nursing information systems*. New York: Springer, 1981.

Hansen, A. C., & Thomas, D. B. A conceptualization of decision making. *Nursing Research*, 1968, *17*, 436–443.

Harmer, B., & Henderson, V. *The principles and practice of nursing* (4th ed.). New York: Macmillan, 1939.

Harmer, B., & Henderson, V. *The principles and practice of nursing* (5th ed.). New York: Macmillan, 1955.

Healy, E. E., & McGurk, W. Effectiveness and acceptance of nurses' notes. *Nursing Outlook*, 1966, *14*(3), 32–34.

Hefferin, E. A., & Hunter, R. E. Nursing assessment and care plan statements. *Nursing Research*, 1975, *24*, 360–366.

Henderson, V. The nursing process—Is the title right? *Journal of Advanced Nursing*, 1982, *7*, 103–109.

Higgins, P. G. Measuring nurses' accuracy of estimating blood loss. *Journal of Advanced Nursing*, 1982, *7*, 157–162.

Holzemer, W. L., Schleutermann, J. A., Farrand, L. L., & Miller, A. G. A validation study: Simulations as a measure of nurse practitioners' problem-solving skills. *Nursing Research*, 1981, *30*, 139–144.

Horn, B. J., & Swain, M. A. *Development of criterion measures of nursing care: Reliability test results and instrument of health status measures* (Vol. 1) (DHEW Publication No. HRA 77–16). University of Michigan, Department of Health Administration, Ann Arbor, Mich., February 1977. (NTIS No. PB-267 005)

Howland, D., & McDowell, W. E. The measurement of patient care: A conceptual framework. *Nursing Research*, 1964, *13*, 4–7.

Kelly, K. An approach to the study of clinical inference in nursing: Part 1. Introduction to the study of clinical inference in nursing. *Nursing Research*, 1964, *13*, 314–315.

Kelly, K. Clinical inference in nursing: 1. A nurse's viewpoint. *Nursing Research*, 1966, *15*, 23–26.

Ketefian, S. Critical thinking, educational preparation, and development of moral judgment. *Nursing Research*, 1981, *30*, 98–103. (a)

Ketefian, S. Moral reasoning and moral behavior. *Nursing Research*, 1981, *30*, 171–176. (b)

Kim, M. J., & Moritz, D. A. (Eds.). *Classification of nursing diagnoses*. Proceedings of the Third and Fourth National Conferences. New York: McGraw-Hill, 1981.

Kraus, V. L. Preinformation—Its effect on nurses' descriptions of a patient. *Journal of Nursing Education*, 1976, *15*(5), 18–26.

Lagina, S. M. A computer to diagnose anxiety levels. *Nursing Research*, 1971, *20*, 484–492.

Matthews, C. A., & Gaul, A. L. Nursing diagnosis from the perspective of concept attainment and critical thinking. *Advances in Nursing Science*, 1979, *2*(1), 17–26.

McCain, R. F. Nursing by assessment—Not intuition. *American Journal of Nursing*, 1965, *65*, 82–84. (a)

McCain, R. F. Systematic investigation of medical-surgical nursing content. *Journal of Nursing Education*, 1965, *4*(2), 23–31. (b)

McLaughlin, F. E., Cesa, T., Johnson, H., Lemons, M., Anderson, S., Larson, P., & Gibson, J. Nurses' and physicians' performance on clinical simulation test: Hypertension. *Research in Nursing and Health*, 1979, *2*, 61–72.

Mickey, J. E. Studying extra-hospital nursing needs: A preliminary report. *American Journal of Public Health*, 1958, *48*, 885–886.

Moreland, H. J., & Grier, M. R. Telephone consultation in care of the older adult. *Geriatric Nursing*, in press.

National League for Nursing. *The problem-oriented system—A multidisciplinary approach*. New York: Author, 1974.

National League of Nursing Education. *Curriculum guide for schools of nursing*. New York. Author, 1937.

Neal, M. V. Conceptualizing a data base for nursing practice. In H. H. Werley & M. R. Grier (Eds.), *Nursing information systems*. New York: Springer, 1981.

Nightingale, F. Training of nurses. In M. A. Nutting & L. A. Dock (Eds.), *History of nursing* (Vol. 2). New York: G. P. Putnam & Sons, 1907 (Reprinted from R. Quain (Ed.). *Dictionary of medicine*. London: Longman's, Green, 1894.)

Orem, D. E. *Nursing: Concepts of practice*. New York: McGraw-Hill, 1971.

Orlando, I. *The dynamic nurse-patient relationship*. New York: Putnam, 1961.

Padilla, G. V., & Grant, M. M. Quality assurance programme for nursing. *Journal of Advanced Nursing*, 1982, *7*, 135–145.

Phaneuf, M. C. Analysis of a nursing audit. *Nursing Outlook*, 1968, *16*(1), 57–60.

Rausch, T., & Rund, D. Nurses' clinical judgments. *Nursing Management*, 1981, *12*(12), 24–26.

Ravensborg, M. R. Empirical validation of automated nursing notes: Informational utility. *Psychological Reports*, 1970, *26*, 279–282.

Romano, C., McCormick, K. A., & McNeely, L. D., Nursing documentation: A model for a computerized data base. *Advances in Nursing Science*, 1982, *4*(2), 43–56.

Roose, J. A. Interpretation of rest by doctors and nurses. *Nursing Research*, 1963, *12*, 111–113.

Rosenberg, M., Glueck, Jr., B. C., Strachel, C. F., Reznikoff, M., & Ericson, R. P. Comparison of automated nursing notes as recorded by psychiatrists and nursing service personnel. *Nursing Research*, 1969, *18*, 350–357.

Rosenberg, M., Reznikoff, M., Stroebel, C. F., & Ericson, R. P. Attitudes of nursing students toward computers. *Nursing Outlook*, 1967, *15*(7), 44–46.

Simmons, D. A. *A classification scheme for client problems in community health nursing* (DHHS Publication No. HRA 80–16). Visiting Nurse Association of Omaha, Nebr., June 1980. (NTIS No. HRP–0501501)

Simon, J. R. Systematic ratings of patient welfare. *Nursing Outlook*, 1961, *9*, 432–436.

Simon, J. R., & Chastain, S. S. Take a systematic look at your patients. *Nursing Outlook*, 1960, *8*, 509–512.

Sparks, R. K. Problem solving ability of graduates from associate and baccalureate degree nursing programs (Doctoral dissertation, University of Minnesota,

1979). *Dissertation Abstracts International,* 1979, *40,* 678B. (University Microfilms No. 83-29-507)

Startsman, T. S., & Robinson, R. E. The attitudes of medical and paramedical personnel toward computers. *Computers and Biomedical Research,* 1972, *5,* 218–227.

Steckel, S. B. Utilization of reinforcement contracts to increase written evidence of the nursing assessment. *Nursing Research,* 1976, *25,* 58–61.

Stein, R. F. An exploratory study in the development and use of automated nursing reports. *Nursing Research,* 1969, *18,* 14–21.

Suhayda, R., & Kim, M. J. Documentation of the nursing process in critical care. In M. J. Kim, G. K. McFarland, and A. M. McLane (Eds.), *Classification of nursing diagnoses: Proceedings of the Fifth National Conference.* St. Louis, Mo.: Mosby, in press.

Sullivan, M. J. Reflections of the nursing process in two methods of recording nurses' notes. In H. H. Werley & M. R. Grier (Eds.), *Nursing information systems.* New York: Springer, 1981.

Swets, J. A., & Pickett, R. M. *Evaluation of diagnostic systems: Methods from signal detection theory.* New York: Academic Press, 1982.

Takacs, K. M., & Valenti, W. M. Temperature measurement in a clinical setting. *Nursing Research,* 1982, *31,* 368–370.

Taylor, D. B., & Johnson, O. H. *Systematic nursing assessment* (DHEW Publication No. HRA 74–17). Washington D.C.: U.S. Government Printing Office, 1974.

Thies, J. B. Hospital personnel and computer based systems: A study of attitudes and perceptions. *Hospital Administration,* 1975, *20,* 17–26.

Thomas, D. B., & Hansen, A. C. Multiple discriminant analysis of public health nursing decision responses. *Nursing Research,* 1969, *18,* 145–153.

Verhonick, P. J. Decubitus ulcer observations measured objectively. *Nursing Research,* 1961, *10,* 211–214.

Verhonick, P. J. Nichols, G. A., Glor, B. A. K., & McCarthy, R. T. I came, I saw, I responded: Nursing observation and action survey. *Nursing Research,* 1968, *17,* 38–44.

Wald, F., & Leonard, R. Towards development of nursing practice theory. *Nursing Research,* 1964, *13,* 309–313.

Walker, C., & Deuble, H. A schema for analysis of accident prevention activities in public health nurses' records. *Nursing Research,* 1968, *17,* 408–414.

Walker, V. H., & Selmanoff, E. D. A study of the nature and uses of nurses' notes. *Nursing Research,* 1964, *13,* 113–121.

Werley, H. H., & Grier, M. R. Research directions. In H. H. Werley & M. R. Grier (Eds.), *Nursing information systems.* New York: Springer, 1981.

Wilcox, J. Observer factors in the measurement of blood pressure. *Nursing Research,* 1961, *10,* 4–20.

Wolfe, H. Can nonnurses make qualitative observations of nursing care? *Nursing Outlook,* 1965, *13,* 309–313.

Yura, H., & Walsh, M. B. *The nursing process.* New York: Appleton-Century-Crofts, 1973.

PART V

Other Research

CHAPTER 12

Nursing Research and the Study of Health Policy

Nancy Milio
SCHOOL OF NURSING AND SCHOOL OF PUBLIC HEALTH
UNIVERSITY OF NORTH CAROLINA AT CHAPEL HILL

CONTENTS

This chapter includes a review and assessment of the contribution of nursing research to the field of policy studies. First, terms of reference are defined, with particular distinctions made between policy analysis and policy research. Guided by these terms, the search of the nursing literature is described and the results are reported. Then follows a brief state-of-the-art discussion of the field of policy studies, and a summary of what might make health policy studies a more useful endeavor for the creation of policy. The chapter closes with suggestions about how nurse researchers might use their special competence to strengthen policy studies and so make them more useable to policymakers.

TERMS OF REFERENCE

Policy is a governmental statement that defines a course of action which will attain or preserve some desired or acceptable state of affairs. The purpose is to alter, within the scope of human initiative, what would occur otherwise. Embodied in legislation and regulations, policy serves as a guide to current and future program and operational decisions. It may emphasize ends or means, or may include both.

Of necessity, the study of policy is a multidisciplinary field, drawing methods and concepts from both academic and applied disciplines. These disciplines include economics, political science and other social sciences, mathematics, planning, and public administration. The aims of policy studies are to observe, describe, explain, analyze, predict, apply, and evaluate policies. The focus may be either the substance of a particular policy or the processes by which policies are actually formulated, implemented, maintained, or changed. The ultimate purpose is to help policy-makers define and resolve policy problems more effectively.

Within the field of policy studies, policy implies *public* (i.e., governmental) policy, not policy set by groups for their own nonprofit or for-profit organizations. The policy perspective is therefore for "society as a whole," a concern for the general or public interest, often with selected analytic emphases on consequences for subgroups, including demographic, private interest groups, or government agencies.

Public policy that has an impact on people's health, directly or indirectly, may be considered health policy. As most commonly used by nurses and others, however, the term health policy usually implies health *services* policy (Milio, 1981).

Although research plays only a small role in the real world of policy-making, it does have some influence, especially in new or controversial areas of public policy. As the pace of social and technological change quickens, and new situations not amenable to the wisdom of experience arise, the necessity for policy-relevant research is increasing and will continue to increase. At the same time, however, new, unprecedented circumstances also will make prediction more tenuous. Nonetheless, this somewhat paradoxical situation is and will be the reality of the climate surrounding policy making.

To make a useful contribution in this environment, nurses can engage in what may be regarded as a spectrum of policy-relevant research. The span runs from the most broad and complex, explicit, government-commissioned *policy analysis* research, to more focused, program-evaluating *policy research,* to the most removed and theoretical or experimental *disciplinary research* that may have policy implications.

Cutting across this spectrum at any point are the uses to which all interested groups, public and private, may put the findings as they seek to influence the development of public policy. Thus, all policy-relevant research, whether or not it includes systematic study of specific policies, may contribute in one or more of several ways to the policy development process. Specifically, these ways include monitoring the course of events that might be relevant to policy; forecasting emergent problems prior to their recognition; identifying and analyzing problem-raising situations; critiquing current policies where they are based on a poor understanding of the problem; redefining the problem; and analyzing the policy-making process itself, including initiation, development, implementation, outcome, and feedback (Vickers, Note 1).

For purposes of this review, the nursing literature was explored for policy-relevant studies primarily in the policy research and policy analysis part of the spectrum, with a secondary focus on disciplinary research that may have policy implications. Before proceeding with the review findings, these terms are defined as they were used in the policy studies field (Coleman, 1981). In effect, the terms set the parameters within which nursing's policy studies are assessed below, the consequent gaps are identified, and future directions for research are implied.

The purpose of *policy analysis research* is perhaps its most distinguishing aspect, one from which other characteristics flow. It is done explicitly to help policymakers make the choices that guide social action (Vickers, 1981).

Because it is intended to assist policymakers, policy analysis is time-bound to the requirements of decision making in legislatures, public bureaucracies, and sometimes the courts. Analysts therefore draw on existing data, including relevant empirical studies, and the judgments of experts and others, evaluating these and any other forms of information that can reveal the pros and cons of alternative choices of action (Klarman, 1980; Shortell & Solomon, 1982). The focus is on probable futures resulting from maintaining, modifying, ending, or initiating policies for given problems.

By contrast, *policy research* is an empirical investigation of the application of a policy in specific situations in order to uncover some of its effects. Thus the scope is confined. The focus is on past events, and there is more use of primary data, with less reliance on value judgments. Policy research therefore may or may not reach the eyes of policy analysts or policymakers. If it does, it may become one piece among many types of information that are taken into account in policy formulation.

Evaluation research is sometimes policy research. An example might be a study of the cost effectiveness of increased Medicare coverage of in-home services in a sample of home health agencies. By contrast, a fuller policy analysis might use such findings to help answer a broader policy question concerning whether Medicare should cover more in-home services. Ideally for such analysis, investigators also would include other studies and views in order to specify all of the expected benefits and costs (both monetary and other); identify alternative actions or means to achieve the same results along with their costs and benefits; address any ethical issues that might be involved; and discuss the findings, limitations, and implications for policy and program decisions (Milio, 1981; Office of Technology Assessment, Note 2).

Because of differing purposes, scope, and time constraints, the methods of policy analysis are more diverse than the approximations of traditional scientific experimental designs used in policy research. They include not only the compilation of previous research but also of surveys (demographic, epidemiological, public opinion, historical), cost-benefit and risk-benefit analyses, operations research techniques, systems analyses, simulation, trend extrapolation, field investigation, the use of expert panels, and Delphi techniques, among others.

Needless to say, policy analysis—because of the intended audience— often is reported and disseminated differently from other kinds of research. The reports often include executive summaries, audiovisual materials, and press summaries. They contain less jargon and theory, and usually are more readable in language and format.

In sum, the definition of questions for investigation in policy analysis comes from the needs of policymakers, stated in terms that are meaningful for future policy decisions, using variables that can be influenced by policy choices. The questions are sufficiently broad in scope to capture the full range of effects (empirically measurable or not) of a given policy, rather than confined, as policy research is, to some limited effects of policy implementation in a specific site.

Still further removed from policy development, *disciplinary* researchers (as in nursing or sociology) work to develop and test theory in a substantive area, and so seek conclusions that are relevant to the discipline's problem foci. They do not make their findings immediately useful to decision makers. Their focus is on complete and precise information, ideally unfettered by time constraints and wed to experimental designs rather than the socially given situations of policy research (Bice, 1980). Researchable questions and appropriate variables are selected and defined according to their theoretical importance, not by the need to evaluate policy or to emphasize those variables that can be manipulated by policy, as required of policy research and policy analysis. Disciplinary research may of course have policy implications and so be drawn on by policy analysts. Most disciplinary research, whether of an experimental or evaluative nature, however, does not focus on the policy implications of findings (Gortner & Nahm, 1977).

POLICY STUDIES IN THE NURSING RESEARCH LITERATURE

Methods of Search

The search for policy studies by nurses was guided by the above definitions of policy research and policy analysis. The following procedures were used. Two MEDLINE computerized bibliographical searches consisted of (a) these descriptors under nursing: research and health, health policy, health planning, legislation, and cost-benefit analysis from 1971 through 1981; and (b) all publications of the National League for Nursing and the Division of Nursing, United States Department of Health and Human Services, limited to available citations dated betwen July 1976 and October 1981. In addition, recent publications of the American Academy of Nursing, 1980 to 1982, were reviewed.

Direct inspections also were made of the *International Nursing Index*, 1972 through 1981, and, for further assurance, selected years of *Nursing Research* (1977, 1978, 1980). The *Index* review included more than 20 terms such as health, health care delivery, organization, financing; legislation, regulation, policy, economics; nutrition, smoking, prevention, environmental policy; social policy; public policy; employment, political processes, decision making; and government. The same descriptors were used in the review of the annual *Nursing Research* indexes, which contained abstracts of articles in other journals and dissertations as well. Finally, nurse researchers interested in policy in the United States and England were contacted regarding their awareness of policy analysis studies done by nurses.

Results

This search of nursing literature revealed that although policy issues are receiving increased attention, approximations of policy research are sparse, and no policy analysis research was done by nurses. A general impression from direct inspection of the indexes is that the predominant focus of the literature was on proximate and personal or individual sources (causes) of health problems and solutions. Perhaps as a consequence, the researchers often do not attend to the broader environmental, population-oriented, policy-manipulable variables that affect health or health care.

Understandably, most nursing research was focused on the problems of the discipline in nursing practice and education. In some, such as Lubic's

(1981) evaluation of a maternity center, the policy implications of the program were discussed. The research methods used, however, were traditional descriptive patient and cost statistics rather than more complex policy study methods. The investigator was well aware of these limitations.

Other evaluative studies, for example, the Spitzer and Grace (1981) analysis of the impact of cost containment on nursing service and education come closer to policy research as defined here. This one fell short in that the authors did not state the particular policy or set of policies contained under the rubric "cost containment." Also, these policies seemed to be institutional rather than governmental. The authors, however, placed their discussion within the context of public policies.

Kos and Rothberg (1981) were all too aware of the problems in doing a cost effectiveness analysis of a free standing nurse clinic. They were able, however, to manipulate a variety of data sources to provide a useful evaluation. Their focus was more on the problems of evaluation than on the policy implications of their findings. Thus, although this study had policy implications, it too fell short of policy research in that the authors neither made its policy importance explicit nor purported to evaluate the application of a particular policy.

Another and more complex example of policy-relevant research involving nurses was the study of the hospital nursing shortage by Aiken, Blendon, and Rogers (1981), who were able to draw on the resources of the Robert Wood Johnson Foundation. This study may be viewed as a successful attempt to provide a plausible redefinition of an issue of importance to nurses. As such, it allowed the restatement of a national policy problem, namely, the maintenance of adequate hospital nursing staff. The authors turned the question into: How may nurses' salaries be maintained adequately, instead of, how can the supply of nurses be increased? In turn, the revised policy problem statement invited the exploration of new policy solutions, which may or may not be within the scope of public policy.

In a policy-related paper, Fagin (1982a) also brought to bear empirical data in an effort to redefine the nursing shortage issue in policy terms. This time it was redefined within the framework and language of competition as the current practical political currency of the 1980 to 1984 Reagan Administration.

Reif and Estes (1982) attempted a redefinition of sorts of a national policy problem. They sought to help nurses see a broad policy issue—how best to provide long-term care—as relevant to nurses, a policy problem to which nurses might contribute solutions. In so doing, they analyzed the problem in its wider political, economic, demographic, and epidemiological facets and showed how policy solutions affected nursing practice. They also called upon nurses, and nurse researchers in particular, to attend to health policy issues beyond those that directly affect nurses, including public policy that indirectly affects health, such as income maintenance, nutrition, and housing policies.

In a recent review of nursing research in gerontology, Kayser-Jones (1981) showed no work was done on policy. Other disciplinary studies with explicit policy implications were done on nursing-specific issues—for example, the Division of Nursing reports on *The Geographic Distribution of Nurses and Public Policy* (Sloan, 1975) and *Analysis and Planning for Improved Distribution of Nursing Personnel and Services* (Elliot & Kearns, 1978). The stated purposes of such studies were often methodological and they were addressed to nurses in particular and interested individuals in general. Furthermore, it is characteristic of Division of Nursing studies that, while some would qualify as policy analysis, such as *The Impact of Health System Changes on the Nation's Requirements for Registered Nurses in 1985* (Doyle, Cooper, & Anderson, 1978), these were not done by nurses. The analysts were primarily economists.

Policy-relevant papers from the National League for Nursing included *The Health Manpower Dilemma* (1971), *Community Health Administration in a Cost Containment Era* (1978), and *Health Policy Making in Action: The Passage and Implementation of the National Health Planning and Resources Development Act of 1974* (1975). These collections addressed policy issues, although they cannot be regarded as policy analysis research, because either (a) policy analysis (as defined here) was not their purpose; or (b) their intended audience, and thus the perspective of their discussion, was the nursing profession, not public policymakers; and (c) the scope of variables or effects addressed were not comprehensive. Other reviews of nursing research on administrative (i.e., institutional) policy (Krueger, 1980) indicated similar nonpolicy purposes, a narrow scope of variables, and nurses as the intended audience. These papers are nonetheless relevant to policymakers in that they expressed the views of those who were affected by certain policies.

Only limited attention (Milio, Note 3) has as yet been given to the systematic analysis of policy-making processes, although such research was urged by Lubic (1981). The Division of Nursing's publication *Nursing Involvement in the Health Planning Process* (Kalisch & Kalisch, 1977) laid the groundwork for such analyses in one area of policy making.

Summary

In sum, the growing interest in health policy among nurses is clear. Increasingly, issues of traditional concern to nurses—the supply and quality of nursing care, the financing of care and economic position of nurses, the education and roles of nurses—are being framed in policy-relevant terms. Much of the analytic work to date focused on redefining policy problems, either within the profession, or in an effort to influence policymakers' perceptions of the policy problems.

The overriding concern as revealed in the literature was on how to influence policy making (Aiken, 1982; American Academy of Nursing, 1981) rather than on emphasizing the substance of alternative policies and analyzing the actual or potential effects. It is, therefore, the uses to which policy studies can be put that currently commands most attention among nurse analysts.

In any case, systematic studies must be done well if they are to be useful to the profession or to policymakers. Most policy-relevant papers done by nurses may be regarded as prepolicy studies. That is, while they may have contributed to policy development processes in a broad social sense, they were focused mainly on defining, analyzing, or redefining the policy issue. They included presentation of policy solutions as general recommendations but did not include systematic analysis of explicit policy proposals either in their application in limited settings (policy research) or in terms of broad, clearly defined health, economic, social, and political consequences (policy analysis research). Furthermore, when some conventional methods of policy studies were discussed, such as cost-benefit analysis, they seemed not to be defined in the terms advised by the recent state-of-the-art evaluation of methodologies by the Office of Technology Assessment (Note 4). Such discrepancies might limit the contributions nurses could make to the field of policy studies in the future.

POTENTIAL CONTRIBUTION OF NURSES TO POLICY STUDIES

Nursing leaders called for research on both the substance of policies (Aiken, 1982) and on the processes of policy making (Lubic, 1981). They were, in effect, asking for policy research, (e.g., the effects of third-party reimbursement for nurses in a particular setting), not policy analysis (e.g., the broad economic, social, and health consequences of a direct and indirect nature if third party reimbursement were to be applied as a national policy.)

The nursing profession's capability for doing policy studies is gradually increasing as research resources develop and perspectives widen in the arenas of education, practice, administration, and professional organizations. In this sense, the increased priority within the American Academy of Nursing of promoting interest in policy issues (Aiken, 1981; Aiken & Gortner, 1982; American Academy of Nursing, 1981) may be seen as supportive of policy studies. Many Division of Nursing publications may also be regarded as resources for supporting policy research or policy analysis on nursing-related issues. These resources include literature reviews, bibliographies, and classification systems, as well as surveys, performance studies, and reports to Congress. An additional and more specific resource would be a detailed and comprehensive literature survey in order to compile nursing research on (a) disciplinary issues, with implicit or explicit policy implications; (b) policy research; (c) policy analysis; (d) other policy-relevant papers; (e) policy process studies; and (f) methodologies used in each of these investigations. Bibliographic summaries of comparable work in the general field of policy studies would also be an important additional resource.

At least one concerted effort is being undertaken to enhance nursing's organizational capacity for policy analysis. At this writing, a feasibility study is underway in England to establish a university-based unit that, independently or by commission, would conduct policy studies. Under a nurse director, the unit investigators would analyze current and proposed health policies for their impact, directly and indirectly, on the nation's nursing resources (broadly defined) from the point of view of the public interest (White, Note 5). Fagin (1982b) called for this kind of analysis, although not necessarily to be done by nurses.

PROBLEMS IN THE POLICY STUDIES FIELD

Nursing may have special contributions to make, not only in policy research, but also in health policy analysis. This type of policy investigation—virtually nonexistent in nursing research—is in any case relatively new as a field of formal study, one still seeking its parameters and appropriate methodologies. While there is general agreement on what an analysis *should* include, very few comprehensive health policy analyses actually were done (National Heart and Lung Institute, Note 6; Texas Technical University, Note 7; Futures Group, Note 8).

The most common form of health policy analysis is technology assessment. It is intended to provide legislative, fund granting, and regulatory policymakers with information on policy options by setting forth the impacts (including short- and long-term; unintended, indirect, or delayed; societal, economic, legal, and ethical consequences) of the use of health technologies, both preventive and curative, environmental, and personal (Banta & Behney, 1981).

More limited studies of health technology assessment, which may be considered forms of policy research, are those testing efficacy, safety, or effectiveness. In recent years, the most common method used for these was randomized controlled trials. Of more than 750 trials conducted by the National Institutes of Health (1977) in 1975, the majority were for drugs (400), followed by diagnostic technologies (85), and surgical procedures (25). Very few involved screening or early detection procedures. Trials to test primary prevention strategies were rare (Banta & Behney, 1981). As noted, nurse researchers are beginning to make contributions in policy research.

Another increasingly common method of health policy research is the cost effectiveness study of health technologies. Such studies were reported less than a dozen times a year in the 1960s, but increased to several dozen annually by the end of the 1970s (Office of Technology Assessment, Note 4). Again, however, most attention was given to the tools for diagnosis and treatment, although early studies were more concerned with preventive technologies.

Somewhat conceptually broader cost-benefit analyses were attempted for a few health technologies. However, there are continuing, if not growing, doubts about the usefulness of this form of analysis for health policy, because of potentially misleading assumptions inherent in conventional cost-benefit techniques, especially with respect to placing monetary values on human life (Rice & Hodgson, 1982; Office of Technology Assessment, Note 4) and on restricted living (Milio, 1981).

In sum, the most common forms of health policy research, studying the efficacy, safety, effectiveness, or efficiency of particular health enhancing techniques—whether hardware (physical artifacts) or software (social and informational tools)—are increasing in number. Their limitations for use in health policy analysis include the assumptions inherent in their methods of measurement, and their focus on single hardware and postprevention technologies rather than software and primary prevention strategies. Nonetheless, they are incorporated in policy analyses.

The limitations of these studies are not necessarily insurmountable. Many of the typical limitations were overcome to some extent in one of the few comprehensive attempts at health policy analysis, e.g., one dealing with means to control hypertension (Weinstein & Stason, 1976). The study may be taken as a model. The explicit purpose was to illuminate policy choices for a national hypertension control strategy, and the perspective taken was that of the public, including varying effects on demographic subgroups. The analysis included measures of efficacy, effectiveness, efficiency, and acceptability across the spectrum of preventive and treatment modes of care. The authors also introduced a "quality of life" technique for estimating benefits derived from early diagnosis and treatment, in addition to dollars saved from reductions in death and disability. They then developed alternate policy choices concerning resource allocation, including program priorities for public funds, and alternate means of delivery (e.g., direct services or fiscal incentives and regulation). They further explicated the ethical issues involved, the limitations of the methods, and their point of view. Finally, the analysts considered administrative feasibility, legislative impact, national priorities, and effects on other diseases and policies, as recommended by critics of policy analysis (Milio, 1981; Acton, Note 9).

In short, Weinstein and Stason advanced the state of the art of policy analysis by incorporating the rigor of policy research (in its measures of efficacy, effectiveness, and efficiency) into the breadth of perspective required for policy-making choices. They provided this scope by including a spectrum of preventive and therapeutic tools, also soft and hard technologies; by estimating outcomes; and by suggesting the impacts of different policy options on related health problems, policies, and social and political processes.

Nursing researchers have not yet engaged in this kind of endeavor. In one recent study, however, attempts were made with secondary data to estimate the health and economic impacts of certain primary and secondary prevention strategies, also taking into account monetary and quality of life effects and social and political considerations (Milio, 1983).

SPECIAL CONTRIBUTIONS BY NURSES

Because the field of health policy analysis is relatively new, still evolving and expanding, nurses are in a position to make special contributions, in collaboration with other disciplines, and especially in certain substantive and methodological areas.

Health policy analysis can contribute to more informed choices by policymakers if the health effects of a broader array of policies are made available to them (and to the public). As described here, the policy problems typically analyzed concern the development and use of medical care strategies, and sometimes traditional public health strategies, such as regulation of air or water pollution. Yet there is evidence that a broad spectrum of other policies had an impact on health that may be even larger than conventional health policies. Among these were employment, energy, income maintenance, agricultural, and food policies (Milio, 1981).

Because nurses are situated in such a variety of settings and sites, urban and rural, workplaces and households, institutions and community, they collectively have the experience to identify the potential health consequences of policies. They thus have the potential to formulate new or previously neglected questions for policy research and policy analysis. For example, what happens to health in rural communities when subsidies for home heating fuel are withdrawn?

Further, the interrelated effects of apparently separate policies were rarely analyzed. Nurses, because of their diversity of practice settings, are in a position to raise and study such policy-relevant questions as: What is the relative impact on low birthweight and infant mortality of a policy that provides regional perinatal care centers, as compared with policies that guarantee prepregnancy food, income maintenance, family planning, and prenatal care? Are some subgroups burdened inequitably by certain mixes of policy choices, and if so, how can they be protected by alternate or supplemental policies?

Nurse researchers can also help focus attention on policy issues within the personal health care system that received little attention but are of increasing importance. What, for example, are the health, economic, and family impacts of government financing of limited home health services as compared with broad in-home, long-term care services? What are the effects on health, costs, client access, and professional relationships under fee-for-service reimbursement as compared with capitation for midlevel practitioners? What are the effects on healing (among other impacts) resulting from policies that encourage patient monitoring by electronic instrumentation instead of by direct, personal observation?

Beyond contributing to a more health-oriented framing of timely policy questions, giving attention to the interrelationships of policies, and adding interpersonal variables to the analysis of policy impacts, nurses may also help solve the methodological problems of policy analysis. Here, the identification and measurement of nonquantifiable costs, benefits, or other consequences of alternate health policy choices are especially relevant and may be within the special competence of nurses to investigate. Of what, for example, do changes in "quality of life" consist when health problems are prevented, as compared with occasions when they are treated by various medical strategies? How can differences in such consequences as pain, loss, comfort, stigma, hope, perceived opportunities, and leisure be estimated? What are the ethical questions involved when alternate health important policy choices are being made?

CONCLUSIONS AND RESEARCH DIRECTIONS

Timely research that is focused on publicly defined problems will have a role of increasing importance in policy-making arenas. These policy studies may be either empirically based policy research or broader policy analyses. They may be substantively oriented, or aimed at policy making processes.

The nursing literature revealed a great deal of general interest in health policy. Yet nurse researchers are just beginning to develop and mobilize their capacity to undertake policy studies, as these are usually understood by students in the policy field.

There are many opportunities for contributions to this young field in substantive areas of health policy, in the processes of policy making, and in methodology. The nature of the nursing enterprise suggests the potential of nurse researchers for doing useful analyses of neglected but increasingly important policy problems and devising methodologies that will strengthen and illuminate policy analyses.

REFERENCE NOTES

1. Vickers, G. *Science and the regulation of society*. Printed lecture. New York: Columbia University Institute for the Study of Science in Human Affairs, 1970.
2. Office of Technology Assessment. *The implications of cost effectiveness analysis of medical technology*. Policy paper. Washington, D.C.: U.S. Congress, 1980.
3. Milio, N. *The policy development process and economic effects of federal austerity for community health policy, 1972–82*. Seminar presentation. The Research School of Social Sciences, Australian National University, Canberra, April 11, 1983.

4. Office of Technology Assessment. *The implications of cost effectiveness analy-sis of medical technology. Background paper #1. Methodological issues and literature review.* Washington, D.C.: U.S. Congress, 1980.
5. White, R. Personal communication, July 23, 1982.
6. National Heart and Lung Institute. *The totally implantable artificial heart.* Report of the artificial heart assessment panel. Washington, D.C.: National Institutes of Health, U.S. Department of Health, Education, and Welfare, 1973.
7. Texas Technical University. *Human rehabilitation techniques: A technology assessment.* Report prepared for the National Science Foundation. Lubbock, Texas: Author, 1977.
8. Futures Group. *A study of life-extending technologies.* Report prepared for the National Science Foundation. Glastonbury, Conn.: Author, 1977.
9. Acton, J. *Measuring the social impact of heart and circulatory disease pro-grams: Preliminary framework and estimates.* Report prepared for the National Heart and Lung Institute. Santa Monica, Calif.: Rand Corporation, April 1975.

REFERENCES

Aiken, L. (Ed.). *Health policy and nursing practice.* New York: McGraw-Hill, 1981.
Aiken, L. The impact of federal health policy on nurses. In L. Aiken & S. Gortner (Eds.), *Nursing in the 1980s.* Philadelphia: Lippincott, 1982.
Aiken, L., Blendon, R., & Rogers, D. The shortage of hospital nurses: A new perspective. *American Journal of Nursing,* 1981, *81,* 1612–1618.
Aiken, L., & Gortner, S. (Eds.). *Nursing in the 1980s.* Philadelphia: Lippincott, 1982.
American Academy of Nursing. *The impact of changing resources on health policy.* Kansas City, Mo.: Author, 1981.
Banta, H., & Behney, C. Policy formulation and technology assessment. *Milbank Memorial Fund Quarterly,* 1981, *59,* 445–479.
Bice, T. Social science and health services research: Contributions to public policy. *Milbank Memorial Fund Quarterly,* 1980, *58,* 173–200.
Coleman, J. Problems of conceptualization and measurement in studying policy impacts. In A. Crichton (Ed.), *Health policy making.* Ann Arbor, Mich.: Health Administration Press, 1981.
Doyle, T., Cooper, G., & Anderson, R. *The impact of health system changes on the nation's requirements for registered nurses in 1985* (DHEW Publication No. [HRA] 78–9). Division of Nursing, Bureau of Health Manpower, Health Resources Administration, Department of Health, Education, and Welfare. Washington, D.C.: U.S. Government Printing Office, 1978.
Elliot, J. E., & Kearns, J. *Analysis and planning for improved distribution of nursing personnel and services* (DHEW Publication No. [HRA] 79–16).

Division of Nursing, Bureau of Health Manpower, Health Resources Administration, Hyattsville, Md.: U.S. Department of Health, Education, and Welfare, 1978.

Fagin, C. M. The national shortage of nurses: A nursing perspective. In L. Aiken & S. Gortner (Eds.), Nursing in the 1980s. Philadelphia: Lippincott, 1982. (a).

Fagin, C. M. Nursing's pivotal role in American health care. In L. Aiken & S. Gortner (Eds.), Nursing in the 1980s. Philadelphia: Lippincott, 1982. (b).

Gortner, S., & Nahm, H. An overview of nursing research in the United States. Nursing Research, 1977, 26, 10–33.

Kalisch, P., & Kalisch, B. Nursing involvement in the health planning process (DHEW Publication No. [HRA] 78–25). Division of Nursing, Health Resources Administration, U.S. Department of Health, Education, and Welfare. Washington, D.C.: U.S. Government Printing Office, 1977.

Kayser-Jones, J. S. Gerontological nursing research revisited. Journal of Gerontological Nursing, 1981, 7, 217–223.

Klarman, H. Observations on health services research and health policy analysis. Milbank Memorial Fund Quarterly, 1980, 58, 201–215.

Kos, B., & Rothberg, J. Evaluation of a free standing nurse clinic. In L. Aiken (Ed.), Health policy and nursing practice, New York: McGraw-Hill, 1981.

Krueger, J. Establishing priorities for evaluation and evaluation research: A nursing perspective. Nursing Research, 1980, 29, 115–118.

Lubic, R. Evaluation of an out-of-hospital maternity center for low risk patients. In L. Aiken (Ed.), Health policy and nursing practice. New York: McGraw-Hill, 1981.

Milio, N. Promoting health through public policy. Philadelphia: F. A. Davis, 1981.

Milio, N. Primary care and the public's health: Judging impacts, goals, and policies. Lexington, Mass.: Heath, 1983.

National Institutes of Health. NIH inventory of clinical trials: Fiscal year 1975 (Vols. 1 & 2). Bethesda, Md.: U.S. Department of Health, Education, and Welfare, 1977.

National League for Nursing. The health manpower dilemma (NLN Publication No. 20–1421). New York: Author, 1971.

National League for Nursing. Health policy making in action: The passage and implementation of the national health planning and resources development act of 1974 (NLN Publication No. 41–1600). New York: Author, 1975.

National League for Nursing. Community health administration in a cost containment era (NLN Publication No. 21–1743). New York: Author, 1978.

Reif, L., & Estes, C. L. Long term care: New opportunities for professional nursing. In L. Aiken & S. Gortner (Eds.), Nursing in the 1980s. Philadelphia: Lippincott, 1982.

Rice, D., & Hodgson, T. The value of human life revisited. American Journal of Public Health, 1982, 72, 536–537.

Shortell, S., & Solomon, M. Improving health care policy research, Journal of Health Policy, Politics, and Law, 1982, 6, 684–702.

Sloan, F. The geographic distribution of nurses and public policy (DHEW Publication No. [HRA] 75–53). Division of Nursing, Bureau of Health Manpower, Health Resources Administration, Bethesda, Md.: U.S. Department of Health, Education, and Welfare, 1975.

Spitzer, B., & Grace, H. Cost and containment: Impact on nursing service and nursing education. In American Academy of Nursing, *The impact of changing resources on health policy*. Kansas City, Mo.: American Academy of Nursing, 1981.

Vickers, G. The poverty of problem solving. *Journal of Applied Systems Analysis*, 1981, *8*, 15–18.

Weinstein, M., & Stason, W. *Hypertension: A policy perspective*. Cambridge, Mass.: Harvard University Press, 1976.

CHAPTER 13

Nursing Research in Scotland: A Critical Review

LISBETH HOCKEY
NURSING STUDIES RESEARCH UNIT
UNIVERSITY OF EDINBURGH, SCOTLAND
AND
MARGARET O. CLARK
SCOTTISH HOME AND HEALTH DEPARTMENT
EDINBURGH, SCOTLAND

CONTENTS

British spellings have been retained in this chapter at the authors' request. In regard to the Nursing Studies Research Unit, Department of Nursing Studies, acknowledgment with gratitude is expressed to the Scottish Home and Health Department for financial support of the research effort, to the Nursing Studies Research Unit's Advisory Committee for advice and support over the years, to the Research Unit Staff for hard work and commitment, to the Health Services personnel for access to the clinical areas, and to the Nursing Schools for access to nurse learners.

307

CENTRAL POLICY ON NURSING RESEARCH

Background

The responsibility for the provision of health care in Scotland rests with the Secretary of State for Scotland who is a member of the Cabinet of the Government of the United Kingdom. Monies for the provision of health services are allocated from the Exchequer of the Central Government, and responsibility for the administration of the service is delegated by the Secretary of State to Health Boards. Scotland has 15 Health Boards that are determined geographically; they provide the whole range of health services for the country.

The Secretary of State retains responsibility for the determination of policy. A team of civil servants working at the central department in Edinburgh assists him. Some of these civil servants are from different health professions, including medicine and nursing. During the 1960s these professional staff members recognised a need to stimulate research in nursing. In the absence of any existing mechanism for doing this, a central policy aimed at facilitating and promoting research in nursing was adopted.

By and large, nurse education in Scotland was not undertaken within a university. Where universities had nursing degree programmes, the resources of time and personnel were not sufficient to permit the required concentrated efforts needed for development of research in nursing. For these reasons little research was being undertaken and few nurses received training in research methods.

The initial step toward introduction of the policy aimed at promotion of research in nursing was to attempt to redress these deficiencies. First, in 1967, a Nursing Research Training Fellowship scheme was introduced and second, in 1971, a Nursing Studies Research Unit was established within the Department of Nursing Studies at the University of Edinburgh. Both of these developments are being supported financially from Central Government monies.

The purpose of the Nursing Research Training Fellowship scheme is to enable registered nurses to leave their posts in the Health Service for a period of two years to enable them to learn about research methods by undertaking a study of their own choice. The nurses are located within a suitable department in any university in Scotland where supervision, appropriate to the subject, can be provided for the research and also where nurses are enabled to attend relevant university classes on subjects appropriate to research or to the area of their study. The students can register for a higher degree if they chose to do so. The award of the Fellowship is not contingent upon the applicant having a first degree, that is, the student is not required to have been in a university programme of any kind to be accepted as a Training Fellow.

The conditions of the Fellowship are summarized as follows:

1. Students continue to receive their salary at the same level it would have been had they remained within the Health Service.
2. University fees are paid by the government department.
3. An allowance is made to enable them to attend conferences relevant to their work during the study period.
4. The costs incurred in planning and conducting the research are met by the government department.

The scheme continues to operate in the way in which it was established. The only difference is that three Fellowships now are awarded annually, compared to only two annually for the first few years.

On completion of the Fellowship, students are expected to return to work in the Health Service for a minimum of two years. In practice, the majority remain longer than this. One of the aims of the Fellowship scheme was achieved in that there is now a cadre of people within the Health Service in Scotland who are equipped to guide, advise, and stimulate others who are interested in conducting research. The second major outcome arising from the central policy was the establishment of the Nursing Studies Research Unit within the Department of Nursing Studies at the University of Edinburgh. Details of this Research Unit are discussed in a subsequent section. There is continued financial support from Central Government funds for both the Unit and the Nursing Research Training Fellowship scheme.

In addition to the above-mentioned initiatives, the Scottish Home and Health Department is one of the major sources for funding research of any kind within the Health Service in Scotland. Nurses, alone or in collaboration with staff from other disciplines, can apply for financial support to conduct research. The awarding of financial support is dependent upon the relevance of the proposed research to the National Health Service and upon the scientific merit of the proposal, as determined by the committee awarding the grant. To date there have been few spontaneous applications from nurses.

The majority of the research projects conducted by nurses alone took place within the aegis of the Nursing Studies Research Unit at the University of Edinburgh. Other projects in which nurses were involved usually were developed on a multidisciplinary basis, probably because of the way in which the Health Service in Scotland is organized. Care is viewed as a team effort, and there is a ready willingness on the part of persons from relevant disciplines to be involved.

One example of this joint approach being enabled by the way in which the Service is organized was a study to develop a programme for the routine screening of elderly patients living in their own homes (Barber & Wallis, 1976). This was carried out by a general medical practitioner in conjunction with a nurse health visitor, and the findings were incorporated into practice. The subjects in the study were patients registered with a general medical practitioner, but who were not presenting themselves for diagnosis or treatment. The aim of the project was to identify and treat early symptoms of medical, nursing, or social problems, preventive services which should allow the individual to enjoy a better quality of life. Another outcome was a reduction of the need for help from the Health Service at subsequent stages of the problem.

Another example of this multidisciplinary approach to health research was demonstrated in 1976 when nurses and bioengineers conducted a study in Glasgow to determine the prevalence of patients with decubiti (Clark, Barbanel, Jordan, & Nicol, 1978). This study involved a census of 10,500 patients receiving care in a hospital or at home on a single day. Although nurses were at the forefront of pressure sore prevention by their determination of appropriate nursing practice, other issues such as the physical and mental state of the patient or equipment used cannot be ignored.

A nurse and two surgeons (Dale, Ruckley, & Harper, 1983) recently described the various methods used in the treatment of recurring and nonhealing leg ulcers. This study was viewed as the first stage of a larger experimental project, with the ultimate aim of providing research-based guidance about the optimum treatment of leg ulcers. Only a few examples of multidisciplinary research have been provided. Other publications are listed in the *Nursing Research Abstracts* (published quarterly), along with publications emanating from England, Ireland, and Wales.

The Present Position

Despite the policy initiatives described above, nursing research in Scotland is still young. The majority of student nurses continue to receive training in the traditional apprenticeship model. While aspects of this model may be commended, the emphasis remains more on training than on education. In addition, formal continuing education programmes are not a regular feature within the Health Service in the United Kingdom. These circumstances continue to perpetuate a somewhat ritualistic approach to the practice of nursing, where acceptance of routine predominates over the development of a more questioning and analytical approach. Much activity is currently underway to introduce a more systematic approach to the planning and delivery of nursing. It is hoped that this initiative will lead to questioning of much of the ritual.

The mechanism exists for funding nursing research. The paucity of research applications is the main reason for little research being undertaken. It is unlikely and possibly unrealistic to expect a major change to occur in the immediate future. Therefore, considerable emphasis presently is being placed on developing research-mindedness among registered nurses. It is hoped that this will stimulate nurses to question, have an awareness of published research, be able to evaluate published research, and perhaps will persuade a few nurses to undertake small local studies that may identify from practise areas those topics requiring greater in-depth study.

It is not possible to assess objectively the effect of these initiatives, but there can be no doubt that research interest and awareness are growing, particularly among practising nurses. We hope to capitalize on this and look for ways of providing maximum support and encouragement to those who wish to develop further. The Central Government of Scotland is committed to continuing support of research in nursing. While funding still may come from Central Government monies, it is hoped that the next stage in nursing's development will be a transfer of initiative for stimulating research away from the Government Department to the nursing profession. Only when the nursing profession begins to question and seek answers to the questions can nurses be sure that progress toward a research-based profession has begun.

As background, an overview of the management of nursing research in Scotland has been presented rather than an evaluation of specific research efforts. The historical perspective is essential before the speed and quality of research development can be evaluated. As stated earlier, the Nursing Studies Research Unit within the Department of Nursing Studies represents one of the government's major initiatives in promoting nursing research in Scotland. Its work is outlined below by its first director, Lisbeth Hockey.

THE NURSING STUDIES RESEARCH UNIT, DEPARTMENT OF NURSING STUDIES, UNIVERSITY OF EDINBURGH

Structure and Early Development

The Nursing Studies Research Unit was established in October 1971 and was funded by the Scottish Home and Health Department, through the mechanism of the Chief Scientist Organisation, the official sponsor of government-funded research. The Unit represents a partnership between the University of Edinburgh and the Government of Scotland.

The establishment of a Nursing Studies Research Unit in Scotland was an innovation for the whole of the United Kingdom. The idea of creating a centre for nursing research was new and so was its administrative and financial structure. It was a scientific advance as far as the nursing profession was concerned, and although by the time this volume is published the Unit will be a vigorous adolescent, this is the first mention of it in this series of Annual Reviews.

It is also relatively recent that nurse researchers in Scotland have attempted to evaluate research systematically and to develop critical skills in this area. The research activities of the Nursing Studies Research Unit are described in this section from an evaluative perspective. Such an evaluation of a research programme has to take into account the administrative framework in which it is conducted. The research programme, rather than isolated studies, is the focus of this review.

In the absence of commonly agreed-upon indicators of value, evaluation is an ambiguous term. Its nature is determined by the evaluator and the purpose of the evaluation; other factors, such as ethical and legal constraints, also may play an important part. The well-known Donabedian (1976, 1978) triad of structure, process, and outcome can be applied to the evaluation of a research programme. In fact, it also can be used to advantage for the assessment of individual research projects; it is a simple and helpful framework for evaluation.

Werley and Shea (1973), in their article on The First Center for Research in Nursing, stressed the importance of a suitable administrative and operational framework in the development of a research programme. The difficulties outlined in that paper were almost identical with those experienced in the Edinburgh Nursing Research Unit. The Unit's Director would have been reassured by the Werley and Shea article had it been available in 1971 to 1973. Although some of the initial problems were overcome successfully, it is not prudent to evaluate the subsequent work without some reference to the early developmental period. The study on Women in Nursing (Hockey, 1976) was initiated and completed during that period. In any future account of nursing research in Scotland, it will not be necessary to retrace the early steps. Also, similar to Werley's experience, the Research Unit's Director was keenly aware of the other envisaged functions of the new Unit, namely, creating greater research awareness among nurses generally, teaching research methodology, and disseminating research-related information.

APPLICATION OF DONABEDIAN'S EVALUATIVE FRAMEWORK TO THE WOMEN IN NURSING STUDY

The Research Unit's first study on Women in Nursing (Hockey, 1976) is used to demonstrate the application of Donabedian's triad to research projects. Review of this study is necessary since it was the basis for the ensuing core programme of research in the Unit between 1975 and 1982.

Structure

The structure in this context refers to the administrative framework that included financial support and staff involved. At the beginning of the study, the Research Unit was at an early developmental stage, with only half its total staff complement employed; the staff included the director, one research associate, and one research assistant. Staffing strategy suggested that the position of research associate should be a teaching post for research, whereas the position of research assistant should be a learning post. The two positions were assigned together for the pursuit of a specific project. During the period of the study more staff were appointed.

Although the Unit's budget dictated to some extent the type and magnitude of the first study to be launched, it was not a constraining factor at any time. There were three major constraints: (a) the relative difficulty in staff recruitment; (b) the need to negotiate research access and, if possible, develop a mechanism for such access in the future; and (c) the director's eagerness to pay due attention to the other objectives of the Unit's work. It

314   OTHER RESEARCH

is relevant to note that the Unit's first research associate was a graduate in sociology who had good research experience but no nursing qualification, and the first research assistant was a qualified nurse who had good nursing experience but was not a university graduate and had no knowledge of research methods. Clearly, the way in which a research project is planned is determined, to a major extent, by the interests and expertise of the responsible personnel. Although the director had overall responsibility for all the work of the Unit, the plan was to allow the research associates to assume the day-to-day control of a specific project with apprentice-type help from the research assistant.

Process

The research process refers to each step of a project. It includes the generation of an idea, formulation of the idea into a researchable question or a testable hypothesis, operationalization of the idea, data collection, data analysis and interpretation, and writing a report and journal articles for dissemination of the findings. Any evaluation of process must include the assessment of each of the preceding steps. There should be particular reference to the scientific merit, such as the theoretical background and framework, the suitability of the data collection method in relation to the questions to be answered, the appropriateness of the analysis and interpretation, as well as the clarity and integrity of presentation in the report and professional or scientific articles.

The study, *Women in Nursing,* was very much a consumer-generated project. It arose from informal documented discussions with different types and levels of nurses in many parts of Scotland. The discussions were analyzed by a research assistant who identified a common core of content. The main focus for inquiry was twofold: (a) problems related to a predominantly female work force for whom family commitments may have interfered with health service needs, and (b) problems related to being a female worker with family commitments to children or dependent adults. Other themes also were pursued in the study. At the time, it was believed important for the first major research project to be totally relevant to the nursing profession in Scotland. The investigators did not claim to use an objective, scientific approach. The study was a naive version of a first-stage delphi technique; informed hindsight has suggested that a more sophisticated research design might have been useful.

For this descriptive study, personal interviews and self-report questionnaires were used for data collection. In spite of careful pilot work, the research tools were wanting, although not too seriously. For example, one or two questions were not quite clear to every respondent. Looking at the problem in a positive way, mistakes afforded excellent learning opportunities. The data analysis was simple and appropriate for the purpose. Interpretation of the data was facilitated by the interdisciplinary team who formed the Unit staff at that stage of the study. The two research associates were not nurses and, therefore, were more detached and less likely to be influenced by circumstances and problems known to exist but not demonstrated by the research.

The benefits derived from the multidisciplinary nature of the team for purposes of analysis and of the data interpretation were offset by some difficulties, as in preparing the report. The plan was to report the study as a whole, in a book, with individual staff members contributing the parts for which they had been responsible. The two learner members were given some experience in writing for publication. It was not easy to achieve sufficient uniformity in presentation to preserve the continuity of a book. Therefore, a considerable part of the report had to be edited substantially or rewritten, and, even so, fragmentation was discernible.

Outcome

It is in relation to outcome that the purpose of the evaluation plays the most important part. For the *Women in Nursing* study, one could judge outcome in terms of scientific merit and the contribution to knowledge, practical usefulness to the profession, and having contributed to the learning and maturing experiences of research workers. These outcomes are not mutually exclusive; research findings that are not credible are not useful.

There were many positive outcomes from this first major Unit project. It certainly proved to be an excellent learning experience for everyone involved and highlighted some general problems which the Research Unit staff had to overcome. Its usefulness to the profession became more apparent as time progressed. Because the book reporting the study was written with the added objective of helping novice researchers, its use was increased and it began to appear on reading lists for postbasic nursing courses. Many nurses who were respondents in the study showed increased research awareness by writing for more information, by active participation in feedback sessions, and by applying for places at the Unit's summer school sessions, which were held two or three times a year for the purpose of meeting the Unit's educational objective. The study contributed to knowledge through the validation of a job satisfaction measure for nurses, which had been designed originally (Brayfield & Rothe, 1951) for other occupational groups. This instrument was used by other researchers in both the United Kingdom and other countries.

Through the honest presentation of problems, difficulties, and mistakes in conducting research, other researchers were made aware of potential hazards. As with most research, the study raised more questions than it answered, but this is the way in which knowledge grows. Three subsequent studies were generated on the basis of the findings. Regrettably, only two of them were completed, and they were published as reports for the sponsors and for limited domestic circulation as a basis for discussion. The third study was intended to identify patients' fears and worries after admission to a hospital and raised some important methodological problems which were published (French, 1981).

APPLICATION OF DONABEDIAN'S
EVALUATIVE FRAMEWORK
TO THE CORE PROGRAMME OF RESEARCH

A programme of research connotes a progression of studies or parallel studies that are developed under a predetermined theme. While the original intention was to allow the findings of one study to generate the next, the Chief Scientist Organization, established two years after the Research Unit, asked for the identification of a research programme, a theme, before the logical progression could occur. By that time, the full complement of six research workers were employed. A programme acceptable to all and appropriate for their potential contributions had to be developed if their expertise and their services were to be retained. Moreover, it was essential that the programme be relevant to the nursing profession, especially to the practice of nursing in the care of patients.

Space does not allow detailed presentation of the discussions and thought processes that took place over the period of gestation, although the evaluation of the final programme should be made in that context. Therefore, in the following section the global aspects of the programme are referred to, using again the structure-process-outcome framework.

Communication in Nursing was the theme finally identified as worthy of a long-term research programme. It was chosen because communication was seen as an activity that can be initiated and controlled by nurses, and it forms an essential and all-pervasive aspect of nursing.

Structure

Six staggered projects were planned, each dealing with a different aspect of communication and each being the responsibility of one or two staff members. The projects were staggered to achieve some evenness in work pressures, especially for the part-time statistician-computing adviser, and the typists. Staggering also allowed staff to help each other at field work peak periods. The six projects were:

1. Communication with Patients for the Purpose of Information Giving,
2. Attitudes of Senior Nursing Staff toward Information Giving by Nurses,
3. Student Nurses' Perception of Communication with Patients as Part of Nursing,
4. The Disabled Patient as a Communicator of His Own Needs,
5. Communication as Part of Top Administration in Nursing,
6. The Communication of Research to the Profession.

In addition, a study of communication as part of the nursing care of patients with a mastectomy and two parallel studies focused on communication between the hospital and community nursing service in relation to the elderly were identified and planned, for the future. As some of the studies were implemented, their emphasis was changed slightly, although the central foci of communication were retained.

By December 1982, when there was a change of the Unit Director, Studies 3 and 6 were completed. Studies 4 and 5 were in the publication stage, and Studies 1 and 2 were in the final analysis stage. The study of communication with patients who had a mastectomy was at an early stage of analysis. Pilot studies on the topic of communication between the hospital and community nursing services in relation to the elderly were completed, and decisions regarding further work were pending. The way in which the results of a pilot study were utilized in further planning was of utmost importance and should form an integral part of any evaluation of the whole.

Process

Now that the theme underpinning the research programme has been explained, it is appropriate to comment on the thrust of the individual studies. Why would one wish to undertake further work on communication with patients for information-giving before surgery when the benefits of such communication had been demonstrated and reported? The reason was a practical one which deserved serious consideration not only in relation to this study but also in any research that is aimed at some change in practice. All previous studies found in the literature were controlled experiments with a research worker giving specific information to one group of patients and placebo information to a control group. Our objective was to ascertain whether similar beneficial patient outcomes would be obtained if the nurse caring for the patients rather than a research worker were to give the information. Only if the findings were positive could one expect nursing practice to be changed to ensure that the giving of specific information would become part of the standard procedure of preparing a patient for surgery and/or other potentially threatening events.

Thus, the method for Study 1, Communication with Patients for the Purpose of Information Giving (Davis, 1981), was also a controlled experiment. The patients were undergoing gastric or biliary surgery, and the independent variable was a "package" of specific information provided by the ward nurse. At a later stage, this information was reinforced by a purpose-designed booklet. The dependent variables were a set of relevant patient outcomes, including sleep, pain, food intake, elimination, and nausea. Baseline data were obtained at an early exploratory stage of the study from careful daily observation of a group of patients in three hospitals. Although the method adopted for the study and the pragmatic framework in which it was undertaken seemed perfectly appropriate and defensible, the major weakness lay in the lack of practical control over the independent variable, the information to be given by nurses. This problem of reconciling rigorous scientific control with the normal work pattern remains to be resolved.

Linked with the preceding problem was the discovery that administrative nursing personnel sometimes seemed reluctant to allow nursing staff to give to patients the type of information designed for this study. That was considered a responsibility of the medical staff. For this reason, Study 2, Attitudes of Senior Nursing Staff toward Information Giving by Nurses, was mounted. The project leader for both studies was the Unit's Deputy Director, a psychology graduate particularly interested in exploring attitudes. He developed a Likert-type questionnaire that was distributed to various professional groups, such as nurses at different levels of the hierarchical structure, medical personnel, physiotherapists, and occupational therapists. The respondents were asked to indicate their view on the giving of certain types of information to patients in relation to information content and the information giver. Inter- and intraprofessional congruence or discrepancy were explored. Regrettably, the results were not available for inclusion in this chapter. Further information on studies mentioned may be obtained from the present Unit Director.

The idea for Study 4, The Disabled Patient as a Communicator of His Own Needs, was generated by a disabled person's pressure group, the Scottish Council on Disability, whose members were dismayed about the experiences of severely disabled persons requiring care in an acute hospital ward for a condition unrelated to their disability. From an evaluative perspective it was relevant for researchers to be sensitive to such indicators and to be willing to explore them in a systematic, scientific manner. Such action would give nursing research more professional credibility because the topics studied were more clearly relevant to nursing and to the care of patients.

The project leader for this work was a graduate in social administration, with an interest in sociological theory. He selected role theory as a conceptual framework and designed a comparative study, using carefully selected samples of disabled patients and matched control normal patients. The concept of disability was based on nationally accepted criteria. The method of data collection was a purpose-designed interview guide. Patients were interviewed in the hospital and in their home after discharge. The aim was to compare disabled with nondisabled patients in relation to objective measures such as length of hospital stay, but also in relation to patient satisfaction. Communication was featured prominently as an indicator of satisfaction, and preliminary findings suggested that inadequate communication correlated positively with almost every other dissatisfaction expressed by both groups of patients. Most research methods have inherent problems, and in this study, the matching of patients on even the simplest variables such as age, sex, ward, and reason for hospitalization, was difficult. Therefore, it took longer than anticipated to obtain the necessary sample size of 100 patients (Atkinson, 1981).

The study of nursing and of communication within it lends itself to a variety of research approaches, and for Studies 3 and 5 investigators used a qualitative design. Although for the study of student nurses the investigators set out to explore communication as part of nursing, it soon became apparent that discussion about communication per se resulted in standard text book comments, seen by the students as being proper answers.

Study 3 was developed into PhD research on Student Nurses Accounts of Their Work and Training (Melia, 1981, 1982, 1983), and the title showed how the study was changed and extended far beyond communication. The qualitative design was based on the work of Glaser and Strauss (1967) in that it had an inductive rather than a deductive approach.

Theoretical rather than statistical sampling was used as propounded by Glaser and Strauss, and the final sample consisted of 40 student nurses. Data were obtained through informal interviews, which were tape recorded and transcribed. Six conceptual categories emerged from the study which demonstrated the way in which student nurses perceived their world (Melia, 1982). In terms of using a qu⌐litative design, the study could be viewed as a change for nursing, which has tended to favour the quantitative approach to research, generally considered to have greater scientific credibility. In this study, credibility was derived from the face validity of the findings. Evaluatively, the various audiences to whom the study was presented recognized the reality of the nursing world in the findings.

A qualitative design was adopted for Study 5, Communication as Part of Top Administration in Nursing, for two reasons. First, it was thought that the data obtained would be richer than if they were collected within the constraints of a structured questionnaire. Secondly, the total population of top administrators in Scotland was considered far too small for quantitative analysis. Informal interviews were conducted and notes made by the interviewer, who was the Unit Director. Tape recording was considered but not pursued. In line with qualitative research methods, the analysis of the data was ongoing, with comments made by one respondent used appropriately, in interviews with others. Thus, specific topics of interest could be pursued as they emerged from the data. On evaluation, this study was not as rigorous as Study 4 in that the documentation at the time of interview inevitably was selective. As the discussions were not tape-recorded, the field notes formed the only record, and it was, therefore, not possible for anyone else to verify the authenticity of the emergent categories. Notwithstanding this weakness, it seemed at this writing that the face validity of the findings would be confirmed.

A simple survey method was used for Study 6, The Communication of Research to the Profession; it served two purposes. First, it provided learning opportunities in survey design for a research student and a newly appointed and inexperienced staff member, and second, it filled a gap in the knowledge available on the communication of research to the nursing profession at large. A snowball technique was used to locate potential respondents. Names of eligible individuals were obtained from respondents through a final question: Do you know anyone else who . . . ? Please provide his/her name and address if you consider it appropriate for us to contact them. The major weakness of this method was that one could not make any claims for the quality of the sample. The investigator did not know if the total population was reached, or if the sample obtained was in any way representative of the total population. However, in the absence of any form of register for use as a sampling frame, the snowball technique seemed the only alternative (Hockey, Johnson, & Laing, 1983; Laing & Johnson, 1982).

The initial stages of the study of patients who had a mastectomy were particularly rewarding. In terms of process, the design was innovative in that it entailed collaboration with another Nursing Research Unit in London and with another leading nurse researcher in London whose work on patients who had a hysterectomy was to be replicated, at least in part. The intention was to introduce collaborative research, thereby making it possible to achieve greater generalizability of findings. Demonstrating the benefits of replication in contrast to its relatively low prestige value in the academic world was another intended outcome.

Mounting this complex study presented many problems. It was impossible to control the field work in London, and very soon it emerged that the Scottish and London patients were inherently different. Therefore, any possibility of true comparison or of merging the groups was discarded. It was decided that the groups would be studied as separate samples, looking for pointers rather than conclusive findings. The study had a descriptive design with an experimental and an evaluative component. The experimental variable was an information booklet for patients and the evaluative component concerned the role of a clinical nurse specialist. Patients were interviewed in their home at four weeks and at four months after surgery, with a brief postal questionnaire at ten weeks after surgery. The interview guide covered many physical, emotional, and social aspects of life; it was semistructured, and the many open-ended questions resulted in rich data, which presented inevitable analysis problems. The pilot study for this work was used toward a Master of Philosophy degree, and a preliminary paper was published (Johnson & Laing, 1982). As indicated earlier, two additional studies on communication in relation to the elderly were in the preliminary pilot stages at the end of 1982. For both, a qualitative design was used.

Outcome

As far as it was possible to ascertain, the collective outcomes from the research programme related more to the learning experiences provided than to findings that had a potential for implementation. As explained, different methods were used and all had their strengths and weaknesses. They were appropriate for the problems under study. Three members of the research team were awarded intermediate or higher research degrees—M Phil (Master of Philosophy) and PhD (Doctor of Philosophy)—and two further awards are expected. Two temporary members of the staff developed enthusiasm for research, which led them into other positions with some responsibility for research. Important outcomes also were seen in the involvement of nurses outside the Research Unit. Interest undoubtedly was generated, and the first two studies led to requests for short courses on social skill training.

Not many research projects in nursing lead to direct implementation of their findings, either because they are small studies from which generalization is not possible, or because they are not initiated to generate change. Researchers attempted to shed light on various aspects of nursing and, possibly, to add an understanding of reality. The research programme reviewed in this chapter followed this pattern. The respective studies within the programme were small. Studies 1 and 2 could have stimulated change as far as information giving was concerned, but it seemed that conventional attitudes may have blocked this. As a result of Study 3, nurses may have felt that communication with patients was worth pursuing more seriously, but the findings had no prescriptive power. The study of student nurses should cause teaching and clinical staff to give serious thought to the students' perceived experience and to attempt a more humane approach. The findings themselves did not suggest how this might be done or whether any change would result in different outcomes. The same is true for findings from the other studies reviewed.

SUMMARY

Hindsight is always clearer than foresight and, if given another chance to develop a research programme, one probably would have taken a different direction. In such an event, a framework for a coherent programme would be laid down, although the coherence itself might not be as rigorous as envisaged.

There is an inherent problem in making a rigid underlying structure compatible with the interests and abilities of individual members of a research staff and with the requirements of originality expected of higher-degree work. An advanced degree is the goal of many nurses at this stage of the development of academic nursing in the United Kingdom. It is possible that a future generation of research workers will have fulfilled their academic aspirations and, therefore, would be more amenable to an imposed structure; the converse is equally possible. The future alone will shed light on this dilemma.

As explained, the research programme outlined above was only a part of the Unit's activities. Detailed reports of the total work were published at roughly two-year intervals, the sixth and most recent report in December 1982 (Nursing Research Unit, 1973, 1975, 1977, 1979, 1981, 1982). On January 1, 1983, Sister Penny Prophet was appointed as Director of the Nursing Research Unit. She must be consulted about future directions.

REFERENCES

Atkinson, F. I. Physically disabled patients in hospital: The development of a research project. *Nursing Times*, 1981, *77*, 744–745.
Barber, J. H., & Wallis, J. B. An information system on the needs of the elderly. *Health Bulletin*, 1976, *34*, 324–330. (Published by Scottish Home and Health Department, Edinburgh.)
Brayfield, A. H., & Rothe, H. F. An index of job satisfaction. *Journal of Applied Psychology*, 1951, *35*, 307–331.
Clark, M. O., Barbanel, J. C., Jordan, M. M., & Nicol, S. M. Pressure sores. *Nursing Times*, 1978, *74*, 363–366.
Dale, J. J., Ruckley, C. V., & Harper, D. R. *Chronic ulcers of the leg: A perennial problem in health care.* Unpublished report to Scottish Home and Health Department, April 1983.
Davis, B. Pre-operative information giving in relation to patient outcome. *Nursing Times*, 1981, *77*, 599–601.
Donabedian, A. A frame of reference. *Quality Review Bulletin*, 1976, *2*(6), 5–8; 30–32.
Donabedian, A. The quality of medical care. *Science*, 1978, *200*, 856–864.
French, K. Methodological considerations in hospital patient opinion surveys. *International Journal of Nursing Studies*, 1981, *18*, 7–32.
Glaser, B., & Strauss, A. L. *The discovery of grounded theory: Strategies for qualitative research.* Chicago: Aldine, 1967.
Hockey, L. (Dir.). *Women in Nursing.* London: Hodder & Stoughton, 1976.
Hockey, L., Johnson, R., & Laing, E. Look, listen, learn. *Nursing Mirror*, 1983, *157*(2), 21–22.
Johnson, R. A., & Laing, E. The nursing contribution to the aftercare of mastectomy patients (Report of pilot study). *In Proceedings of the Rcn Research Society Annual Conference* (Vol. 13, pp. 305–319). London: Royal College of Nursing, 1982.
Laing, E., & Johnson, R. A. Survey of nurses associated with research in the United Kingdom in 1980 (Report of a pilot study). *Proceedings of the Rcn Research Society Annual Conference* (Vol. 13, pp. 321–337). London: Royal College of Nursing, 1982.

Melia, K. M. Student nurses' construction of nursing: A discussion of a qualitative method. *Nursing Times*, 1981, *77*, 697–699.

Melia, K. M. Tell it as it is—Qualitative methodology and nursing research: Understanding the student nurse's world. *Journal of Advanced Nursing*, 1982, *7*, 327–335.

Melia, K. M. Students' views of nursing: Discussion of method. *Nursing Times*, 1983, *79*(20), 24–25.

Nursing Research Abstracts. London: Department of Health and Social Security, Alexander Fleming House, Elephant and Castle (Published quarterly).

Nursing Research Unit. *Biennial report*. Edinburg, Scotland: Nursing Research Unit, Department of Nursing Studies, University of Edinburg, 1973, 1975, 1977, 1979, 1981, 1982.

Werley, H. H., & Shea, F. P. The first center for research in nursing: Its development, accomplishments, and problems. *Nursing Research*, 1973, *22*, 217–231.

Index

Index

ORDER FORM

Save 10% on Volume 3 with this coupon

____Check here to receive a pre-payment invoice with a 10% discount for Volume 3, 1985 of the ANNUAL REVIEW OF NURSING RESEARCH.

Save 10% on all future volumes with a continuation order

____Check here to place your continuation order for the ANNUAL REVIEW OF NURSING RESEARCH. You will receive a pre-payment invoice with a 10% discount upon publication of each new volume, beginning with Volume 3, 1985. You may pay for prompt shipment or cancel with no obligation.

Name _____

Institution _____

Address _____

City/State/Zip _____

Examination copies for possible course adoptions are available to instructors on approval. Write on institutional letterhead, noting course, level, present text, and expected enrollment. (Include $1.60 for postage and handling). Prices slightly higher overseas. Prices subject to change.

Mail this coupon to:
SPRINGER PUBLISHING COMPANY
200 Park Avenue South, New York, N.Y. 10003